D1568172

ANIMAL BREEDING

Modern Genetics
A series of books covering new developments across the entire field of genetics.
Edited by Richard Lathe, Centre for Genome Research, University of Edinburgh,
Kings Buildings, Edinburgh, EH9 3JQ, UK

Volume 1
Embryonal Stem Cells: Introducing Planned Changes into the Animal Germline
Martin L. Hooper

Volume 2
Molecular Genetics of Inherited Eye Disorders
edited by *Alan F. Wright* and *Barrie Jay*

Volume 3
Molecular Genetics of Drug Resistance
edited by *John D. Hayes* and *C. Roland Wolf*

Volume 4
Animal Breeding: Technology for the 21st Century
edited by *A.J. Clark*

Additional volumes in preparation

Signalling Pathways in Apoptosis
edited by *M. Lavin* and *D. Watters*

ANIMAL BREEDING

Technology for the 21st Century

Edited by

A.J. Clark

Roslin Institute
Midlothian
UK

harwood academic publishers
Australia • Canada • China • France • Germany • India • Japan
Luxembourg • Malaysia • The Netherlands • Russia • Singapore
Switzerland • Thailand

Amsteldijk 166
1st Floor
1079 LH Amsterdam
The Netherlands

British Library Cataloguing in Publication Data

A catalogue record for this book is available from the British Library.

ISBN: 90-5702-292-3
ISSN: 1056-4497

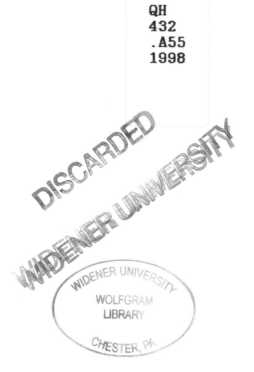

Charles Smith — an appreciation

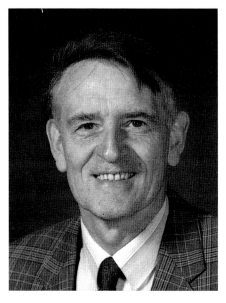

1932–1997

Professor Charles (Charlie) Smith died on 16th of June 1997 in Guelph, Ontario, Canada. Right up until his death he was a leading light in the field of animal breeding.

Charlie Smith was the son of an Aberdeenshire farmer and gained a first class honours degree in Agriculture at Aberdeen University. He then went to Iowa State University where he completed his PhD under Professor J.L. Lush. He returned to Scotland and took up a job at the Animal Breeding Research Organisation in Edinburgh where he focused his attention on pig breeding. His theoretical investigations coupled with practical improvement schemes hastened the adoption of new methodology and in a relatively short time British pig breeding had gained world-wide recognition.

Changing fields in 1968 Charlie moved to the Department of Human Genetics at Edinburgh University. He developed the first registry of Inherited Diseases and developed methods to calculate risk in genetic counselling and worked on the resolution of genetic effects and heterogeneity in familial diseases.

In 1974 he returned to the field of animal breeding taking up the post of Head of Department of Applied Genetics at ABRO where he continued experimental and theoretical work in cattle, sheep and pig breeding. In 1987 he moved to Canada accepting the Chair in Animal Breeding Strategies at the University of Guelph. There he was an influential figure at the Centre for Genetic Improvement of Livestock focusing on both practical and theoretical developments for breeding strategies and breeding objectives.

One of Charlie Smith's greatest strengths was his interest in open mindedness in the development and practical application of new technology in animal breeding. It was in 1983 that he and Frank Nicholas wrote their highly influential paper on the use of MOET (multiple ovulation and embryo transfer) in dairy cattle breeding. This led directly to the establishment of the first MOET nucleus herd, an approach that was then revolutionary in dairy cattle breeding but is widely practised in various forms round the world today. When transgenic technology became available in the 1980s he was one of the first to think about the practical applications and considerations in breeding programmes. Similarly, with the development of genome mapping techniques he was one of the first to recognize that molecular markers might open up new possibilities for animal breeders. It is, therefore, particularly appropriate that Charlie wrote the Introductory Chapter for this volume which is dedicated to his memory.

CONTENTS

PREFACE TO THE SERIES

The Modern Genetics series, established under the editorship of Professor H. John Evans, was intended to cover new developments across the entire field of genetics of plants and animals, including man, and at all levels from the molecule to the population. This aim will be sustained and built upon, with increasing emphasis on the practical applications of the new genetics, be they in agriculture, medicine or biotechnology.

The present volume affords a topical illustration of the meeting point between academic research and practical exploitation. When the basic techniques for modifying and mapping the mammalian genome were first worked out in the research laboratory, there was little anticipation of what the fuller ramifications of this technology might be. Nonetheless, their application to the tailoring of the genomes of farm animals has been swift to follow. It is particularly appropriate that this volume is edited by Dr John Clark, one of the pioneers in this new and expanding field.

R. Lathe

PREFACE

During the latter half of this century, animal breeding has been remarkably successful in improving the efficiency of livestock production. For some traits efficiency gains in the order of 2–3% per annum have been achieved. Such changes are cumulative and permanent and, so, significant benefits have accrued over time. These gains have been achieved with little or no knowledge of the genes underlying the traits. Rather, they have depended upon the phenotypic selection of animals and their relatives allied to increasingly sophisticated statistical and computing methods to estimate the genetic parameters of a particular trait.

Notwithstanding these successes, it is clear that recent advances in both developmental biology and molecular biology are set to revolutionise the practice of animal breeding in the next century. New techniques for acquiring and culturing early embryos will facilitate their propagation as well as underpinning the methods for their manipulation. Cloning from cultured cells by nuclear transfer is already a reality in sheep and, assuming that it can be achieved in other species, will revolutionise the identification, propagation and dissemination of elite embryos throughout the breeding industries. Genome maps have been created for all the major species of livestock and are already being used to locate genes underpinning production traits. Marker assisted selection will enable genetic selection to be carried out on the genotype as well as the phenotype with important consequences for the improvement of sex and age limited traits. The maps are revealing that there is substantial conservation of genome organisation amongst higher vertebrates which means that the extensive information being generated in the Human Genome Project may be exploited for the identification of specific trait genes in livestock. Finally, the combination of embryo manipulation and molecular biology has led to the generation of transgenic livestock. Conventional transgenesis involves the direct addition of new genes by pro-nuclear injection and this has been accomplished in all the major livestock species. As yet, this has not had a major impact on the improvement of conventional production traits. Rather, this technology has been exploited to develop new biomedical uses for farm animals including the production of human therapeutic proteins in milk and the supply of "humanised" organs for xenotransplantation. The ability to generate animals from cells in culture now holds open the possibility of carrying out precise changes to the germline, such as gene knockouts or gene replacements, and will certainly broaden applications for transgenic animals in medicine and, in the longer term, agriculture.

This volume brings together a rich collection of papers by internationally recognised scientists in three areas of research where remarkable progress is being made — embryo manipulation, genome analysis and germline manipulation. These areas are underpinned by a combination of molecular biology, genetics and embryology which when applied to livestock give us a glimpse of how animal breeding will develop in the next century.

CONTRIBUTORS

Andersson, L
Department of Animal Breeding
and Genetics
Swedish University of
Agricultural Sciences
Uppsala Biomedical Centre
Box 597
S-751 24 Uppsala
Sweden

Archibald, A L
Roslin Institute (Edinburgh)
Roslin
Midlothian
EH25 9PS
UK

Campbell, K H S
PPL Therapeutics
Roslin
Midlothian
EH25 9PS
UK

Coleman, A
PPL Therapeutics
Roslin
Midlothian
EH25 9PP
UK

Eyestone, W H
PPL Therapeutics, Inc
Virginia Tech Corporate
Research Center
Blacksburg
VA 24060
USA

Gardner, D K
Institute of Reproduction
and Development
Monash University
Level 5, Monash Medical Centre
246 Clayton Road, Clayton
Victoria 3168
Australia

Garner, I
PPL Therapeutics
Roslin
Midlothian
EH25 9PP
UK

Georges, M
Department of Genetics
Faculty of Veterinary Medicine
University of Liège
20 Bd de Colonster (B43)
4000-Liège (Sart Tilman)
Belgium

Gibson, J P
Centre for Genetic Improvement of
Livestock
Department of Animal and
Poultry Science
University of Guelph
Guelph
Ontario N1G 2W1
Canada

Haley, C S
Roslin Institute (Edinburgh)
Roslin
Midlothian
EH25 9PS
UK

Langford, G
Department of Surgery
Douglas House
18 Trumpington Road
Cambridge
CB2 2AH
UK

Pursel, V G
US Department of Agriculture
Agricultural Research Service
Beltsville Agricultural Research Center
Beltsville
MD 20705
USA

† **Smith, C**
Department of Animal and
Poultry Science
Ontario Agricultural College
University of Guelph
Guelph
Ontario N1G 2W1
Canada

Stice, S L
Advanced Cell Technology
Paige Laboratory
University of Massachusetts
Amherst, MA 01003
USA

Van der Beek, S
Wageningen Agricultural University
PO Box 338
6700 AH Wageningen
The Netherlands

Visscher, P M
University of Edinburgh
Institute of Ecology and
Resource Management
West Mains Road
Edinburgh
EH9 3JG
UK

White, D
Department of Surgery
Douglas House
18 Trumpington Road
Cambridge
CB2 2AH
UK

Wilmut, I
Roslin Institute (Edinburgh)
Roslin
Midlothian
EH25 9PS
UK

INTRODUCTION:
CURRENT ANIMAL BREEDING

CHARLES SMITH *

Animal and Poultry Science, University of Guelph, Guelph, Ontario, Canada N1G 2W1

The purpose of animal breeding is to improve genetically the economic efficiency of livestock production. The main driving force is the competitive position and so the profit of the producer, but in practice the choices are not always rational. The main tool in genetic improvement of economic merit is conventional selection. Annual genetic response rates of 0.5–3% of the mean for different species are possible for single traits over many (10–30) generations. Usually several or many traits (5–30) are involved in economic merit. Selection is on these component traits of merit weighted in a selection index, rather than on profit directly. Sophisticated statistical computing methods are used to estimate the genetic parameters for the traits and to apply them to derive the estimated breeding values of candidates for selection. Selection effects are cumulative and permanent, so large genetic differences and economic benefits can be achieved over time by current breeding methods. Continuing selection efforts are needed to achieve these benefits and to accommodate changes in breeding objectives and production systems.

The various livestock species differ in their organisation and in their agencies for improvement. They also differ in the effectiveness and hence in the improvement made. Most commercial production is from crossbreds, to benefit from breed differences (complementarity) and heterosis, but milk and fine wool production are by purebreds.

The new technologies can change both the rates and systems of genetic change, by increasing accuracy, intensity or timeliness of selection. Use of computer simulation has been of great value in designing and evaluating new breeding strategies and systems. Statistical and computing innovations have been exploited quickly. The use of new reproductive technologies, marker assisted selection, identification of QTL and transgenics have been limited or slower than anticipated due to the difficulties (and costs) of applying the technologies. Current animal breeding systems can be effective and may be hard to improve upon in practice.

KEY WORDS: animal breeding; selection; breeding systems; genetic improvement.

INTRODUCTION

Animal breeding is at a crossroads. A range of new tools and technologies is becoming available and these may change the methods used and the organisation of breeding systems. The objective of this initial chapter is to give a broad outline of animal breeding as it is currently practiced, so as to set the scene for the application of new technologies. An attempt will be made to review the main characteristics of animal genetic improvement and to summarise its potential and its actual effectiveness, and to review its deficiencies. Emphasis will be given to the basic principles, and to the current literature on the topics.

---

* Prof. C. Smith died in June 1997, before this volume was published.

ECONOMIC MERIT

The purpose of animal breeding is to genetically improve the economic merit of farm livestock. The goal for society is to minimise the cost per unit value of product, hence maximising economic efficiency (Dickerson, 1970). Equivalent results were obtained by using "normal" profit (Brascamp et al., 1985) and by "rescaling" production to the same output, input or profit (Smith et al., 1986). However, the driving force in genetic improvement is the producer who buys and uses the improved stock. The choice should be such as to maximise his profit, but the choices are not always rational. Theoretically, economic weights derived from neoclassical production theory and the profit function for the firm (or farm) seem to be the appropriate weights to use (Amer and Fox, 1992; Amer, 1994). In practice, the differences in economic weights from different methods are usually not large (Ponzoni, 1988) and their effect on the rates of economic response through selection indexes combining several traits are usually small (Smith, 1983). Note that a clear evaluation of the breeding goal is essential to all methods of improvement.

Direct selection on profit, though possible (Visscher and Goddard, 1995), is not optimal since it does not allow for differences in heritability and variability of the component traits. The profit function is usually non-linear, but for simplicity and convenience linear profit functions are normally used. Goddard (1983) and Dekkers et al. (1995) have shown that linear functions are good approximations to complex non-linear functions, especially if the economic weights are updated each generation. The linear approximations are good because the rates of genetic change per generation are small. Another useful result dealt with economic weights derived at different finishing points, for example, at a constant age, weight or fatness in beef cattle. Wilton and Goddard (1996) showed equivalence of the economic weights, provided management variables are optimised for the current genotype.

The outlook on economic weights may differ between producers and breeding companies (van der Steen et al., 1994). For example, a company which lags in a trait compared with competitors may put more selection pressure on that trait to catch up (de Vries, 1989) rather than the rational procedure to maximise economic merit.

POSSIBLE SELECTION RESPONSE

The main tool in genetic improvements is selection. A general expression for the predicted equilibrium genetic response, as a percentage of the mean of the trait per year, is given by Smith (1984) as

$$100 \frac{\sigma}{\bar{x}} \frac{h(i_\mathrm{m} r_\mathrm{Gm} + i_\mathrm{f} r_\mathrm{Gf})}{L_\mathrm{m} + L_\mathrm{f}}, \tag{1}$$

where m and f refer to male and female, $\bar{x}$ and σ are the mean and standard deviation of the trait selected, h^2 is the heritability, L is the average age of parents when their offspring are born, i is the selection intensity (the superiority of selected parents) from selection of the best proportion (p) for breeding, and r_G is the correlation of the breeding value of the individual selected and the information used in selection, and measures the accuracy of selection. The expression **(1)** shows the effect and interplay of the various factors affecting the response. If the heritability and correlation apply to the base population, the response is reduced by 22–27% (Dekkers, 1992) in later generations due to the effect of previous selection on the genetic variance in the current generation (Bulmer, 1971). Examples of possible predicted rates of selection response, and the component parts, are given in Table 1 for some relevant traits for the various species of farm livestock. Annual rates of 0.5% to over 3% of the mean are predicted. Note that response rates can be good for traits of low heritability if the coefficient of variation is high, for example, in litter size in pigs. Species with higher reproductive rates and shorter generation intervals tend to have higher possible rates of response.

Table 1 Rates of genetic response possible year for individual traits and livestock types and current selection effort.

	CV (%)	h^2 (%)	L (years)	*Form of selection*			*Selection intensity* $(i_m+i_f)/2$	*Possible genetic response (%/year)*	*Current selection effort*
				Indiv. index	*Family index*	*Progeny test*			
Cattle									
Growth rate	10	40	2.5	x		(x)	0.9	1.4	M
Lean percent	5	30[a]	2.5	x[a]			0.9	0.5	L
Milk yield	15	25	6	x		x	1.5	1.5	H
Sheep									
Growth rate	15	15	1.5	x			0.9	1.4	M
Lean percent	5	30[a]	1.5	x[a]			0.9	0.9	M
Litter size	30	10	1.8	x	(x)		1.4	2.1	L
Pigs									
Growth rate	7	30	1	x			1.3	2.7	H
Lean percent	4	30[a]	1	x[a]			1.3	1.6	H
Litter size	25	10	1	x	(x)		1.4	3.0	M
Chickens									
Growth rate	7	20	1	x			2.2	3.2	H
Lean percent	5	20[a]	1	x[a]			2.2	2.2	M
Egg production	10	8	1	x	(x)		1.8	2.1	H

From Smith (1984): CV — Coefficient of variation; h^2 — heritability; L — generation interval; [a] — allows for indirect measure of lean percent by fat depth; x — most common, (x) also used; i_m, i_f — male and female selection intensity; H — High, M — Moderate, L — Low.

RATES OF RESPONSE ACHIEVED

Sheridan (1988) reviewed selection responses, mainly in laboratory animals, and found a correlation of 0.5 between estimated and realized heritabilities. In the farm livestock experiments, the predicted rates of response overestimated the rates achieved. However, he did not allow for the temporary reduction in genetic variation due to previous selection (Bulmer, 1971). Smith (1984) examined rates of response achieved in selection experiments with farm animals and in industry. He found good rates of improvement in many cases and concluded that selection is effective if it is well applied. A good example of what is possible by selection is given by Havenstein et al. (1994) who compared control line broilers typical of 1957 commercial broilers with current (1991) commercial broilers. The annual rate of genetic change in weight at 12 weeks of age over the 34 years averaged 4.3% of the original mean, or 2.6% per year of the changing mean! Other traits, such as breast shape and muscling, had also been improved. There were some undesirable changes, especially increases in the incidence of leg defects and higher mortality rates, both moderated by husbandry practices. These large genetic changes in growth rate have led to concomitant changes in efficiency and costs of producing poultry meat and to its becoming the dominant meat consumed. Good rates of genetic response have also been obtained by industry in dairy cattle for milk yield (e.g. van Vleck, 1987; Burnside et al., 1992) and these should be spread internationally with multiple-country comparison of dairy sires — MACE (Schaeffer, 1993). Moderate rates of response have been obtained for increased growth and reduced fatness in pigs (e.g. Kennedy et al., 1996). By contrast, genetic changes in beef cattle and sheep have been small because there has been little consistent selection for traits of economic merit.

MULTI TRAIT SELECTION

In practice single trait selection is the exception rather than the rule. Usually several or many traits must be considered. As an example, traits relevant to the improvement of dairy cattle are listed in Table 2 and total 30 to 40. Similar lists could be made for other livestock. With so many traits, the selection pressure on any one trait is decreased, but the selection effort is concentrated on overall economic merit. This requires an evaluation of the economic value of a unit change in each of the traits to weight the traits in the breeding objective for overall merit. The heritabilities of the traits and the correlations among the traits, as well as the economic weights, are all taken into account in deriving the selection index. Theoretically, this maximises the overall genetic response in economic merit. In practice it may be expedient to omit the economically less important traits and concentrate on the most important (Smith, 1983; Sivanadian and Smith, 1997).

Table 2   List of 30–40 traits considered in genetic improvement of dairy cattle.

Vital traits	Viability, Age at sexual maturity, Fertility (male and female), Rebreeding period, Productive herd life (Longevity), Calving ease (calf and cow), Genetic defect free, Semen quality, Semen freezeability
Production traits	Milk yield, Protein yield, Fat yield, Feed intake, Body weight, Persistency, All lactations, Salvage value
Health traits	Reproductive health, Metabolic health (ketosis, milk fever), Udder health (mastitis resistance), Stress resistance
Structural traits	Feet and legs, Udder shape and height, Teat size and placement, Claw quality
Other traits	Temperament, Milking speed, Specific milk proteins (caseins and lactoglobulins)
Dairy type traits	Dairy character, Frame and capacity, Rump, Stature, Chest width, Loin strength, Pin width, Pin setting, Foot angle, Bone quality, Rear leg set, Udder texture, Final class

CROSS BREEDING

Crossbreds are used for commercial production in most species, as shown in Table 3. This is to take advantage of heterosis (hybrid vigour) and to exploit complementary differences between breeds. The exceptions are dairy cattle, fine wool sheep and racing horses, all of which predominantly use a single breed. In crossbreeding, species with higher reproductive rates use three-way and four-way crosses, while sheep and beef cattle use two-way crosses or rotational crosses (e.g. Gama and Smith, 1993). For the two-, three- and four-way crosses, different breeds/lines are needed and combined in an optimum way (Goddard, 1995). Breed lines will be selected for different sets of objectives (specialized lines) depending on their place in the crossing system. Selection is usually for purebred performances, rather than on crossbred performance, or on a combination of the two (Wei and van der Werf, 1994; Armstrong *et al.*, 1994). There is usually a number of breeds to choose from and breeding companies keep a number of different selection lines. This allows choice among them to accommodate changes in production or marketing requirements.

Briefly, there is little heterosis for carcass traits, 2–5% for growth and production traits and 5–10% for survival and reproductive traits, so it is usually worthwhile to utilize crossbreeding. However, unlike selection response, the benefits do not accumulate over generations.

STATISTICS AND COMPUTING

In animal breeding, the earlier methods of least squares analysis have been replaced by best linear unbiased prediction (BLUP) method (Henderson, 1984). This uses the relationships among animals to simultaneously estimate fixed effects and random animal (breeding value) effects needed for selection. With the great increase in computing power, large bodies of data over several generations and for several (multi) traits can be handled. Improved estimates of variance

CHARLES SMITH

Table 3 Current organisation of genetic improvement for the various livestock species showing the agencies and the breeding systems used for commercial production.

| | Genetic Improvement Agency | | | Commercial production | | | | |
	Individual breeders	Co-operative national	Breeding company	Purebred A	Two-way cross AB	Rotation A(B(C...))	Three-way cross A(BC)	Four-way cross AB(CD)
Cattle								
Dairy	+	++	++	+++	+			
Meat	+	+++		+	++	++	++	
Sheep								
Meat	+	+++		+	++		+++	
Wool	++	+		+++	+			
Pigs								
Meat		++	++			+	+++	++
Horses								
Racing	++			+++				
Chickens								
Eggs			+++		++		+++	++
Meat			+++				+++	++
Turkeys								
Meat			+++					+++

After Gama and Smith, 1993. +++ Most common, ++ Common, + Less common, rare if blank.

components can be obtained by iterative procedures such as restricted maximum likelihood (REML) and more recently by Gibbs Sampler methods, which derive marginal posterior distributions of the parameters, based on the data. These methods are enthusiastically received and used by animal breeders (Sorensen *et al.*, 1995), but the extra precision of the estimates of the parameter and of breeding values may be small. Some anomalous results are found, such as high negative genetic correlations between direct and maternal effects in beef cattle (Bailey *et al.*, 1995) and swine (Irgang *et al.*, 1994), and an effect of the number of generations studied affecting the estimates (Jeyaruban and Gibson, 1996). It is argued that the theory and new methodologies have been rather uncritically adopted with few experimental checks or data analyses to confirm the extra value of the more complex new models and methods (Fairfull and Muir, 1996).

Computing power has also led to many computer simulation studies, both deterministic and stochastic, at the expense of theoretical work. Many different models can be used, with a range of parameters and any number of replicates. Thus, many breeding strategies and genetic models can be studied, and copious results produced. Summarizing and synthesising these may be difficult. However, insights may be obtained and a theoretical and general solution derived.

Simulation may anticipate and highlight new problems. For example, selection on BLUP EBV, based on information relatives, results in higher average relationship among selected individuals and increased inbreeding in the progeny, compared to individual selection. Comparing selection schemes at the same level of inbreeding (by varying the number of sires selected) reduces the advantage of the more accurate methods (Quinton *et al.*, 1992; Verrier *et al.*, 1993). Several strategies, taking account of the relationship and merit of selection candidates, have been developed to achieve high rates of genetic response while moderating inbreeding (Brisbane and Gibson, 1995; Wray and Goddard, 1994; Woolliams and Meuwissen, 1993; Grundy *et al.*, 1994; Quinton and Smith, 1995).

GENETIC ARCHITECTURE

Our knowledge of the genetic architecture (number of loci and the distribution of their allelic frequencies and effects) is limited in laboratory animals (Shrimpton and Robertson, 1988; Pomp *et al.*, 1994; Keightley *et al.*, 1996) and is very limited for economic traits of farm livestock. There are a few loci with large effects (e.g. Smith and McMillan, 1989), but these are the exception. Most of the genetic variation is unassigned. The "infinite" locus model, with a large number of effects, is usually used theoretically and in simulation. More recently, models with an exponential distribution (a few with large or moderate effects, and many with small effects) have been used (e.g. Lande and Thompson, 1990). The search for quantitative trait loci (QTL) with moderate or large effects, using microsatellite markers, or directly for "candidate" genes through knowledge of their DNA, is now active. These approaches, allowing for a proportion of false positives, should give a good indication of the nature of the genetic variation. However, loci with large effects cannot be expected because selection would have already used and fixed such loci, unless they had compensating unfavourable effects on other traits. So, the hope is that loci with moderate effects can be reliably found and used to enhance selection methods (e.g. Lande and Thompson, 1990; Kashi *et al.*, 1990). However, if it turns out that most QTL loci have small effects, the benefits from identifying QTL will be small. Note also that the effects of QTL, and of genetic markers associated with them, will have to be estimated for all traits in the breeding goal, not a small task and one introducing estimation errors.

ORGANISATION

There are substantial differences in the organisation and agencies for genetic improvement in the different livestock species. These are outlined in Table 3. In poultry, almost all the improvement is done by competing breeding companies with professional poultry geneticists, and their work is very effective. Pig improvement and dairy cattle have competitive breeding companies, but also have national or farmer-cooperative agencies involved in genetic improvement. The improvement work is well focused on economic objectives and is quite effective. By contrast, sheep breeding and beef cattle breeding are still largely the province of the farmer-breeder, supported by recording schemes either breed or nationally organised. The economic objectives are less clearly defined and the schemes are less effective or ineffective.

DISCUSSION

Conventional selection on phenotypes is effective with rates of response of 0.5–3% of the mean per year, depending on the species and trait. Although modest, the responses are cumulative and become appreciable over time. In practice, they are not often realised because of misdirected selection, poor definition of breeding goals and changing requirements. The breeding goal will usually involve many traits rather than only a few, and needs continuous updating. However, this applies to any improvement method. Thus, conventional selection for economic merit, properly applied, provides both the foundation and the standard from which to measure the benefits of new methods and technologies. These will generally help to improve conventional methods rather than replace them. The value of knowing the genetic architecture of traits, of increasing the reproductive rate and of other technical advances offer improved efficiency in application of selection rather than novel systems. However, some new technologies, such as the development of transgenes, offer the use of new products or processes and these form a different approach. By and large, the early optimism about exploiting the new technologies as expressed in Smith *et al.* (1986) has still to be realised.

REFERENCES

Amer, P.R. (1994) Economic theory and breeding objectives. *5th World Congr. Genet. Appl. Livest. Prod.*, **18**, 197–204.

Amer, P.R. and Fox, G.C. (1992) Estimation of economic weights in genetic improvement using neo-classical production theory: an alternative to rescaling. *Anim. Prod.*, **54**, 341–350.

Armstrong, S.L., Miller, S.P., Wilton, J.W. and Griffiths, S. (1994) Combining purebred and crossbred data in multibreed genetic evaluation of beef cattle. *5th World Congr. Genet. Appl. Livest. Prod.*, **17**, 249–252.

Bailey, D.R.C., Liu, M.F. and Shannon, N.H. (1995) Effects of dietary energy planes on growth and heritability for postweaning growth traits in young beef bulls. *Canad. J. Anim. Sci.*, **75**, 469–472.

Brascamp, E.W., Smith, C. and Guy, D.R. (1985) Derivation of economic weights from profit equations. *Anim. Prod.*, **40**, 175–180.

Brisbane, J.R. and Gibson, J.P. (1995) Balancing selection response and rate of inbreeding by including genetic relationships in selection decisions. *Theor. Appl. Genetics*, **91**, 421–431.

Bulmer, M.G. (1971) The effect of selection on genetic variability. *Amer. Nat.*, **105**, 201–211.

Burnside, E.B., Jansen, G.B., Civati, G. and Dadati, D. (1992) Observed and theoretical genetic trends in a large dairy population under intensive selection. *J. Dairy Sci.*, **75**, 2242–2253.

Dekkers, J.C.M. (1992) Asymptotic response to selection on best linear unbiased predictors of breeding values. *Anim. Prod.*, **54**, 351–360.

Dekkers, J.C.M., Birke, P.V. and Gibson, J.P. (1995) Optimum linear selection indexes for multiple generation objectives with non-linear profit functions. *Anim. Sci.*, **61**, 165–175.

de Vries, A.G. (1989) A method to incorporate competitive position in the breeding goal. *Anim. Prod.*, **48**, 221–227.

Dickerson, G.E. (1970) Efficiency of animal production – molding the biological components. *J. Anim. Sci.*, **30**, 849–859.

Fairfull, R.F. and Muir, W.M. (1996) Selection and breeding of laying hens. Present and future solutions. *Proceedings of the 20th World Poultry Congress*, 395–415.

Gama, L.T. and Smith, C. (1993) The role of inbreeding depression in livestock production systems. *Livest. Prod. Sci.*, **36**, 203–211.

Goddard, M.E. (1983) Selection for non-linear profit functions. *Theor. App. Gen.*, **64**, 339–344.

Goddard, M.E. (1995) Optimal crossbreeding schemes for beef production. *Proc. Aust. Assoc. Anim. Breed. Genetics*, **11**, 434–438.

Grundy, B., Caballero, A., Santiago, E. and Hill, W.G. (1994) A note on using biassed parameter values and non-random mating to reduce the rates of inbreeding in selection programmes. *Anim. Prod.*, **59**, 465–468.

Havenstein, G.B., Ferket, P.R., Scheideler, S.E. and Larson, B.T. (1994) Growth, liveability and feed conversion of 1957 vs 1991 broilers when fed typical 1957 and 1991 broiler diets. *Poultry Sci.*, **73**, 1785–1794.

Henderson, C.R. (1984) *Applications of Linear Models in Animal Breeding*, University of Guelph, Guelph.

Irgang, R., Favero, J.A. and Kennedy, B.W. (1994) Genetic parameters for litter size of different parities in Duroc, Landrace and Large White sows. *J. Anim. Sci.*, **72**, 2237–2246.

Jeyaruban, M.G. and Gibson, J.P. (1996) Estimation of additive genetic variance in commercial layer poultry and simulated populations under selection. *Theor. Appl. Genetics*, **92**, 483–491.

Kashi, Y., Hallerman, E. and Soller, M. (1990) Marker assisted selection of candidate bulls for progeny testing programmes. *Anim. Prod.*, **51**, 63–74.

Keightley, P.D., Hardge, T., May, L. and Bulfield, G. (1996) A genetic map of quantitative trait loci for body weight in the mouse. *Genetics*, **142**, 227–235.

Kennedy, B.W., Quinton, M.A. and Smith, C. (1996) Genetic changes in Canadian performance tested pigs for fat depth and growth rate. *Canadian J. Anim. Sci.*, **76**, 41–48.

Lande, R. and Thompson R. (1990) Efficiency of marker assisted selection in the improvement of quantitative traits. *Genetics*, **124**, 743–756.

Pomp, D., Cushman, M.A., Foster, S.C., Drudik, D.K., Fortman, M. and Eisen, E.J. (1994) Identification of quantitative trait loci for body weight and body fat in mice. *5th World Congr. Genet. Appl. Livest. Prod.*, **21**, 209–212.

Ponzoni, R.W. (1988) The derivation of economic values combining income and expense in different ways: An example with Australian Merino sheep. *J. Anim. Breed. Genet.*, **105**, 143–153.

Quinton, M.A. and Smith, C. (1995) Comparison of evaluation-selection systems for maximising genetic response at the same level of inbreeding. *J. Anim. Sci.*, **73**, 2208–2212.

Quinton, M.A., Smith, C. and Goddard, M.E. (1992) Comparison of selection methods at the same level of inbreeding. *J. Anim. Sci.*, **70**, 1060–1067.

Schaeffer, L.R. (1993) Multicountry comparison of dairy sires. *J. Dairy Sci.*, **77**, 2671–2678.

Sheridan, A.K. (1988) Agreement between estimated and realised genetic parameters. *Anim. Breed. Abstr.*, **56**, 877–889.

Shrimpton, A.E. and Robertson, A. (1988) The isolation of polygenic factors controlling bristle score in Dros. melan. *Genetics*, **118**, 445–459.

Sivanadian, B. and Smith, C. (1997) The effect of adding further traits in index selection. *J. Anim. Sci.*, **75**, 2016–2023.

Smith, C. (1983) Effects of changes in economic weights on the efficiency of index selection. *J. Anim. Sci.*, **56**, 1057–1064.

Smith, C. (1984) Rates of genetic change in farm livestock. *Res. and Devel. in Agric.*, **1**, 79–85.

Smith, C., King, J.W.B. and McKay, J.C. (1986) *Exploiting New Technologies in Animal Breeding: Genetic Developments*. Oxford Science Pub.

Smith, C. and McMillan, I. (1989) The use of identified genes in animal breeding. In *Evolution and Animal Breeding*, edited by W.C. Hill and T.F.C. Mackay, CAB International, pp. 237–243.

Smith, C., James, J.W. and Brascamp, E.W. (1986) On the derivation of economic weights in livestock improvement. *Anim. Prod.*, **43**, 545–551.

Sorensen, D., Andersen, S. and Gianola, D. (1995) Gibbs sampling for likelihood and Bayesian inference in quantitative genetics. *46th Meeting European Assoc. Anim. Prod.*, Prague.

van Vleck, L.D. (1987) Observations on selection advances in dairy cattle. In *Quantitative Genetics*, edited by B.S. Weir, E.J. Eisen, M.M. Goodman and G. Hamburg. Sinauer Associates, Mass., USA.

van der Steen, H.A.M., Knap, P.W. and Bichard, M. (1994) The approach of an international breeding organisation to meet requirements of a national pig industry. *5th World Congr. Genet. Appl. Livest. Prod.*, **17**, 402–405.

Verrier, E., Colleau, J.J. and Foulley, J.L. (1993) Long-term effects of selection based on the animal model BLUP in a finite population. *Theor. Appl. Genet.*, **87**, 446–454.

Visscher, P.M. and Goddard, M.E. (1995) Genetic analysis of profit for Australian dairy cattle. *Anim. Sci.*, **61**, 9–18.

Wei, M. and van der Werf, J.H.J. (1994) Maximising genetic response in crossbreds using both purebred and crossbred information. *Anim. Prod.*, **59**, 401–413.

Wilton, J.W. and Goddard, M.E. (1996) Selection for carcass and feedlot traits considering alternative slaughter endpoints and optimised management. *J. Anim. Sci.*, **74**, 37–45.

Woolliams, J.A. and Meuwissen, T.H.E. (1993) Decision rules and variance of response in breeding schemes. *Anim. Prod.*, **56**, 179–186.

Wray, N.R. and Goddard, M.E. (1994) Increasing long-term response to selection. *Genet. Evol. Sel.*, **26**, 431–451.

Part 1
MANIPULATING THE EMBRYO

1. EMBRYO DEVELOPMENT AND CULTURE TECHNIQUES

DAVID K. GARDNER *

The Center for Reproductive Medicine
799 East Hampden Ave., Suite 300
Englewood, Colorado 80110, United States of America

The mammalian preimplantation/pre-attachment embryo undergoes considerable changes in its physiology and energy metabolism as it proceeds from the zygote to the blastocyst stage. Attempts to culture the mammalian zygote in the 1960s were restricted to a few strains of mice and their F1 hybrids, as the embryos of both sheep and cattle arrested in development at the 8- to 16-cell stage in culture. The introduction of co-culture techniques in the mid 1980s, whereby sheep and cattle embryos were incubated with somatic cells, helped to alleviate the *in vitro* induced arrest at the 8- to 16-cell stage and facilitated blastocyst development. However, such co-culture systems required the use of complex tissue culture media supplemented with serum. Serum has subsequently been shown to be associated with the production of offspring with significantly greater birth weights than normal, leading to both difficulties in managing such pregnancies and an unacceptable frequency of neonatal death. A recent resurgence of interest in mammalian embryo physiology has culminated in the formulation of defined embryo culture media, capable of supporting high levels of viable blastocyst development *in vitro*. Optimal embryo development in culture takes place not in one, but two or more media, each designed to cater for the changing requirements of the embryo as it develops. The ability to maintain the embryos of sheep and cattle in culture without compromising developmental potential will expedite the development and introduction of procedures such as transgenesis and cloning. This chapter reviews the physiology of the mammalian embryo and the subsequent development and application of new defined embryo culture systems for sheep and cattle.

KEY WORDS: cattle; sheep; preimplantation; pre-attachment; metabolism; viability.

INTRODUCTION

In contrast to the embryos of laboratory animals, relatively little is known about the physiology of the sheep and cattle embryo. This has stemmed primarily from the costs associated with the retrieval of such embryos from the female and from the paucity of techniques available for the study of single or small groups of embryos. However, with the advent of *in vitro* maturation and *in vitro* fertilization systems, and the development of more sensitive techniques for biochemical and genetic analysis, there has been an exponential increase in research on the embryos of domestic animals. One of the rate limiting factors to detailed analysis of ruminant embryo development has been the relative inability to maintain the viability of the pre-attachment embryo for extended periods outside of the maternal environment. This chapter therefore reviews present knowledge of the early mammalian embryo and discusses the development of culture systems for

---
* Tel.: 303-788-8300. Fax: 303-788-8310.

the embryos of the sheep and cattle which can maintain the development of the fertilized oocyte up to the hatching blastocyst stage. Furthermore, the possibility of being able to select the most viable embryos for transfer or cryopreservation from within a cohort using physiological markers is discussed.

PHYSIOLOGY OF THE EMBRYO AND FEMALE TRACT

Embryo Development from Zygote to Blastocyst

The physiology of the early embryos of domestic animals is markedly different to that of primates and rodents (Betteridge and Flecon, 1988; Leese, 1991; Parrish and First, 1993). Furthermore, rather than implanting in the endometrium on day-5 to -7 as in the human (Edwards, 1995) or late on day-4 as in the mouse (Pratt, 1987) the blastocysts of domestic animals undergo an extended pre-attachment period, such that apposition and attachment of the chorion to the uterine epithelium does not occur until around day-14 in sheep and around day-19 in cattle (McLaren, 1980; King and Thatcher, 1993). During this period there is extensive elongation of the blastocyst. This distinct difference between species gives rise to the terminologies of preimplantation embryo (for primates and rodents) and pre-attachment embryo (for domestic animals). It is also important to note that the physiology of the adults of different species are very different. The ruminant nature of domestic animals means that the types and levels of nutrients within the blood (Annison and Armstrong, 1970) and plausibly within the fluids of the reproductive tract will be different from that of both primates and rodents. This has implications for the possible nutrients available to the developing embryo.

In vivo, development of the zygote to the blastocyst stage in sheep and cattle takes about 6 days. Prior to the blastocyst stage there is no net growth of the embryo, and the individual cells (blastomeres) undergo restrictive mitoses, referred to as cleavage divisions (hence the term cleavage stage embryo). The cleavage stage embryos of most all mammalian species remain in the oviduct for around three days before entering the uterus. At this time sheep and cattle embryos have reached the 8- to 16-cell stage and are about to undergo the process of compaction. Prior to compaction, the individual blastomeres of the embryo are unattached and are therefore exposed to the maternal environment to the same degree. This has implications for the regulation of intracellular physiology, as each blastomere can be considered as in independent entity, apparently lacking the sophisticated regulatory mechanisms present in a multicellular tissue. Indeed, the homeostatic mechanisms employed by the individual blastomeres of the cleavage stage embryo are somewhat analogous to those used by unicellular organisms. The importance of this observation is evident once an attempt is made to culture these early stages (discussed below). Just prior to compaction, the blastomeres become polarised, marking the beginning of cell allocation within the embryo. The significance of compaction to embryo physiology is that it represents the formation of the first transporting epithelium of the conceptus (the trophectoderm). At this stage the embryo is referred to as a morula. It is the trophectoderm which is responsible for the regulation of the embryo's internal environment which is in turn essential for subsequent development and differentiation. Basolaterally positioned $Na^+/K^+/ATPases$ are thought to generate ion gradients up which fluid flows to create the blastocoel. The formation of such fluid and maintenance of the blastocoel is energetically expensive. The embryo at this stage is known as the blastocyst. The second cell type present in the blastocyst is the inner cell mass, a pluripotent group of cells from which the fetus will develop. These cells derive their nutrients from both the trophectoderm cells and the fluid comprising the blastocoel.

Composition of Oviduct and Uterine Fluids

During the pre-attachment period, the ruminant embryo has access to nutrients within the oviduct and uterine fluids. Analysis of oviduct and uterine fluids from several mammalian species has revealed some interesting observations. Carbohydrate levels do change with the day of oestrous or menstrual cycle. In the human oviduct, glucose levels are at their lowest and pyruvate levels at their highest at the time when the early embryo is present (Gardner et al., 1996a). In the uterus, glucose is present at relatively high levels, whilst pyruvate and lactate levels are significantly lower than in the oviduct. Similarly in the pig, glucose levels in the ampulla of the oviduct are significantly lower after mating than during the pre-ovulatory period (Nichol et al., 1992).

Importantly, oviduct and uterine fluids of the mammalian species studied so far are characterised by high levels of free amino acids (Perkins and Goode, 1967; Menezo, 1972; Casslen, 1987; Miller and Schultz, 1987; Gardner and Leese, 1990; Nancarrow et al., 1992; Moses et al., 1997). Specifically the amino acids alanine, aspartate, glutamate, glycine, serine and taurine are present at high concentrations. The fact that both oocytes and embryos possess specific transport systems for amino acids (Van Winkle, 1988), readily take them up from the surrounding culture medium (Partridge et al., 1996), and maintain an endogenous pool (Schultz et al., 1981), indicates that amino acids have a physiological role in the preimplantation/pre-attachment period of mammalian embryo development.

The concentration of all individual components of the fluids of the reproductive tract remains to be fully characterised, but we know that the developing embryo is exposed to ions, carbohydrates, amino acids, fatty acids, ketone bodies, albumin, glycosaminoglycans, glycoproteins and growth factors (Leese, 1988; Hunter, 1994). The precise function of each individual component in embryo development in domestic animals has yet to be elucidated, although many components have been shown to have an increasingly complex and interactive role in the development of the mouse embryo (Gardner and Lane, 1993a; Lane and Gardner, 1994, 1997).

Nutrition and Metabolism of the Embryo

The nutrition and metabolism of the developing mammalian embryo reflects somewhat its changing physiology, and like differences in whole animal physiology, differences in embryo nutrition and metabolism do exist between species. However, there appear to be some common traits among eutherian species, such as their susceptibility to oxidative stress and their requirement for different culture conditions as embryo development proceeds. It must be remembered however, that the available data has been generated from *in vitro* studies and care must therefore be taken when extrapolating to the embryo *in vivo*. Furthermore, the significance of energy metabolism during mammalian embryo development cannot be understated, as impairment of metabolism is associated with developmental delay and arrest (Seshagiri and Bavister, 1991; Gardner and Lane, 1993b; Gardner, 1998). It is evident that successful early embryo development is dependent upon the embryo's ability to generate energy though the appropriate metabolic pathway(s) at specific times during the preimplantation/pre-attachment period.

Unlike most somatic cells in culture, the mammalian embryo does not utilise glucose to a great degree until after compaction. In fact up to this stage of development, in certain culture conditions glucose can actually be detrimental to early mammalian embryo development (Schini and Bavister, 1988; Chatot *et al.*, 1989; Pinyopummintr and Bavister, 1991; Thompson *et al.*, 1992; Matsuyama *et al.*, 1993; Kim *et al.*, 1993a,b; Conaghan *et al.*, 1993). Rather than using this hexose, the early embryo utilises pyruvate, lactate and/or amino acids (Leese, 1991; Gardner and Lane, 1993a; Bavister, 1995) to generate the required energy. Furthermore, it appears that specific amino acids are essential for the maintenance of cellular physiology. Prior to the generation of the first transporting epithelium at compaction, the individual blastomeres of the embryo have limited means of controlling their intracellular environment, and are therefore at the mercy of the surrounding fluids. An adaptive response to this situation faced by unicellular organisms is the use of amino acids to stabilise protein function (Somero, 1986; Kinne, 1993; Ballantyne and Chamberlin, 1995). Amino acids can do this by acting as both osmolytes (Van Winkle *et al.*, 1990; Lawitts and Biggers, 1992; Biggers *et al.*, 1993) to protect against ionic stress and possibly as buffers of intracellular pH (Bavister and McKiernan, 1993). It is therefore proposed that specific amino acids not only serve as a suitable energy source for the embryo (Tiffin *et al.*, 1991; Rieger *et al.*, 1992a,b) but can act as regulators of energy metabolism (Gardner and Lane, 1993b; Gardner *et al.*, 1994) and confer a considerable degree of protection for intracellular function. Such amino acids include, alanine, glycine, glutamine and proline, i.e. those present at high levels in oviduct fluid.

The early embryo is characterised by low levels of oxidative metabolism and low oxygen consumption whilst the later stages (i.e. post-compaction) exhibit both high levels of glycolysis and high oxygen consumption (Mills and Brinster, 1967; Houghton *et al.*, 1996; Thompson *et al.*, 1996). The relatively low level of metabolism in the pre-compacted embryo may well reflect the quiescent state of the oocyte, which remains energetically dormant within the ovary for a considerable time. As the oocyte and zygote have relatively low levels of biosynthesis prior to embryonic genome activation and expression, there will be a high ATP/ ADP ratio within the blastomeres, which will in turn allosterically regulate the flux through the glycolytic pathway (Biggers *et al.*, 1989). As the embryo becomes increasingly transcriptionally active (Telford *et al.*, 1990) and protein synthesis increases (Frei *et al.*, 1989), and as the blastocoel is formed through the action of the basolateral ATPases (Benos and Biggers, 1981; Biggers *et al.*, 1988), the ATP/ ADP ratio will fall due to an increase in energy demand and an increased glycolytic flux will become possible. Indeed, glucose metabolism by both the sheep and cattle embryos increases with development, with the highest rates of utilisation occurring at the blastocyst stage (Tiffin *et al.*, 1991; Rieger *et al.*, 1992a,b; Thompson *et al.*, 1992; Gardner *et al.*, 1993).

The blastocysts of primates and rodents exhibit high levels of glycolysis even in the presence of adequate levels of oxygen for oxidative metabolism, termed "aerobic glycolysis". This has been interpreted as the embryos adaptation to its imminent invasion of the endometrium, which remains avascular for a period of up to 12 h, and will therefore be relatively anoxic (Rogers *et al.*, 1982a,b, 1983). It is likely, therefore, that glycolysis will be the predominant means of generating energy during implantation (Gardner, 1987; Leese, 1989). However, this may not be the sole explanation for the high levels of glycolysis in blastocysts of domestic animals as they do not 'implant' for a further week. An alternative explanation for the metabolism of the ruminant blastocyst is that a high level of aerobic glycolysis is a common characteristic of rapidly dividing cells and tumours, with which the mammalian blastocyst shares several traits (Hume and Weidermann, 1979; Morgan and Faik, 1981; Wenner and Tomei, 1981; Mandel, 1986). As well as being used to generate energy for blastocoel expansion and mitosis, high levels of glucose utilisation will be required for the synthesis of triacylglycerols and phospholipids and to provide precursors for complex sugars of mucopolysaccharides and glycoproteins. Glucose metabolised by the pentose phosphate pathway (PPP) generates ribose moieties required for nucleic acid synthesis and the NADPH required for the biosynthesis of lipids and other complex molecules (Reitzer *et al.*, 1980; Morgan and Faik, 1981). NADPH is also required for the reduction of intracellular glutathione, an important antioxidant for the embryo (Rieger, 1992). The production of nucleic acids is probably an important biosynthetic role of glucose in the blastocyst. Interestingly, although the absolute amount of glucose metabolised through the PPP increases with development (Rieger *et al.*, 1992a), the percentage of the total glucose consumed which is metabolised through this pathway is lowest at the blastocyst stage (Rieger and Guay, 1988). This again raises the question as to why such high levels of aerobic glycolysis are required. It has been proposed that high levels of aerobic glycolysis, such as that observed in the mammalian blastocyst, will ensure that there is sufficient substrate available for biosynthetic pathways, such as DNA replication, RNA transcription and synthesis of new membranes, at the required times during cellular proliferation (Newsholme *et al.*, 1985; Newsholme, 1990). This in turn suggests that there are times within the cell cycle during which the PPP is more active then others. A further explanation could lie in the utilisation of mitochondrial shuttles in the oxidation of hydrogen equivalents formed through glycolysis. Unfortunately, it is not known whether the blastocyst has the ability to transport hydrogen equivalents into the mitochondria via either the glycerol phosphate or malate-aspartate shuttles. Should these shuttles be lacking, then forming lactate from glucose will represent the only means of regenerating the cytoplasmic NAD^+ required for glycolysis to proceed. However, should one of these shuttles be present, then the blastocyst will be able to utilise glucose oxidatively. Interestingly, the malate-aspartate (NADH) shuttle of different tumours can contribute between 20% and 80% of the total respiratory rate (Greenhouse and Lehninger, 1976, 1977). As the mammalian blastocyst has a high respiratory quotient combined with high levels of lactate production, it is plausible that glycolysis is used to derive ATP oxidatively through the NADH shuttle.

   In contrast to the embryos of primates and rodents, the embryos of domestic animals have a considerable potential energy reserve in the form of lipid within the cytoplasm. However, the significance of such an endogenous store to embryo development has yet to be elucidated. *In vitro* studies indicate that exogenous energy substrates are required for cleavage and subsequent development of the cattle zygote (Pinyopummintr and Bavister, 1996a). Although it is feasible that energy-rich lipid reserves are utilised, the total lipid content of the bovine blastocyst actually increases by a factor of 10 from day 7 to day 13 (Menezo *et al.*, 1982), thereby questioning their utilisation as an endogenous energy reserve prior to this time. It is conceivable however that lipids are subsequently used as an energy source and for membrane synthesis during the elongation period.

   An important consideration, especially when one is trying to formulate culture media, is that looking at individual substrates may be misleading, as the embryo will be exposed to and utilises several nutrients at one time, with complicated and important interactions existing between them. Indeed, the mammalian embryo possesses a considerable degree of plasticity and can adapt to the absence of one substrate by increasing its utilisation of others (Gardner and Leese, 1988). Furthermore, inadequate culture conditions *in vitro* induce serious metabolic aberrations in the embryo, whereby the pattern of energy metabolism is significantly different to that of embryos developed *in vivo* (Menke and McLaren, 1970; Gardner and Leese, 1990; Gardner and Sakkas, 1993). It appears that the more unphysiological the culture conditions are, the greater the metabolic stress placed on the embryo, which in turn is associated with loss of developmental competence (Gardner and Lane, 1993b). Further studies on energy metabolism of the embryo will be invaluable in the continual development of more suitable culture media.

USE OF TEMPORARY RECIPIENTS AND CO-CULTURE

If the sheep or cattle embryo is replaced in the uterus prior to compaction, i.e. before the morula stage, embryo survival is low resulting in poor pregnancy rates (Bavister, 1995). This therefore necessitates extended culture of the embryo to facilitate non-surgical embryo transfer.

Species-Specific Blocks in Embryo Development in Culture

Early attempts to culture the mouse zygote to the blastocyst stage *in vitro* were unsuccessful, although it was possible to obtain blastocysts from the 2-cell stage. It became evident that mouse embryos from certain inbred and random-bred strains underwent a 2-cell block in development in culture (Whitten, 1956, 1957; Whittingham 1966). Similarly, attempts to culture the embryos of sheep or cattle resulted in their arrest at the 8- to 16-cell stage (Wright and Bondioli, 1981). Interestingly, both time points correspond to the time at which the embryonic genome is activated (Flach *et al.*, 1982; Telford *et al.*, 1990). Furthermore, for sheep and cattle embryos such blocks occur around the time when the embryo passes from the oviduct to the uterus and when mitochondria mature to adult configuration. It would appear therefore that this is a critical phase in the development of the mammalian embryo and that the embryo is very sensitive to its environment at this time.

Overcoming Developmental Arrest in Culture

A method developed to overcome the 2-cell block in the mouse, was to transfer the zygotes to an explanted mouse oviduct (Whittingham and Biggers, 1967). Although such a system was useful for such short term incubations, problems associated with maintaining a whole organ explant for several days did not make this an option for extended embryo culture.

A viable and successful alternative was the transfer of embryos to recipient animals whose oviducts had been ligated at the uterotubal junction to prevent the entry of embryos into the uterus. Interestingly, the recipient female did not have to be of the same species. This approach has been used successfully for the culture of early sheep and cattle embryos to the blastocyst stage. The rabbit (Lawson *et al.*, 1972; Boland, 1984; Sirard *et al.*, 1985; Iwasaki *et al.*, 1990) and sheep (Willadsen, 1979; Eyestone *et al.*, 1987) have been used as temporary recipients. However, this technique is not without considerable cost, labour and loss of embryos.

Therefore, in an attempt to mimic conditions *in vivo*, Gandolfi and Moor (1987) used a monolayer of oviduct epithelial cells to support the development of *in vivo* fertilised sheep embryos in culture. This co-culture of somatic cells and embryos was successful with 42% of embryos reaching the blastocyst stage after 6 days compared to very poor development (no blastocysts) in the control group. In the same year, Heyman *et al.* (1987) showed that trophoblastic vesicles derived from day-14 cattle and day-12 ewes could increase the number of embryos passing the 16-cell stage in culture. Since then, numerous studies have demonstrated that co-culture with somatic cells, many of which are not necessarily of the female reproductive tract or even the same species, can increase embryo development *in vitro* (Wiemer *et al.*, 1991; Goto *et al.*, 1988, 1994; Rehman *et al.*, 1994; Myers *et al.*, 1994; van Inzen *et al.*, 1995; Reed *et al.*, 1996). Furthermore, medium in which somatic cells have been cultured, termed conditioned medium, can also increase bovine embryo development (Eyestone and First, 1989).

Inherent Problems of Co-Culture

There are two important points to be raised at this time. Firstly, the majority of co-culture studies have employed complex tissue culture media as their standard growth solution. Secondly, co-culture systems invariably include serum. These culture conditions are required for the successful maintenance of the *somatic cells* present in the co-culture system. In the absence of the somatic cells, such media with serum support very low levels of embryo development (Gandolfi and Moor, 1987; Goto *et al.*, 1994). This observation is not totally surprising when one considers that the physiology of the pre-attachment embryo, especially prior to compaction, is very different of that of a somatic cell. The fact that co-culture works at all indicates at the very least that the somatic cells modify the culture medium in a manner consistent with embryo physiology. Recent studies by Rieger *et al.* (1995a) and by Edwards *et al.* (1997) have shown that this appears to be the case, with the somatic cells reducing the concentration of glucose significantly whilst producing favourable levels of lactate and pyruvate. Furthermore, an elegant study by Leppens and Sakkas (1995) showed quite clearly that the success or otherwise of embryo co-culture was dependant upon the base medium used. When a suitably defined embryo culture medium was used in the co-culture system, as opposed to a tissue culture medium, the somatic cells no longer conferred any benefit to the embryo. The actual mechanism(s) by which somatic cells confer their benefit is still a matter of contention (Bongso *et al.*, 1993; Bavister, 1993). Possible modes of action include the production of specific growth factors and proteins; alterations of the metabolite pool in the vicinity of the embryo; and the removal of possible embryo toxins, such as transitional metals. It is plausible that somatic cells could act in more than one way to confer their benefit to the embryo.

More alarming than the relatively low blastocyst development in co-culture however is the observation that when resultant blastocysts are transferred to recipient ewes/cattle the gestation periods are longer than normal. These pregnancies also give rise to some abnormally large offspring, with a 10–25% increase in birth weight (Behboodi *et al.*, 1995; Sinclair *et al.*, 1995). Furthermore, a high percentage of these large calves die (nearly 50%, Behboodi *et al.*, 1995). A possible cause of this may not be the action of the somatic cells per se, but rather the inclusion of serum in the culture medium as the macromolecule. In support of this, Walker *et al.* (1992, 1996) have reported the birth of large lambs after the culture of embryos to the blastocyst stage in synthetic oviduct fluid medium (SOF, Tervit *et al.*, 1972) supplemented with human serum. In this case serum is thought to induce the over expression of growth factors by the embryo. Importantly, mammalian embryos are never exposed to serum *in vivo*, as neither oviduct nor uterine fluids are simple serum transudates (Leese, 1988). Rather, serum is a pathological fluid, the composition of which is greatly undefined and which varies enormously with the source. Furthermore, serum is a vast reservoir for growth factors. Studies using more defined embryo culture systems (outlined below) have shown that the inclusion of serum induces premature blastulation (Walker *et al.*, 1992; Thompson *et al.*, 1995), changes in embryo morphology

(Figure 1.1) (Gardner, 1994; Gardner *et al.*, 1994; Thompson *et al.*, 1995), and perturbations in ultrastructure (Dorland *et al.*, 1994; Thompson *et al.*, 1995) and energy metabolism (Gardner *et al.*, 1994). Using a more defined culture system, SOF medium supplemented with amino acids and 8 mg/ml BSA (SOFaa), Thompson *et al.* (1995) were able to culture sheep zygotes to the blastocyst stage and then transfer them to recipient females. A cohort of zygotes was also cultured to the blastocyst stage in the presence of 20% human serum. When compared to lambs born to a group of naturally-mated ewes, it was found that those blastocysts cultured in the defined culture system (SOFaa) had a similar gestation length (145 ± 1 days) and birth weight (3.5 ± 0.2 kg) to those embryos developed *in vivo* from the zygote (146 ± 1 days and 3.4 ± 0.2 kg, respectively). In contrast, embryos

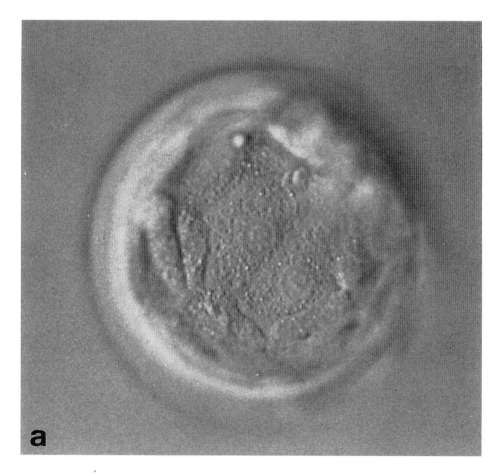

Figure 1.1 (a) Sheep blastocyst cultured from the zygote in synthetic oviduct fluid medium supplemented with all 20 of Eagle's amino acids (SOFaa). Note the translucent appearance of the trophectoderm. (From Gardner, 1994. With permission.)

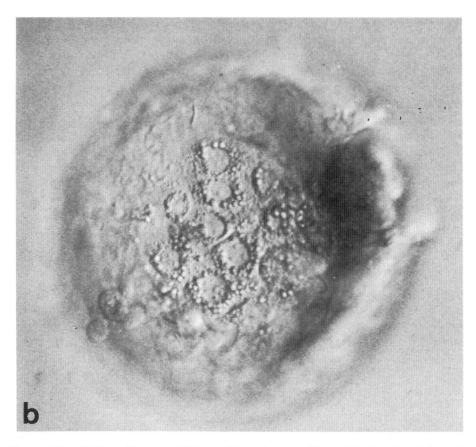

Figure 1.1   (b) Sheep blastocyst (sibling of that shown in Figure 1.1(a)) cultured from the zygote in SOF medium supplemented with 20% human serum. The trophectoderm exhibits many vesicular inclusions which have been shown to be lipid through osmium staining. (From Gardner, 1994. With permission.)

which had been ex- posed to serum in culture were born 2 days late (147 ± 1) and were significantly heavier $(4.2 \pm 0.2\,\mathrm{kg})$. Therefore the use of serum in embryo culture systems and the aetiology of the observed effects warrants consideration and investigation.

DEVELOPMENT OF DEFINED CULTURE SYSTEMS

With the resurgence of interest in the physiology of the sheep and cattle embryo (Rieger and Guay, 1988; Rieger *et al.*, 1992a,b; Tiffin *et al.*, 1991; Thompson *et al.*, 1992, 1993, 1994, 1996; Gardner *et al.*, 1993, 1994, 1996b, 1997a), there has been a dramatic increase in our knowledge regarding embryo nutrition and metabolism, and subsequently in our ability to maintain viable embryos in more defined culture conditions.

Regarding the development of the oocyte matured and fertilized *in vivo*, it appears that in the sheep at least it is possible to culture the zygote to the blastocyst at rates of 95% in 6 days of culture with cell numbers equivalent to those embryos developed *in vivo* (Gardner *et al.*, 1994). More importantly however, the resultant blastocysts had the equivalent viability of blastocysts developed *in vivo* (Gardner *et al.*, 1994). Unfortunately, there is little if any data on the development in culture of *in vivo* matured and fertilized bovine oocytes. As for the development of the fertilized oocyte matured *in vitro*, development in culture is less successful, with only around 50% of the resultant bovine embryos reaching the blastocyst in 6 days of culture (Gardner, 1994; Edwards *et al.*, 1997). However, the viability of these blastocysts is quite respectable, with 55% of those transferred resulting in offspring (Gardner, 1994). Similar rates have also been reported for the sheep (Thompson *et al.*, 1995). It would appear therefore that the process of *in vitro* maturation (IVM) and/or *in vitro* fertilization (IVF) are not optimised, resulting in impaired embryo development. Although it is conceivable that improved culture conditions will further increase embryo development *in vitro* culture (IVC), it is plausible that substantial increases in embryo development will come from improvements in IVM and IVF conditions. However, one must consider the fact that those oocytes matured *in vivo* have been naturally selected, while those oocytes matured *in vitro* are taken from follicles of unknown status.

APPLICATION OF IVM/IVF/IVC

IVM Conditions

Conditions for *in vitro* maturation of sheep and bovine oocytes have remained relatively unchanged since their inception. Follicles of between 2 and 8 mm in diameter are aspirated from the ovary (Pavlok *et al.*, 1992; Blondin and Sirard, 1995; Sirard and Blondin, 1996), and oocytes mature at 39°C in 5% CO_2 for around 24 h. Machatkova *et al.* (1996) reported that for optimal embryo development, oocytes should be collected at the end of the luteal phase (days 14 to 16). Maturation of oocyte–cumulus complexes routinely takes place in tissue culture medium TCM-199 with Earle's salts supplemented with 10% heat-treated fetal calf serum. However, the use of tissue culture media for oocyte maturation is now being questioned. It has been demonstrated that different maturation media affect subsequent embryo development (Bavister *et al.*, 1992; Rose and Bavister, 1992). It is evident that events during maturation *in vitro* have significant effects on subsequent developmental capability of resultant embryos (De Matos *et al.*, 1995, 1996). Follicle stimulating hormone (FSH; around 0.075 units/ml), luteinizing hormone (LH; around 0.075 units/ml) and oestradiol (around 1 µg/ml) are routinely added to the maturation medium employed (Blondin and Sirard, 1995; Thompson *et al.*, 1995). However, the effectiveness of exogenous gonadotrophins in the presence of serum has been questioned (Keefer *et al.*, 1993). Interestingly, the levels of gonadotrophins used in *in vitro* maturation systems are several orders of magnitude greater than physiological concentrations (Bevers *et al.*, 1997). Furthermore, a combination of epidermal growth factor (EGF; 50 ng/ml) and insulin-like growth factor-1 (IGF-1; 100 ng/ml) has been shown to be capable of stimulating nuclear maturation in the absence of serum and gonadotrophins (Rieger *et al.*, 1995b; Gandolfi *et al.*, 1996). Such oocytes gave rise to equivalent percentages of blastocysts as those oocytes matured in the presence of serum and gonadotrophins, i.e. conventional maturation conditions.

Upon maturation, the surrounding cumulus cells undergo expansion as exhibited in Figure 1.2. The cumulus cells surrounding the oocyte are required not only for endocrine support of oocyte maturation, but also serve to produce appropriate energy substrates for the oocyte during maturation, fertilization and subsequent embryo development (Leese and Barton, 1985; Gardner and Leese, 1990; De Loos *et al.*, 1991; Zuelke and Brackett, 1992, 1993; Zhang *et al.*, 1995; Gardner *et al.*, 1996).

Interestingly the optimal oxygen concentration for oocyte maturation and subsequent fertilization is 20% (Pinyopummintr and Bavister, 1995). This is in contrast to the requirements of the embryo, for which the optimal concentration appears to be below 10% (see the section on IVC). Although the optimal oxygen

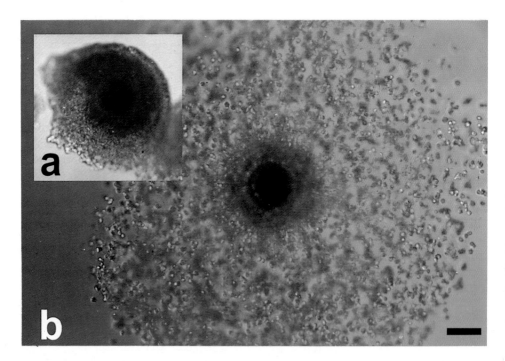

Figure 1.2 (a) Immature cattle oocyte collected from a 6 mm follicle of an excised ovary. (b) The same oocyte as (a) after maturation for 24 h in tissue culture medium 199 supplemented with 0.075 units/ml FSH and LH and 10% fetal calf serum. Note degree of cumulus expansion. Bar is 100 μm.

concentration for oocyte maturation is higher than required for embryo culture, the oocyte itself may not be exposed to 20% oxygen due to the active metabolism of the cumulus cells. The actual concentration of oxygen in the vicinity of the oocyte will realistically be below 20%.

IVF Conditions

Unlike the spermatozoa of humans and rodents which undergo spontaneous capacitation *in vitro*, the spermatozoa of ruminants require exposure to an oviductal environment for capacitation. Analysis of bovine oviduct fluid revealed that a heparin like glycosaminoglycan was the potential capacitating agent for spermatozoa (Parrish *et al.*, 1989a). Therefore, the glycosaminoglycan heparin can be used to capacitate spermatozoa *in vitro* (Parrish *et al.*, 1988). Penicillamine, hypotaurine and epinephrine (PHE) are routinely added to the fertilization medium in order to decrease the time for fertilization to be achieved (Susko-Parrish *et al.*, 1990). However, the mechanism by which PHE assists fertilization remains unknown. Of note is the observation that glucose in the fertilization medium delays capacitation (Parrish *et al.*, 1989b), and therefore it is routinely omitted. The most commonly used fertilization medium is Tyrodes Albumin Lactate Pyruvate medium, referred to as Fert-TALP (Bavister and Yanagamachi, 1977; Bavister, 1989), although modifications of embryo culture media such as SOF can also be used just as successfully for both sheep and cattle (Thompson *et al.*, 1995; Earl *et al.*, 1997). Similarly, Keskintepe and Brackett (1996) have used Brackett and Oliphant's Defined Medium (DM: Brackett and Oliphant, 1975) for bovine sperm preparation and IVF. Insemination times of around 18 to 20 h, a temperature of 39°C in 5% CO_2 in air (20% O_2), and sperm numbers of around 1×10^6/ml are conventionally used.

In Vitro Culture Conditions

Ions

Sodium chloride is the most abundant salt in any culture medium and therefore makes the greatest contribution to the osmolarity of the medium. Although oviduct fluid has been reported to be hyperosmotic (around 360 mOsmol: Borland *et al.*, 1977, 1980), mammalian embryo development in culture is higher at reduced osmolarities (around 250–270 mOsmol: Whitten and Biggers, 1968; Lawitts and Biggers, 1991; Liu and Foote, 1996). High concentrations of sodium chloride appear to be especially detrimental to embryo development in culture (Lawitts and Biggers, 1992; Lim *et al.*, 1994).

Carbohydrates

Pinyopummintr and Bavister (1991) obtained limited development of bovine embryos to the blastocyst after 8 days of culture in hamster embryo culture medium (HECM), which had no pyruvate or glucose. Rosenkrans *et al.* (1993) subsequently showed that in the absence of pyruvate it was possible to get bovine blastocyst development, albeit at very low percentages. However, as pyruvate, lactate and glucose are all present in the mammalian oviduct and uterus (Carlson *et al.*, 1970; Casslen and Nilsson, 1984; Leese, 1988; Gardner and Leese, 1990; Nichol *et al.*, 1992; Gardner *et al.*, 1996a), it is more physiological to include all of the carbohydrates in the culture medium. Among the highest reported rates of both sheep and cattle embryo development have occurred when embryos were cultured in the presence of 0.33 mM pyruvate, 3.3 mM lactate and 1.5 mM glucose (Gardner *et al.*, 1994; Keskintepe *et al.*, 1995; Edwards *et al.*, 1997).

Amino Acids

Amino acids are now acknowledged as important regulators of early mammalian embryo development in culture (Bavister and McKiernan, 1993; Bavister, 1995; Gardner and Lane, 1993a,c, 1996, 1997; Gardner, 1994; Lane and Gardner, 1994, 1997; McKiernan *et al.*, 1995). With the exception of taurine those amino acids at high concentrations in oviduct fluid bear a striking homology to those amino acids present in Eagle's (Eagle, 1959) non-essential amino acids. Gardner and Lane (1993c) demonstrated that while Eagle's non-essential amino acids and glutamine increased development of the cleavage stage mouse embryo, Eagle's essential amino acids actually impaired early embryo development in culture. Gardner *et al.* (1994) subsequently showed that the inclusion of Eagle's amino acids in SOF medium, significantly increased the development of *in vivo* fertilized sheep zygotes to the blastocyst stage in culture. In this study it was possible to obtain 95% blastocyst formation on day-6 of culture compared with 67% when the SOF medium lacked amino acids and was supplemented with 20% human serum. Furthermore 79% of the blastocysts developed in SOFaa medium hatched, and the mean blastocyst cell numbers (173 ± 6) were equivalent to *in vivo* developed control blastocysts (160 ± 9). The viability of such blastocysts was equivalent to that of *in vivo* developed embryos. When this culture system was employed for the development of IVM/IVF cattle embryos, around 50% of fertilised oocytes reached the blastocyst stage after just 6 days of culture (Gardner, 1994; Edwards *et al.*, 1997; Tables 1.1 and 1.2). Figure 1.3 shows the typical morphology of cattle embryos cultured from the zygote to the hatching blastocyst stage in SOFaa medium, complete development *in vitro* occurring in 6 days of culture. Similarly, Rosenkrans and First (1994), found that the addition of the amino acids present in either Eagle's basal medium of Eagle's minimum essential medium to the embryo culture medium CR1 increased cattle embryo development to the blastocyst stage *in vitro*, although embryo development in this medium appears relatively low (Table 1.2). Liu and Foote (1995), using the culture medium KSOM (Lawitts and Biggers, 1993) as the base, found that Eagle's non-essential amino acids with essential amino acids (at half the concentration used by Eagle) gave highest blastocyst development. Interestingly at the concentration used by Eagle, essential amino acids were reported to be inhibitory to embryo development,

Table 1.1 Composition of embryo culture media for sheep and cattle embryos.

Component	SOF[a]	KSOM[b]	CR1aa[c]	mHECM-3[d]
NaCl	107.7	95	114.7	113.8
KCl	7.16	2.5	3.1	3.0
KH_2PO_4	1.19	0.35	—	—
$CaCl_2 \cdot 2H_2O$	1.71	1.71	—	1.90
$MgCl_2 \cdot 6H_2O$	0.49	—	—	0.46
$MgSO_4 \cdot 7H_2O$	—	0.2	—	—
$NaHCO_3$	25.1	25.0	26.2	25.0
Na pyruvate	0.33	0.20	0.40	—
Na lactate	3.3	10.0	—	3.5
Ca lactate	—	—	5.0	—
Glucose	1.5	0.20	—	—
Gln	1.0	1.0	1.0	@
Non-essential amino acids	Yes	Yes	Yes	@
Essential amino acids (minimum essential medium)	Yes	Yes (at half concentration)	No	@
Essential amino acids (basal medium eagle)	No	No	Yes	No
EDTA	0.1	0.01	0	0
BSA (mg/ml)	8	#	3	—
PVA (mg/ml)	#	1	—	0.1

[a] Gardner, 1994; Gardner et al., 1994, 1997a; Keskintepe et al., 1995; Thompson et al., 1995.
[b] Liu and Foote, 1995.
[c] Rosenkrans and First, 1994.
[d] Pinyommintr and Bavister, 1996a.
BSA and/or PVA have also been used.
@ 11 amino acids present in HECM-6; McKiernan et al., 1995.

a finding reported previously in the mouse (Gardner and Lane, 1993c). Consistent with the beneficial effects of non-essential amino acids on the embryo, are the findings of Moore and Bondioli (1993) and Lee and Fukui (1996), that glycine and alanine stimulate cattle embryo development. However, of all the amino acids glutamine has received most attention. Not only is this amino acid metabolised by the cattle embryo throughout development (Rieger et al., 1992a,b) but has been shown to be as effective as groups of amino acids in stimulating the development of the cleavage stage cattle embryo (Pinyopummintr and Bavister, 1996b; Steeves and Gardner, 1997).

Interestingly, the mammalian embryo appears to undergo a switch in its amino acid requirement as development proceeds. In both cattle and mice, pre-compacted embryo development is faster in the presence of Eagle's non-essential amino acids and glutamine (Lane and Gardner, 1997; Steeves and Gardner,

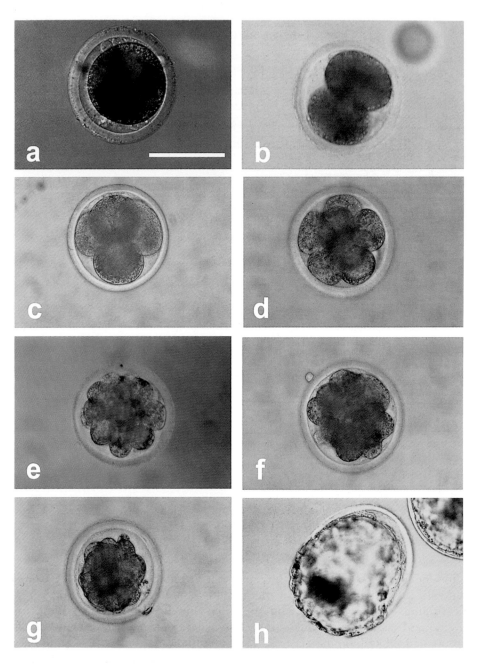

Figure 1.3 Temporal development of cattle embryos in culture. Embryos were grown in medium SOFaa. (Gardner, 1994) (a) Denuded fertilised oocyte 20 h post insemination (PI). Bar is 100 μm. (b) 2-cell embryo, at 32 h PI. (c) 4-cell embryo at 44 h PI. (d) 8-cell embryo at 68 h PI. (e) 16-cell embryo at 92 h PI. (f) 16- to 32-cell embryo undergoing the intial phase of compaction around 116 h PI. (g) morula at 140 h PI. (h) Expanded hatching blastocyst at 168 h PI (6 days of culture from the zygote). Note the inner cell mass in the bottom left of the blastoyst.

Table 1.2 Development of *in vitro* produced cattle embryos in different culture systems.

Culture system	Reference	% Blastocyst from cleaved oocytes	Blastocyst cell number	Number of days in culture
Co-culture with bovine oviduct epithelial cells and serum	Wiemer *et al.* (1991)	47	nd	8
HECM	Pinyommintr and Bavister (1991)	10	119	8
SOFaa with BSA	Gardner (1994)	45	123	6
	Edwards *et al.* (1997)	64	97	6
SOFaa with PVA	Keskintepe *et al.* (1995)	50	nd	6
CR1aa with BSA	Rosenkrans and First (1994)	29	nd	6
KSOM with PVA. First 48 h in KSOM with no amino acids followed by culture in KSOM with amino acids for 6 days	Liu and Foote (1995)	41	nd	8
mHECM-3 with lactate, 11 amino acids and PVA for 2 days followed by culture in TCM 199 + 10% bovine serum	Pinyommintr and Bavister (1996a)	41	nd	8

1997). Beneficial effects of this group of amino acids, which also contains alanine and glycine, may well be attributable to their protective role in maintaining cellular function (described above). After compaction, embryo development is enhanced by the inclusion of all 20 amino acids. It has been shown in the mouse that while the non-essential amino acids stimulate the trophectoderm and glutamine stimulates hatching, the inclusion of essential amino acids causes an increase in the number of inner cell mass cells (Lane and Gardner, 1997).

A cautionary note when dealing with amino acids in embryo culture media is that they are highly labile in solution at $37°C$, the result of which is the release of ammonium into the medium (Gardner and Lane, 1993c). This ammonium is toxic to the early embryo and can even induce birth defects in the mouse (Lane and Gardner, 1994). It is therefore very important that this toxicity is alleviated for optimal embryo growth to occur. This can be achieved in one of two ways; either the medium can be renewed every 48 h (mouse and human) and 72 h (sheep and cattle), or the ammonium can be transaminated *in situ* to form the non-toxic product glutamate (Lane and Gardner, 1995).

Vitamins

Although the role of vitamins in rabbit embryo development has been thoroughly investigated (Kane, 1987), there have been relatively few studies on their role in either sheep (Gardner *et al.*, 1994) or cattle embryo development (Rosenkrans and First, 1994). The reason for this may lie in the fact that ruminant blastocysts will develop readily in culture in the absence of vitamins providing amino acids are present. However, vitamins do stimulate cattle blastocyst expansion post-hatching in culture when added after compaction (Gardner, unpublished observations).

Proteins and Other Macromolecules

The source and type of protein to which embryos are exposed in culture has significant effects on embryo development. Pinyopummintr and Bavister (1991) demonstrated a biphasic response of the cattle embryo to serum, with serum inhibiting development at or before the first cleavage whilst stimulating blastocyst formation when added prior to compaction. Subsequently, Pinyopummintr and Bavister (1994) showed that different serum types such as bovine calf and fetal calf affected embryo development and that heat inactivation of serum was not necessary. In the case of serum albumin there is not only considerable variation between sources but even between lot numbers (Batt *et al.*, 1991; McKiernan and Bavister, 1992; Rorie *et al.*, 1994). This variation in both serum and serum albumin has led to the call for protein-free culture media, in which alternative, more defined macromolecules are used. Two candidates include polvinyl alcohol (PVA, Bavister, 1981) and a more physiological macromolecule, the glycosaminoglycan hyaluronate (HA, Furnus *et al.*, 1996; Gardner *et al.*, 1997b). From *in vitro* studies it is evident that serum is not required for blastocyst development in the ruminant embryo, blastocysts developing in the presence of either BSA, PVA or HA in such media as SOF (Gardner, 1994; Gardner *et al.*, 1994; Keskintepe *et al.*,1995, 1996; Thompson *et al.*, 1995; Furnus *et al.*, 1996) or KSOM (Liu and Foote, 1995), supplemented with amino acids.

Growth Factors

It is known that the mammalian embryo produces the transcripts for specific growth factors during development (Watson *et al.*, 1992, 1994). Indirect evidence for the role of endogenous growth factors has come from the observations that embryo development in culture was increased when embryos were cultured in reduced volumes and/or in groups (Wiley *et al.*, 1986; Paria and Dey, 1990; Lane and Gardner, 1992; Gardner *et al.*, 1994; Keefer *et al.*, 1994). More importantly, culturing mouse embryos in reduced incubation volumes and in groups increased viability after transfer (Lane and Gardner, 1992). It has since been shown that an increase in cell number and viability stems from a specific increase in inner cell mass size when embryos are cultured in groups (Gardner *et al.*, 1997c). Interestingly, grouping embryos in the same drop of medium had no effect on trophectoderm cell numbers, implying a cell specificity for the factor. This finding has since been repeated in cattle (Gardner and Ahern, unpublished observations). Subsequently, there has been much interest in identifying such factors so that they can be added to the culture medium (Schultz *et al.*, 1992; Heyner *et al.*, 1993; Stewart, 1994; Harvey *et al.*, 1995). A limited number of exogenous growth factors, such as platelet derived growth factor (PDGF) (Larson *et al.*, 1992a; Thibodeaux *et al.*, 1993), transforming growth factor β and basic fibroblast growth factor (Larson *et al.*, 1992b) have been tried in cattle embryo culture and shown to increase embryo development beyond the 8- to 16-cell stage. Although conferring limited benefit on their own, combinations of growth factors may well have synergistic effects on embryo development.

Gas Phase

The oxygen concentration within the lumen of the female reproductive tract has been measured in several species and two important observations have been reported. Firstly the concentration of oxygen within the female tract (3–9%; Bishop, 1965; Mastroianni and Jones, 1965; Ross and Graves, 1974; Fischer and Bavister, 1993) is significantly less than that present in air (20%). Secondly, the oxygen concentration tends to be lower in the uterus than oviduct (Fischer and Bavister, 1993), as low as 1.5% in the monkey uterus. In line with these physiological data, development of mammalian embryos in culture is significantly increased when the oxygen concentration is between 5% and 10% compared to 20% (air) (Quinn and Harlow, 1976; Thompson *et al.*, 1990; Batt *et al.*, 1991; Bernadi *et al.*, 1996; Gardner and Lane, 1996). From such observations it has been proposed that the mammalian embryo is susceptible to oxidative stress (Johnson and Nasr-Esfahini, 1994). It is plausible therefore that as ruminant embryos have a higher lipid content compared to mouse embryos (Leese, 1991) that they will be more susceptible to oxidative damage *in vitro*. The inclusion of specific antioxidants in the culture medium may therefore serve to improve ruminant embryo development. Indeed, it has been reported that the inclusion of 1 mM glutathione significantly improved development of the cattle embryo to the blastocyst (Luvoni *et al.*, 1996). Interestingly, pyruvate which is present in all embryo culture media for sheep and cattle, acts as an antioxidant being able to reduce intracellular levels of hydrogen peroxide in the embryo (Kouridakis and Gardner, 1995).

Requirement for Quality Control

In order to successfully develop and use defined embryo culture media it is paramount that the laboratory has a most rigorous quality control system in place. In a co-culture system both the somatic cells and serum undoubtedly help to mop up any toxins present, thereby conferring a greater degree of tolerance to the system. Until the time when defined media become commercially available it is essential to run bioassays on each new component of the culture system. The most suitable bioassay for any media is the cell type that one is trying to grow. However, in the case of domestic animal embryos this is not always feasible or economic. Therefore, an alternative is the use of a mouse embryo bioassay (Gardner and Lane, 1993a). In such a bioassay each medium component can be screened for toxicity by culturing mouse zygotes in protein-free medium for 4 days, by which time greater than 80% of the embryos should have reached the expanded blastocyst stage.

Comparison of Culture Systems

The problem with most all studies on the cattle embryo is that few, if any, studies have involved embryo transfers, i.e. determination of viability. This makes a true evaluation and comparison of culture systems very difficult. Tables 1.1 and 1.2 show the composition of several embryo culture media and their ability to support the development of *in vitro* produced cattle embryos. Interestingly, it would appear that SOFaa medium is superior to both KSOM and HECM media supplemented with specific amino acids, in its ability to support cattle embryo development to the blastocyst stage.

FUTURE DEVELOPMENTS

Use of Lambs and Calves as Oocyte Donors

With the advent and increasing success of IVM, IVF and IVC procedures, one of the rate limiting factors in assisted breeding technology is the time taken for any progeny to reach sexual maturity. However, prepuberal calves have been used successfully as oocyte donors, thereby greatly reducing generation intervals (Armstrong *et al.*, 1992). Oocytes can be collected either by laparoscopy, laparotomy or transvaginal ultrasound. It is therefore possible to mature and fertilize oocytes from a prepuberal calf, transfer the resultant embryos to recipients and obtain live offspring before the oocyte donor has herself reached sexual maturity. However, there appears to be variations in the ability of laboratories to culture the embryos of calves younger than 6 months old (Revel *et al.*, 1995; Duby *et al.*, 1996; Tervit, 1996). Similarly, in the sheep Earl *et al.* (1995) have demonstrated that it is feasible to obtain large numbers of viable oocytes from 8 to 9 week old lambs. Clearly ongoing research in this area will culminate in the dramatic reduction in generation intervals.

Sequential Culture Media/Perfusion Culture

The mammalian embryo is exposed to a changing environment as it progresses through the female reproductive tract. Furthermore, the embryo itself undergoes significant changes in its physiology and requirements. Therefore, it is not realistic to talk about developing the optimal culture medium when in effect optimal embryo development requires the use of two or more media, each formulated to meet the changing requirements of the embryo. In the mouse

(Gardner *et al.*, 1997d; Lane and Gardner, 1997) and human (Barnes *et al.*, 1995; Gardner and Lane, 1997; Gardner *et al.*, 1997d) it has been demonstrated that using specifically formulated sequential media significantly increased both embryo development in culture and viability after transfer. An alternative to using sequential media, whereby the embryos are physically placed in different culture conditions on successive days, is the use of perfusion culture (Wilson *et al.*, 1992; Gardner, 1994; Thompson, 1996; Reggio *et al.*, 1996). The development of a suitable perfusion system has the advantage that not only can the embryo be exposed to a potent- ially infinite number of nutrient gradients, but all potentially harmful end-products of metabolism such as ammonium can be readily removed. Furthermore, the embryo can be exposed to specific growth factors at the appropriate time during development and one need not be concerned about the half life of such factors.

Selection of Viable Embryos Prior to Transfer

Assessment of viable embryos in culture remains notoriously subjective, gross embryo morphology being used as the most common method of selecting embryos for transfer. Development of suitable and practical tests of embryo viability will increase the overall success of assisted reproductive procedures by identifying those embryos with little developmental potential prior to transfer or cryopreservation. There are several comprehensive reviews on the suitability of viability tests for embryos (Rieger, 1984; Gardner and Leese, 1993; Overstrom, 1996). In the following section, the most promising candidates for means of identifying viable embryos will be discussed.

Nutrient Uptake/Energy Metabolism

In 1980 Renard *et al.* (1980), demonstrated that day-10 cattle blastocysts which had a glucose uptake higher than 5 µg/h developed better both in culture and *in vivo* after transfer than those blastocysts with a glucose uptake below this value. Unfortunately, due to the insensitivity of the spectrophotmetric method employed it was not possible to quantitate glucose uptake by earlier embryos. Following on from this work, Rieger (1984) showed that morphologically normal day-7 cattle blastocysts took up significantly more radiolabelled glucose that degenerating ones. Rieger (1984) went on to propose that embryonic metabolism may well be a suitable method of assessing viability prior to transfer. Using a similar approach, Rondeau *et al.* (1995), demonstrated that utilisation of radiolabelled substrates by mouse morulae in culture was correlated with embryo morphology. With the development of non-invasive microfluorescence however, it became possible to quantitate glucose uptake by individual day-4 mouse blastocysts prior to transfer to recipient females (Gardner and Leese, 1987). It was found that those embryos which went to term had a significantly higher glucose uptake in culture than those embryos which failed to develop after transfer. Unfortunately, all of these studies were retrospective and as such could not conclusively demonstrate whether it was possible to identify viable embryos prior to transfer using metabolism as a marker. However, a study on the metabolism of day-7 cattle blastocysts before and after cryopreservation showed that it was possible to identify those blastocysts capable of re-expansion in the hours immediately post thaw. Those blastocysts which survived the freeze-thaw procedure had a significantly higher glucose uptake and lactate production than those embryos which did not re-expand and subsequently died (Gardner et al., 1996b). Of greater significance however, was the observation that there was no overlap in the distribution of glucose uptake by the *viable* and *non-viable* embryos, suggesting that it may therefore be possible to use metabolic criteria for prospective selection of viable embryos (Gardner et al., 1996b). Following on from this study, Lane and Gardner (1996) performed a prospective trial in which day-5 mouse blastocysts were classified as either viable or non-viable according to their glycolytic activity. It was found that those blastocysts which exhibited a pattern of glycolytic utilisation similar to that of embryos developed *in vivo* had a developmental potential of 80%, whilst those blastocysts which exhibited an excessive lactate production (i.e. aberrant glycolytic activity), had a developmental potential of only 6%. As such, this data supports the hypothesis proposed by Rieger (1984) that embryonic metabolism can be used to successfully identify viable embryos in culture prior to transfer, thereby significantly increasing pregnancy rates.

Oxygen Uptake

With the advent of multichannel embryo microrespiration systems (Overstrom, 1987, 1996; Overstrom et al., 1992) and fluorometric assays (Houghton et al., 1996; Thompson et al., 1996), it is now possible to non-invasively quantitate oxygen consumption by individual and small groups of cattle embryos. These procedures will be invaluable in elucidating mammalian embryo metabolism/respiration. Whether oxygen consumption by embryos is correlated with developmental potential has yet to be determined.

Enzyme Leakage

A tangible marker of plasma membrane integrity, and therefore cellular viability, is the leakage of specific cytosolic enzymes, such as lactate dehydrogenase (LDH), into the surrounding medium. Johnson et al. (1991) used this approach to assess the developmental capacity of day 6.5 to 7.5 *in vivo* produced cattle embryos after 24 h in culture. There was a significant inverse relationship between the appearance of the enzyme LDH in the medium and embryo development, i.e. those embryos which failed to develop released significantly more enzyme into the surrounding culture medium. Whether this approach can be used prospectively to select viable embryos has yet to be determined.

Hormone/Growth Factor Production

Hernandez-Ledezma et al. (1993) have shown that the production of trophoblast interferon by cattle blastocysts was determined by both the developmental stage and quality of the embryo. It is most likely, therefore, that the ability to detect such factors in the culture medium will be of great value in determining the viability of an embryo.

Sexing

Different rates of development according to the sex of an embryo was first reported in the mouse by Tsunoda *et al.* (1985), who observed that male embryos developed to the blastocyst stage faster than females *in vitro*. This observation was subsequently confirmed by Gardner and Leese (1987). Physiological differences between male and female embryos may stem from the fact that female embryos have twice the activity of X-linked genes over males during the preimplantation/ pre-attachment period (Adler *et al.*, 1977; Epstein *et al.*, 1978; Monk and Harper, 1979; West, 1982; Williams, 1986). Tiffin *et al.* (1991) determined differences in energy metabolism between male and female cattle embryos. Subsequently, Xu *et al.* (1992) observed that male cattle embryos tended to develop to more advanced stages in culture than female embryos during the first 8 days after insemination. Yadav *et al.* (1993) later found that of the early cleaving embryos that reached the 8-cell stage, more were likely to be male. Whether rates of embryo development in culture, or assays of X-linked enzymes, can be used to prospectively select for sex has yet to be determined. However, it is evident that the ability to select for sex prior to transfer has enormous implications for animal breeding programs.

CONCLUSIONS

The mammalian preimplantation/pre-attachment embryo undergoes considerable changes in its physiology and energy metabolism as it proceeds from the zygote to the blastocyst stage. Attempts to culture the mammalian zygote in the 1960s were restricted to a few strains of mice and their F1 hybrids, as the embryos of both sheep and cattle arrested development at the 8- to 16-cell stage. The introduction of co-culture in the mid 1980s of sheep and cattle embryos with somatic cells helped to alleviate this *in vitro* induced arrest, although such co-culture systems required the use of complex tissue culture media supplemented with serum. Serum has subsequently been shown to be associated with the production of offspring with significantly greater birth weights, leading to both difficulties in managing such pregnancies and an unacceptable frequency of neonatal death. The resurgence of interest in mammalian embryo physiology has culminated in the formulation of defined embryo culture media, capable of supporting high levels of viable blastocyst development *in vitro*. Optimal embryo development in culture takes place not in one, but two or more media, each designed to cater for the changing requirements of the embryo as it develops. The ability to maintain the embryos of sheep and cattle in culture without compromising developmental potential will greatly expedite the development and introduction of procedures such as transgenesis and cloning.

ACKNOWLEDGEMENTS

Sincerest thanks to my friends and colleagues Drs. Michelle Lane, Don Rieger and Jeremy Thompson for their comments on this manuscript and numerous discussions over the years. Should we all have agreed at the same time it would have been a miracle. Thanks also to Tracey Steeves for her valuable comments on the manuscript.

REFERENCES

Adler, D.A., West, J.D. and Chapman, V.E. (1977) Expression of α-galactosidase in preimplantation mouse embryos. *Nature*, **267**, 838–839.

Annison, E.F. and Armstrong, D.G. (1970) Volatile fatty acid metabolism and energy supply. In *Physiology of Digestion and Metabolism in the Ruminant*, edited by A.T. Phillipson, pp. 422–437. Newcastle: Oriel Press.

Armstrong, D.T., Holm, P., Irvine, B., Petersen, B.A., Stubbings, R.B., McLean, D., Stevens, G. and Seamark, R.F. (1992) Pregnancies and live birth from *in vitro* fertilization of calf oocytes collected by laparoscopic follicular aspiration. *Theriogenology*, **38**, 667–678.

Ballantyne, J.S. and Chamberlin, M.E. (1995) Regulation of cellular amino acid levels. In *Cellular and Molecular Physiology of Cell Volume Regulation*, edited by K. Strange, pp. 111–122. Boca Raton: CRC Press.

Barnes, F.L., Crombie, A., Gardner, D.K., Kausche, A., Lacham-Kaplan, O., Suikkari, A.-M., Tiglias, J., Wood, C. and Trounson, A. (1995) Blastocyst development and pregnancy after *in vitro* maturation of human primary oocytes, intracytoplasmic sperm injection and assisted hatching. *Hum. Reprod.*, **10**, 3243–3247.

Batt, P.A., Gardner, D.K. and Cameron, A.W.N. (1991) Oxygen concentration and protein source affect the development of preimplantation goat embryos *in vitro*. *Reprod. Fert. Devel.*, **3**, 601–607.

Bavister, B.D. (1981) Substitution of a synthetic polymer for protein in a mammalian gamete culture system. *J. Exp. Zool.*, **217**, 45–51.

Bavister, B.D. (1989) A consistently successful procedure for *in vitro* fertilization of golden hamster eggs. *Gamete Res.*, **23**, 139–158.

Bavister, B.D. (1993) Response to the use of co-culture for embryo development. *Hum. Reprod.*, **8**, 1152–1162.

Bavister, B.D. (1995) Culture of preimplantation embryos: facts and artifacts. *Hum. Reprod., Update*, **1**, 91–148.

Bavister, B.D. and McKiernan, S.H. (1993) Regulation of hamster embryo development *in vitro* by amino acids. In *Preimplantation Embryo Development*, edited by B.D. Bavister, pp. 57–72. New York: Springer-Verlag.

Bavister, B.D. and Yanagamachi, R. (1977) The effects of sperm extracts and energy sources on the motility and acrosome reaction of hamster spermatozoa *in vitro*. *Biol. Reprod.*, **16**, 228–237.

Bavister, B.D., Rose-Hellekant, T.A. and Pinyopummintr, T. (1992) Development of *in vitro* matured/ *in vitro* fertilised bovine embryos into morulae and blastocysts in defined culture media. *Theriogenology*, **37**, 127–146.

Behboodi, E., Anderson, G.B., BonDurant, R.H., Cargill, S.L., Kreuscher, B.R., Medrano, J.F. and Murray, J.D. (1995) Birth of large calves that developed from *in vitro*-derived bovine embryos. *Theriogenology*, **44**, 227–232.

Benos, D. and Biggers, J.D. (1981) Blastocyst fluid formation. In *Fertilization and Embryonic Development In Vitro*, edited by L. Mastroianni, Jr. and J.D. Biggers, pp. 283–297. New York, Plenum Press.

Bernardi, M.L., Flechon, J.-E. and Delouis, C. (1966) Influence of culture system and oxygen tension on the development of ovine zygotes matured and fertilized *in vitro*. *J. Reprod. Fertil.*, **106**, 161–167.

Betteridge, K.J. and Flechon, J.-E. (1988) The anatomy and physiology of pre-attachment bovine embryos. *Theriogeneology*, **29**, 155–187.

Bevers, M.M., Dieleman, S.J., van der Hurk, R. and Izadyar, F. (1997) Regulation and modulation of oocyte maturation in the bovine. *Theriogenology*, **47**, 13–22.

Biggers, J.D., Bell, J.E. and Benos, D.J. (1988) The mammalian blastocyst: transport functions in a developing epithelium. *Am. J. Physiol.*, **255**, C419–432.

Biggers, J.D., Gardner, D.K. and Leese, H.J. (1989) Control of carbohydrate metabolism in preimplantation mammalian embryos. In *Regulation of Growth in Development*, edited by I.Y. Rosenblum and S. Heyner, pp. 19–32. Boca Raton: CRC Press.

Biggers, J.D., Lawitts, J.A. and Lechene, C.P. (1993) The protective action of betaine on the deleterious effects of NaCl on preimplantation mouse embryos *in vitro*. *Mol. Reprod. Dev.*, **34**, 380–390.

Bishop, D.W. (1965) Oxygen concentration in the rabbit female genital tract. *Proc. Int. Cong. Anim. Reprod. Art. Insem.*, **1**, 53.

Blondin, P. and Sirard, M.A. (1995) Oocyte and follicular morphology as determining characteristics for developmental competence in bovine oocytes. *Mol. Reprod. Dev.*, **41**, 54–62.

Boland, M.P. (1984) Use of the rabbit oviduct as a screening tool for the viability of mammalian eggs. *Theriogenology*, **21**, 126–137.

Bongso, A., Fong, C.-Y., Ng, S.-C. and Ratnam, S. (1993) The search for improved *in-vitro* systems should not be ignored: embryo co-culture may be one of them. *Hum. Reprod.*, **8**, 1155–1160.

Borland, R.M., Hazra, S., Biggers, J.D. and Lechene, C.P. (1977) The elemental composition of the environment of the gametes and preimplantation embryo during the initiation of pregnancy. *Biol. Reprod.*, **16**, 147–157.

Borland, R.M., Biggers, J.D., Lechene, C.P. and Taymour, M.L. (1980) Elemental composition of fluid in the human fallopian tube. *J. Reprod. Fertil.*, **58**, 479–482.

Brackett, B.G. and Oliphant, G. (1975) Capacitation of rabbit spermatozoa *in vitro*. *Biol. Reprod.*, **12**, 260–274.

Carlson, D., Black, D.L. and Howe, G.R. (1970) Oviduct secretions in the cow. *J. Reprod. Fertil.*, **22**, 549–552.

Casslen, B.G. (1987) Free amino acids in human uterine fluid possible role of high taurine concentration. *J. Reprod. Med.*, **32**, 181–184.

Casslen, B.G. and Nilsson, B. (1984) Human uterine fluid, examined in undiluted samples for osmolarity and the concentrations of inorganic ions, albumin, glucose and urea. *Am. J. Obstet. Gyn.*, **150**, 877–881.

Chatot, C.L., Ziomek, C.A., Bavister, B.D., Lewis, J.L. and Torres, I. (1989) An improved culture medium supports development of random-bred I-cell mouse embryos *in vitro*. *J. Reprod. Fertil.*, **86**, 679–688.

Conaghan, J., Handyside, A.H., Winston, R.M.L. and Leese, H.J. (1993) Effects of pyruvate and glucose on the development of human preimplantation embryos *in vitro*. *J. Reprod. Fertil.*, **99**, 87–95.

De Loos, F., Kastrop, P., Van Maurik, P., Van Beneden, Th.H. and Kruip, Th.A.M. (1991) Hetero-logous cell contacts and metabolic coupling in bovine cumulus oocyte complexes. *Mol. Reprod. Dev.*, **28**, 255–259.

De Matos, D.G., Furnus, C.C., Moses, D.F. and Baldassarre, H. (1995) Effect of cyteamine on glutathione level and developmental capacity of bovine oocyte matured *in vitro*. *Mol. Reprod. Dev.*, **42**, 432–436.

De Matos, D.G., Furnus, C.C., Moses, D.F., Martinez, A.G. and Matkovic, M. (1996) Stimulation of glutathione synthesis of *in vitro* matured bovine oocytes and its effects on embryo development and freezability. *Mol. Reprod. Dev.*, **45**, 451–457.

Dorland, M., Gardner, D.K. and Trounson, A. (1994) Serum in synthetic oviduct fluid causes mitochondrial degeneration in ovine embryos. *J. Reprod. Fertil. Abstract Series*, **13**, 70.

Duby, R.T., Damiani, P., Looney, C.R., Fissore, R.A. and Robl, J.M. (1996) Prepuberal calves as oocyte donors: promises and problems. *Theriogenology*, **45**, 121–130.

Eagle, H. (1959) Amino acid metabolism in mammalian cell cultures. *Science*, **130**, 423–437.

Earl, C.R., Irvine, B.J., Kelly, J.M., Rowe, J.P. and Armstrong, D.T. (1995) Ovarian stimulation protocols for oocyte collection and *in vitro* embryo production from 8 to 9 week old lambs. *Theriogenology*, **43**, 203.

Earl, C.R., Kelly, J., Rowe, J. and Armstrong, D.T. (1997) Glutathione treatment of bovine sperm enhances *in vitro* blastocyst production rates. *Theriogenology*, **47**, 255.

Edwards, L.E., Batt, P.A., Gandolfi, F. and Gardner, D.K. (1997) Modifications made to culture medium by bovine oviduct epithelial cells: changes to carbohydrates stimulate bovine embryo development. *Mol. Reprod. Devel.*, **46**, 146–154.

Edwards, R.G. (1995) Implantation and early pregnancy after assisted conception. In *Principles and Practice of Assisted Human Reproduction*, edited by R.G. Edwards and S.A. Brody, pp. 555–605. Philadelphia: Saunders.

Epstein, C.J., Smith, S., Travis, B. and Tucker, G. (1978) Both X chromosomes function before visible X-chromosome inactivation in female mouse embryos. *Nature*, **274**, 500–503.

Eyestone, W.H., Leibfriend-Rutledge, M.L., Northey, D.L., Gilligan, B.G. and First, N.L. (1987) Culture of one- and two-cell bovine embryos to the blastocyst stage in the ovine oviduct. *Theriogenology*, **28**, 1–7.

Eyestone, W.H. and First, N.L. (1989) Co-culture of early cattle embryos to the blastocyst stage with oviductal tissue or in conditioned medium. *J. Reprod. Fertil.*, **85**, 715–720.

Fischer, B. and Bavister, B.D. (1993) Oxygen tension in the oviduct and uterus of rhesus monkeys, hamsters and rabbits. *J. Reprod. Fertil.*, **99**, 673–679.

Frei, R.E., Schultz, G.A. and Church, R.B. (1989) Qualitative and quantitative changes in protein synthesis occur at the 8-16-cell stage of embryogenesis in the cow. *J. Reprod. Fertil.*, **86**, 637–641.

Flach, G., Johnson, M.H., Braude, P.R., Taylor, R.A.S. and Bolton, V.N. (1982) The transition from maternal to embryonic control in the 2-cell mouse embryo. *EMBO J.*, **1**, 681–686.

Furnus, C.C., deMatos, D.G., Martinez, A.G. and Matkovic, M. (1996) Effect of hyaluronic acid on development of IVM/IVF bovine embryos. *Proc. Int. Cong. An. Rep.*, P22-3.

Gandolfi, F. and Moor, R.M. (1987) Stimulation of early embryonic development in the sheep by co-culture with oviduct cells. *J. Reprod. Fertil.*, **81**, 23–28.

Gandolfi, F., Pocar, P., Luciano, A.M. and Rieger, D. (1996) Effects of EGF and IGF-1 during *in vitro* maturation of cattle oocytes on subsequent embryo development and metabolism. *Theriogenology*, **45**, 277.

Gardner, D.K. (1987) The nutrition and energy metabolism of the preimplantation mouse embryo. Ph.D. Thesis, University of York, York.

Gardner, D.K. (1994) Culture of mammalian embryos in the absence of serum and somatic cells. *Cell Biology International*, **18**, 1163–1179.

Gardner, D.K. (1998) Changes in requirements and utilization of nutrients during mammalian preimplantation embryo development and their significance in embryo culture. *Theriogenology* (in press).

Gardner, D.K. and Lane, M. (1993a) Embryo culture systems. In *Handbook of In Vitro Fertilization*, edited by A. Trounson and D.K. Gardner, pp. 85–114. Boca Raton: CRC Press.

Gardner, D.K. and Lane, M. (1993b) The 2-cell block in CF1 mouse embryos is associated with an increase in glycolysis and a decrease in tricarboxylic acid (TCA) cycle activity: alleviation of the 2-cell block is associated with the restoration of *in vivo* metabolic pathway activities. *Biol. Reprod.*, **49**, Suppl. 1, 152.

Gardner, D.K. and Lane, M. (1993c) Amino acids and ammonium regulate the development of mouse embryos in culture. *Biol. Reprod.*, **4**, 377–385.

Gardner, D.K. and Lane, M. (1996) Alleviation of the "2-cell block" and development to the blastocyst of CF1 mouse embryos: role of amino acids, EDTA and physical factors. *Hum. Reprod.*, **11**, 2703–2712.

Gardner, D.K. and Lane, M. (1997) Culture and selection of viable blastocysts: A feasible proposition for human IVF? *Hum. Reprod.*, update (in press).

Gardner, D.K. and Leese, H.J. (1987) Assessment of embryo viability prior to transfer by the non-invasive measurement of glucose uptake. *J. Exp. Zool.*, **242**., 103–105.

Gardner, D.K. and Leese, H.J. (1988) The role of glucose and pyruvate transport in regulating nutrient utilization by preimplantation mouse embryos. *Development*, **104**, 423–428.

Gardner, D.K. and Leese, H.J. (1990) Concentrations of nutrients in mouse oviduct fluid and their effects on embryo development and metabolism *in vitro*. *J. Reprod. Fertil.*, **88**, 361–368.

Gardner, D.K. and Leese, H.J. (1993) Assessment of embryo metabolism and viability. In *Handbook of In Vitro Fertilization*, edited by A. Trounson and D.K. Gardner, pp. 195–211. Boca Raton: CRC Press.

Gardner, D.K. and Sakkas, D. (1993) Mouse embryo cleavage, metabolism and viability: role of medium composition. *Hum. Reprod.*, **8**, 288–295.

Gardner, D.K., Lane, M. and Batt, P.A. (1993) The uptake and metabolism of pyruvate and glucose by individual pre-attachment sheep embryos developed *in vivo*. *Mol. Reprod. Devel.*, **36**, 313–319.

Gardner, D.K., Lane, M., Spitzer, A. and Batt, P.A. (1994) *In vivo* rates of cleavage for sheep zygotes cultured to the blastocyst stage *in vitro* in the absence of serum and somatic cells: amino acids, vitamins and increased embryo density stimulate development. *Biol. Reprod.*, **50**, 390–400.

Gardner, D.K., Lane, M., Calderon, I. and Leeton, J. (1996a) The environment of the human embryo *in vivo*: Analysis of oviduct and uterine fluids during the menstrual cycle and metabolism of cumulus cells. *Fertil. Steril.*, **65**, 349–353.

Gardner, D.K., Pawelczynski, M. and Trounson, A. (1996b) Nutrient uptake and utilisation can be used to select viable day-7 bovine blastocysts after cryopreservation. *Mol. Reprod. Dev.*, **44**, 472–475.

Gardner, D.K., Lane, M.W. and Lane, M. (1997a) Bovine blastocyst cell number in increased by culture with EDTA for the 72 hours of development from the zygote. *Theriogenology*, **47**, 278.

Gardner, D.K., Lane, M. and Rodriguez-Martinez, H. (1997b) Fetal development after transfer is increased by replacing protein with the glycosaminoglycan hyaluronate for embryo culture. *Hum. Reprod.*, **12**: Abstract Book 1, 0–215.

Gardner, D.K., Lane, M.W. and Lane, M. (1997c) Development of the inner cell mass in mouse blastocysts is stimulated by reducing the incubation volume embryo ratio. *Hum. Reprod.*, **12**: Abstract Book 1, p-132.

Gardner, D.K., Lane, M., Kouridakis, K. and Schoolcraft, W.B. (1997d) Complex physiologically based serum-free culture media increase mammalian embryo development. In *In Vitro Fertilization and Assisted Reproduction*, edited by V. Gomel and P.C.K. Leung, pp. 187–191. Bologna: Monduzzi Editore.

Goto, K., Kajihara, Y., Kosaka, S., Koba, M., Nakanishi, Y. and Ogawa, K. (1988) Pregnancies after co-culture of cumulus cells with bovine embryos derived from *in-vitro* fertilization of *in-vitro* matured follicular oocytes. *J. Reprod. Fertil.*, **83**, 753–758.

Goto, K., Iwai, N., Ide, K., Takuma, Y. and Nakanishi, Y. (1994) Viability of one-cell bovine embryos cultured *in vitro*: comparison of cell-free culture with co-culture. *J. Reprod. Fert.*, **100**, 239–243.

Greenhouse, W.V.V. and Lehninger, A.L. (1976) Occurrence of malate-aspartate shuttle in various tumour types. *Cancer Res.*, **36**, 1392–1396.

Greenhouse, W.V.V. and Lehninger, A.L. (1977) Magnitude of malate-aspartate reduced nicotinamide adenine dinucleotide shuttle activity in intact respiring tumour cells. *Cancer Res.*, **37**, 4173–4181.

Harvey, M.B., Leco, K.J., Arcellana-Panlilio, M.Y., Zhang, X., Edwards, D.R. and Schultz, G.A. (1995) Roles of growth factors during peri-implantation development. *Mol. Hum. Reprod.*, **10**, 712–718.

Hernandez-Ledmezma, J.J., Mathialagan, N., Villanueva, C., Sikes, J.H. and Roberts, R.M. (1993) Expression of bovine trophoblast interferons by *in vitro*-derived blastocysts is correlated with their morphological quality and stage of development. *Mol. Reprod. Dev.*, **36**, 1–6.

Heyman, Y., Menezo, Y., Chesne, P., Camous, S. and Garnier, V. (1987) *In vitro* cleavage of bovine and ovine early embryos: improved development using coculture with trophoblastic vesicles. *Theriogenology*, **27**, 59–68.

Heyner, S., Shah, N., Smith, R.M., Watson, A.J. and Schultz, G.A. (1993) The role of growth factors in embryo production. *Theriogenology*, **39**, 151–161.

Houghton, F.D., Thompson, J.G., Kennedy, C.J. and Leese, H.J. (1996) Oxygen consumption and energy metabolism of the early mouse embryo. *Mol. Reprod. Devel.*, **44**, 476–485.

Hume, D.A. and Weidemann, M.J. (1979) Role and regulation of glucose metabolism in proliferating cells. *J. Natl. Cancer Inst.*, **62**, 3–8.

Hunter, R.H.F. (1994) Modulation of gamete and embryonic microenvironments by oviduct glyco-proteins, *Mol. Reprod. Devel.*, **39**, 176–181.

Iwasaki, S., Yoshiba, N., Ushijima, H., Watanabe, S. and Nakahara, T. (1990) Morphology and proportion of inner cell mass of bovine blastocysts fertilized *in vitro* and *in vivo*. *J. Reprod. Fertil.*, **90**, 279–284.

Johnson, M.H. and Nasr-Esfahini, M.H. (1994) Radical solutions and cultural problems: Could free oxygen radicals be responsible for the impaired development of preimplantation mammalian embryos *in vitro*? *BioEssays*, **16**, 31–38.

Johnson, S.K., Jordan, J.E., Dean R.G. and Page, R.D. (1991) The quantification of bovine embryo viability using a bioluminescent assay for lactate dehydrogenase. *Theriogenology*, **35**, 425–433.

Kane, M.T. (1987) *In vitro* growth of preimplantation rabbit embryos. In *The Preimplantation Embryo*, edited by B.D. Bavister, pp. 193–217. New York: Plenum Press.

Keefer, C.L., Stice, S.L. and Dobrinsky, J. (1993) Effect of follicle-stimulating hormone and luteinizing hormone during bovine *in vitro* maturation on development following *in vitro* fertilization and nuclear transfer. *Mol. Reprod. Dev.*, **36**, 469–474.

Keefer, C.L., Stice, S.L., Paprocki, A.M. and Golueke, P. (1994) *In vitro* culture of bovine IVM-IVF embryos: Cooperative interaction among embryos and the role of growth factors. *Theriogenology*, **41**, 1323–1331.

Keskintepe, L., Burnely, C.A. and Brackett, B.G. (1995) Production of viable bovine blastocysts in defined *in vitro* conditions. *Biol. Reprod.*, **52**, 1410–1427.

Keskintepe, L. and Brackett, B.G. (1996) *In vitro* developmental competence of *in vitro*-matured bovine oocytes fertilized and cultured in completely defined media. *Biol. Reprod.*, **55**, 333–339.

Kim, J.H., Funahashi, H., Niwa, K. and Okuda, K. (1993a) Glucose requirement at different developmental stages of *in-vitro* fertilised bovine embryos cultured in semi-defined medium. *Theriogenology*, **39**, 875–886.

Kim, J.H., Niwa, K., Lim, J.M. and Okuda, K. (1993b) Effects of phosphate, energy substrates, and amino acids on development of *in vitro*-matured, *in vitro*-fertilized bovine oocytes in a chemically defined, protein-free culture medium. *Biol. Reprod.*, **48**, 1320–1325.

King, G.J. and Thatcher, W.W. (1993) Pregnancy. In *Reproduction in Domestic Animals*, edited by G.J. King, pp. 229–269. Amsterdam: Elsevier.

Kinne, R.K.H. (1993) The role of organic osmolytes in osmoregulation: from bacteria to mammals. *J. Exp. Zool.*, **265**, 346–355.

Kouridakis, K. and Gardner, D.K. (1995) Pyruvate in embryo culture media acts as an antioxidant. *Proc. Fert. Soc. Aus.*, **14**, 29.

Lane, M. and Gardner, D.K. (1992) Effect of incubation volume and embryo density on the develop-ment and viability of mouse embryos *in vitro*. *Hum. Reprod.*, **7**, 558–562.

Lane, M. and Gardner, D.K. (1994) Culture of preimplantation mouse embryos in the presence of amino acids increases post-implantation development whilst the concomitant production of ammonium induces birth defects. *J. Reprod. Fertil.*, **102**, 305–312.

Lane, M. and Gardner, D.K. (1995) An enzymatic method of removing embryo-toxic ammonium from culture medium: effect on development of mouse embryos *in vitro* and *in vivo*. *J. Exp. Zool.*, **271**, 356–363.

Lane, M. and Gardner, D.K. (1996) Selection of viable mouse blastocysts prior to transfer using a metabolic criterion. *Hum. Reprod.*, **11**, 1975–1978.

Lane, M. and Gardner, D.K. (1997) Differential regulation of mouse embryo development and viability by amino acids. *J. Reprod. Fertil.* **109**, 153–164.

Larson, R.C., Ignotz, G.G. and Currie, W.B. (1992a) Platelet derived growth factor (PDGF) stimulates development of bovine embryos during the fourth cell cycle. *Development*, **115**, 821–826.

Larson, R.C., Ignotz, G.G. and Currie, W.B. (1992b) Transforming growth factor-β and basic fibroblast growth factor synergistically promote early bovine embryo development during the fourth cell cycle. *Mol. Reprod. Dev.*, **33**, 432–435.

Lawitts, J.A. and Biggers, J.D. (1991) Optimisation of mouse embryo culture media using simplex methods. *J. Reprod. Fertil.*, **91**, 543–556.

Lawitts, J.A. and Biggers, J.D. (1992) Joint effects of sodium chloride, glutamine, and glucose in mouse preimplantation embryo culture media. *Mol. Reprod. Dev.*, **31**, 189–194.

Lawitts, J.A. and Biggers, J.D. (1993) Culture of preimplantation embryos. *Methods of Enzymology*, **225**, 153–164.

Lawson, R.A.S., Rowson, L.E.A. and Adams, C.E. (1972) The development of cow eggs in the rabbit oviduct and their viability after re-transfer to heifers. *J. Reprod. Fertil.*, **28**, 313–315.

Lee, E.-S. and Fukui, Y. (1996) Synergistic effect of alanine and glycine on bovine embryos cultured in a chemically defined medium and amino acid uptake by *in vitro* produced bovine morulae and blastocysts. *Biol. Reprod.*, **55**, 1383–1389.

Leese, H.J. (1988) The formation and function of oviduct fluid. *J. Reprod. Fertil.*, **82**, 843–856.

Leese, H.J. (1989) Energy metabolism of the blastocyst and uterus at implantation. In *Blastocyst Implantation*, edited by K. Yoshinaga, pp. 39–44. Boston: Adams Publishing.

Leese, H.J. (1991) Metabolism of the preimplantation mammalian embryo. In *Oxford Reviews of Reproductive Biology*, 13, edited by S.R. Milligan, pp. 35–72. London: Oxford University Press.

Leese,H.J. and Barton, A.M. (1985) Production of pyruvate by isolated mouse cumulus cells. *J. Exp. Zool.*, **234**, 231–236.

Leppens, G. and Sakkas, D. (1995) Differential effect of epithelial cell-conditioned medium fractions on preimplantation mouse embryo development. *Hum. Reprod.*, **10**, 1178–1183.

Lim, J.M., Kim, J.H., Okuda, K. and Miwa, K. (1994) The importance of NaCl concentration in a chemically defined medium for the development of bovine oocytes matured and fertilized *in vitro*. *Theriogenology*, **42**, 421–432.

Liu, Z. and Foote, R.H. (1995) Effects of amino acids on the development of *in-vitro* matured/*in-vitro* fertilization bovine embryos in a simple protein-free medium. *Hum. Reprod.*, **11**, 2985–2991.

Liu, Z. and Foote, R.H. (1996) Sodium chloride, osmolyte, and osmolarity effects on blastocyst formation in bovine embryos produced by *in vitro* fertilization (IVF) and cultured in simple serum-free media. *J. Assist. Reprod. Genet.*, **13**, 562–568.

Luvoni, G.C., Keskintepe, L. and Brackett, B.G. (1996) Improvement of bovine embryo production *in vitro* by glutathione-containing medium. *Mol. Reprod. Dev.*, **43**, 437–443.

Machatkova, M., Jokesova, E., Petelikova, J. and Dvoracek, V. (1996) Developmental competence of embryos derived from oocytes collected at various stages of the estrous cycle. *Theriogenology*, **45**, 801–810.

Mandel, L.J. (1986) Energy metabolism of cellular activation, growth, and transformation. *Curr. Top. Memb. Trans.*, **27**, 261–291.

Mastroianni, L., Jr. and Jones, R. (1965) Oxygen tension within rabbit fallopian tube. *J. Reprod. Fertil.*, **9**, 99–102.

Matsuyama, K., Miyakoshi, H. and Fukui, Y. (1993) Effect of glucose during the *in vitro* culture in synthetic oviduct fluid medium on *in vitro* development of bovine oocytes matured and fertilized *in vitro*. *Theriogenology*, **40**, 595–605.

McKiernan, S.H. and Bavister, B.D. (1992) Different lots of bovine serum albumin inhibit or stimulate *in vitro* development of hamster embryos. *In Vitro Cell. Dev. Biol. Anim.*, **28**A, 154–156.

McKiernan, S.H., Clayton, M. and Bavister, B.D. (1995) Analysis of stimulatory and inhibitory amino acids for development of hamster one-cell embryos *in vitro*. *Mol. Reprod. Dev.*, **42**, 188–199.

McLaren, A. (1980) Fertilization, cleavage and implantation. In *Reproduction in Farm Animals*, edited by E.S.E. Hafez, pp. 226–246. Philadelphia: Les and Febiger.

Menezo, Y.J.R. (1972) Amino constituents of tubal and uterine fluids of the oestrous ewe: comparison with blood serum and ram seminal fluid. In *The Biology of Spermatozoa*, edited by E.S.E. Hafez and C.G. Thibault, pp. 174–181. New York: Basel Press.

Menezo, Y., Renard, J.-P., Delobel, B. and Pageaux, J.F. (1982) Kinetic study of fatty acid composition of day 7 to day 14 cow embryos. *Biol. Reprod.*, **26**, 787–790.

Menke, T.M. and McLaren, A. (1970) Mouse blastocysts grown *in vivo* and *in vitro*: carbon dioxide production and trophoblast outgrowth. *J. Reprod. Fertil.*, **23**, 117–127.

Mills, R.M. and Brinster, R.L. (1967) Oxygen consumption of pre-implantation mouse embryos. *Exp. Cell Res.*, **47**, 337–344.

Miller, J.G.O. and Schultz, G.A. (1987) Amino acid content of preimplantation rabbit embryos and fluids of the reproductive tract. *Biol. Reprod.*, **36**, 125–129.

Monk, M. and Harper, M.I. (1979) Sequential X chromosome inactivation coupled with cellular differentiation in early mouse embryos. *Nature*, **281**, 311–313.

Moore, K. and Bondioli, K.R. (1993) Glycine and alanine supplementation of culture medium enhances development of *in vitro* matured and fertilized cattle embryos. *Biol. Reprod.*, **48**, 833–840.

Morgan, M.J. and Faik, P. (1981) Carbohydrate metabolism in cultured animal cells. *Biosci. Rep.*, **1**, 669–686.

Moses, D.F., Matkovic, M., Cabrera Fisher, E. and Martinez, A.G. (1997) Amino acid contents of sheep oviductal and uterine fluids. *Theriogenology*, **47**, 336.

Myers, M.W., Broussard, J.R., Menezo, Y., Prough, S.G., Blasckwell, J., Godke, R.A. and Thibodeaux, J.K. (1994) Established cell lines and their conditioned media support bovine embryo development during *in-vitro* culture. *Hum. Reprod.*, **9**, 1927–1931.

Nancarrow, C.D., Hill, J.L. and Connell, P.J. (1992) Amino acid secretion by the ovine oviduct. *Proc. Aust. Soc. Reprod. Biol.*, **24**, 71.

Newsholme, E.A. (1990) Application of metabolic-control logic to the requirements for cell division. *Biochem. Soc. Trans.*, **18**, 78–80.

Newsholme, E.A., Crabtree, B. and Ardawi, M.S.M. (1985) The role of high rates of glycolysis and glutamine utilization in rapidly dividing cells. *Bioscience Reports*, **5**, 393–400.

Nichol, R., Hunter, R.H.F., Gardner, D.K., Leese, H.J. and Cooke, G.M. (1992) Concentration of energy substrates in porcine oviduct fluid and blood plasma during the peri-ovulatory period. *J. Reprod. Fert.*, **96**, 699–707.

Overstrom, E.W. (1987) *In vitro* assessment of blastocyst differentiation. In *The Mammalian Preimplantation Embryo*, edited by B.D. Bavister, pp. 95–116. New York: Plenum Press.

Overstrom, E.W. (1996) *In vitro* assessment of embryo viability. *Theriogenology*, **45**, 3–16.

Overstrom, E.W., Duby, R.T., Dobrinsky, J., Roche, J.F. and Boland, M.P. (1992) Viability and oxidative metabolism of the bovine blastocyst. *Theriogenology*, **37**, 269.

Paria, P.C. and Dey, S.K. (1990) Preimplantation embryo development *in vitro*: cooperative interactions among embryos and role of growth factors. *Proc. Natl. Acad. Sci. USA*, **87**, 3756–2760.

Parrish, J.J. and First, N.L. (1993) Fertilization. In *Reproduction in Domestic Animals*, edited by G.J. King, pp. 195–227. Amersterdam: Elsevier.

Parrish, J.J., Susko-Parrish, J., Winer, M.A. and First, N.L. (1988) Capacitation of bovine sperm by heparin. *Biol. Reprod.*, **38**, 1171–1180.

Parrish, J.J., Susko-Parrish, J., Handrow, R.R., Sims, M.M. and First, N.L. (1989a) Capacitation of bovine spermatozoa by oviduct fluid. *Biol. Reprod.*, **40**, 1020–1025.

Parrish, J.J., Susko-Parrish, J. and First, N.L. (1989b) Capacitation of bovine sperm by heparin: inhibitory effect of glucose and role of intracellular pH. *Biol. Reprod.*, **41**, 683–699.

Partridge, R.J., Pullar, D., Wrathall, A.E. and Leese, H.J. (1996) Consumption of amino acids by *in vivo* and *in vitro*-derived bovine embryos. *Theriogenology*, **45**, 181.

Pavlok, A., Lucas-Hahn, A. and Niemann, H. (1992) Fertilization and developmental competence of bovine oocytes derived from different categories of antral follicles. *Mol. Reprod. Dev.*, **31**, 63–67.

Perkins, J.L. and Goode, L. (1967) Free amino acids in the oviduct fluid of the ewe. *J. Reprod. Fertil.*, **14**, 309–311.

Pinyopummintr, T. and Bavister, B.D. (1991) *In vitro* matured/*in vitro* fertilized bovine oocytes can develop into morulae/blastocysts in chemically defined, protein-free culture media. *Biol. Reprod.*, **45**, 736–742.

Pinyopummintr, T. and Bavister, B.D. (1994) Development of bovine embryos in a cell-free culture medium: effects of type of serum, timing of its inclusion and heat inactivation. *Theriogeneology*, **41**, 1241–1249.

Pinyopummintr, T. and Bavister, B.D. (1995) Optimum gas atmosphere for *in vitro* maturation and *in vitro* fertilization of bovine oocytes. *Theriogenology*, **44**, 471–477.

Pinyopummintr, T. and Bavister, B.D. (1996a) Energy substrate requirements for *in vitro* development of early cleavage-stage bovine embryos. *Mol. Reprod. Dev.*, **44**, 193–199.

Pinyopummintr, T. and Bavister, B.D. (1996b) Effects of amino acids on development *in vitro* of cleavage stage bovine embryos into blastocysts. *Reprod. Fertil. Dev.*, **8**, 835–841.

Pratt, H.P.M. (1987) Isolation, culture and manipulation of preimplantation mouse embryos. *In Mammalian Development A Practical Approach*, edited by M. Monk, pp. 13–42. Oxford: IRL Press.

Quinn, P. and Harlow, G.M. (1976) The effect of oxygen on the development of preimplantation mouse embryos. *J. Exp. Zool.*, **206**, 73–80.

Reed, W.A., Suh, T.-K., Bunch, T.D. and White, K.L. (1996) Culture of *in vitro* fertilized bovine embryos with bovine oviduct epithelial cells, buffalo rate liver (BRL) cells, or BRL-cell-conditioned medium. *Theriogenology*, **45**, 439–449.

Reggio, B.C., Lim, J.M., Hansel, W. and Godke, R.A. (1996) Developing a dynamic culture system for bovine embryos: Effects of chamber size and tubing type on preimplantation development of 8-cell embryos. *Theriogenology*, **45**, 200.

Rehman, N., Collins, A.R., Suh, T.K. and Wright, R.W. Jr. (1994) Development of IVM-IVF produced 8-cell bovine embryos in simple, serum-free media after conditioning or co-culture with buffalo rat liver cells. *Molec. Reprod. Dev.*, **38**, 251–255.

Reitzer, L.J., Wice, B.M. and Kennel, D. (1980) The pentose cycle: control and essential function in HeLa cell nucleic acid synthesis. *J. Biol. Chem.*, **255**, 5616–5626.

Renard, J.P., Philippon, A. and Menezo, Y. (1980) *In vitro* glucose uptake of glucose by bovine blastocysts. *J. Reprod. Fertil.*, **58**, 161–164.

Revel, F., Mermillod, P., Peynot, N., Renard, J.P. and Heyman, Y. (1995) Low developmental capacity of *in vitro* matured and fertilized oocytes from calves compared with that of cows. *J. Reprod. Fertil.*, **103**, 115–120.

Rieger, D. (1984) The measurement of metabolic activity as an approach to evaluating viability and diagnosing sex in early embryos. *Theriogenology*, **21**, 138–149.

Rieger, D. (1992) Relationship between energy metabolism and development of the early embryo. *Theriogenology*, **37**, 75–93.

Rieger, D. and Guay, P. (1988) Measurement of the metabolism of energy substrates in individual bovine blastocysts. *J. Reprod. Fertil.*, **83**, 585–591.

Rieger, D., Loskutoff, N.M. and Betteridge, K.J. (1992a) Developmentally related changes in the metabolism of glucose and glutamine by cattle embryos produced and co-cultured *in vitro*. *J. Reprod. Fertil.*, **95**, 585–595.

Rieger, D., Loskutoff, N.M. and Betteridge, K.J. (1992b) Developmentally related changes in the uptake and metabolism of glucose, glutamine and pyruvate by cattle embryos produced *in vitro*. *Reprod. Fertil. Dev.*, **4**, 547–557.

Rieger, D., Grisart, B., Semple, E., Van Lengendonckt, A., Betteridge, K.J. and Dessy, F. (1995a) Comparison of the effects of oviductal co-culture and oviductal cell-conditioned medium on the development and metabolic activity of cattle embryos. *J. Reprod. Fertil.*, **105**, 91–98.

Rieger, D., Luciano, A.M., Modina, S., Pocar, P., Lauria, A. and Gandolfi, F. (1995b) The effect of EGF and IGF-1 on metabolism and nuclear maturation of cattle oocytes. *J. Reprod. Fertil. Abstract Series*, **15**, 73.

Rogers, P.A.W., Murphy, C.R. and Gannon, B.J. (1982a) Absence of capillaries in the endometrium surrounding the implanting rat blastocyst. *Micron*, **13**, 373–374.

Rogers, P.A.W., Murphy, C.R. and Gannon, B.J. (1982b) Changes in the spatial organisation of the uterine vasculature during implantation in the rat. *J. Reprod. Fertil.*, **65**, 211–214.

Rogers, P.A.W., Murphy, C.R., Rogers, A.W. and Gannon, B.J. (1983) Capillary patency and permeability in the endometrium surrounding the implanting rat blastocyst. *Int. J. Microcirc. Clin. Exp.*, **2**, 241–249.

Rondeau, M., Guay, P., Goff, A.K. and Cooke, G.M. (1995) Assessment of embryo potential by visual and metabolic evaluation. *Theriogenology*, **44**, 351–366.

Rorie, R.W., Miller, G.F., Nasti, K.B. and McNew, R.W. (1994) *In vitro* development of bovine embryos as affected by different lots of bovine serum albumin and citrate. *Theriogenology*, **42**, 397–403.

Rose, T.A. and Bavister, B.D. (1992) Effect of maturation medium on *in vitro* development of *in vitro* fertilized bovine embryos. *Mol. Reprod. Dev.*, **31**, 72–77.

Ross, R.N. and Graves, C.N. (1974) O_2 levels in the female rabbit reproductive tract. *J. Anim. Sci.*, **39**, 994.

Rosenkrans, C.F. Jr., Zeng, G.Q., McNamara, G.T., Schoff, P.K. and First, N.L. (1993) Development of bovine embryos *in vitro* as affected by energy substrates. *Biol. Reprod.*, **49**, 459–462.

Rosenkrans, C.F. Jr. and First, N.L. (1994) Effect of free amino acids and vitamins on cleavage and developmental rate of bovine zygotes *in vitro*. *J. Anim. Sci.*, **72**, 434–437.

Schini, S.A. and Bavister, B.D. (1988) Two-cell block to development of cultured hamster embryos is caused by phosphate and glucose, *Biol. Reprod.*, **39**, 1183–1192.

Schultz, G.A., Kaye, P.L., McKay, D.J. and Johnson, M.H. (1981) Endogenous amino acids pool sizes in mouse eggs and preimplantation embryos. *J. Reprod. Fertil.*, **61**, 387–393.

Schultz, G.A., Hogan, A., Watson, A.J., Smith, R.M. and Heyner, S. (1992) Insulin, insulin-like growth factors and glucose transporters; temporal patterns of gene expression in early murine and bovine embryos. *Reprod. Fertil. Dev.*, **4**, 361–371.

Seshagiri, P.B. and Bavister, B.D. (1991) Glucose and phosphate inhibit respiration and oxidative metabolism in cultured hamster eight-cell embryos: evidence for the "Crabtree effect", *Mol. Reprod. Devel.*, **30**, 105–111.

Sinclair, K.D., Broadbent, P.J. and Doman, D.F. (1995) *In vitro* produced embryos as a means of achieving pregnancy and improving productivity in beef cattle. *Anim. Sci.*, **60**, 55–64.

Sirard, M.A. and Blondin, P. (1996) Oocyte maturation and IVF in cattle. *Anim. Reprod. Sci.*, **42**, 417–426.

Sirard, M.A., Lambert, R.D., Menard, D.P. and Bedoya, M. (1985) Pregnancies after *in vitro* fertilization of cow follicular oocytes, their incubation in rabbit oviduct and transfer to the cow uterus. *J. Reprod. Fertil.*, **75**, 551–556.

Somero, G. (1986) Protons, osmolytes, and fitness of internal milieu for protein function. *Am. J. Physiol.*, **251**, R197–R213.

Steeves, T.E. and Gardner, D.K. (1997) Temporal and differential effects of amino acids on bovine embryo development in culture. *Biol. Reprod.*, **56**, suppl. 1, 25.

Stewart, C.L. (1994) Leukaemia inhibitory factor and the regulation of pre-implantation development of the mammalian embryo. *Mol. Reprod. Dev.*, **39**, 233–238.

Susko-Parrish, J.L., Wheeler, M.B., Ax, R.L., First, N.L. and Parrish, J.J. (1990) The effect of penicillamine, hypotaurine, epinephrine and sodium metabisulfite, on bovine *in vitro* fertilization. *Theriogenology*, **33**, 333.

Telford, N.A., Watson, A.J. and Schultz, G.A. (1990) Transition from maternal to embryonic control in early mammalian development: a comparison of several species. *Mol. Reprod. Devel.*, **26**, 90–100.

Tervit, H.R. (1996) Laparoscopy/laparotomy oocyte recovery and juvenile breeding. *Anim. Reprod. Sci.*, **42**, 227–238.

Tervit, H.R., Whittingham, D.G. and Rowson, L.E.A. (1972) Successful culture *in vitro* of sheep and cattle ova. *J. Reprod. Fertil.*, **30**, 493–497.

Thibodeaux, J.K., Del Vecchio, R.P. and Hansel, W. (1993) Role of platelet-derived growth factor in development of *in vitro* matured and *in vitro* fertilized bovine embryos. *J. Reprod. Fertil.*, **98**, 61–66.

Thompson, J.G. (1996) Defining the requirements for bovine embryo culture. *Theriogenology*, **45**, 27–40.

Thompson, J.G.E., Simpson, A.C., Pugh, P.A., Donnelly, P.E. and Tervit, H.R. (1990) Effect of oxygen concentration on *in-vitro* development of preimplantation sheep and cattle embryos. *J. Reprod. Fertil.*, **89**, 573–578.

Thompson, J.G., Simpson, A.C., Pugh, P.A. and Tervit, H.R. (1992) Requirement for glucose during *in vitro* culture of sheep preimplantation embryos. *Mol. Reprod. Dev.*, **31**, 253–257.

Thompson, J.G., Bell, A.C.S., Pugh, P.A. and Tervit, H.R. (1993) Metabolism of pyruvate by pre-elongation sheep embryos and effect of pyruvate and lactate concentrations during *in vitro* culture. *Reprod. Fertil. Dev.*, **5**, 417–423.

Thompson, J.G., Tervit, H.R., Pugh, P.A. and Gardner, D.K. (1994) Development of a cell-free defined sheep embryo culture system. *Proc. Int. Sym. Reprod. Dom. Animals*, **4**, 41.

Thompson, J.G., Gardner, D.K., Pugh, P.A., McMillan, J. and Tervit, R.H. (1995) Lamb birth weight following transfer is affected by the culture system used for pre-elongation development of embryos. *Biol. Reprod.*, **53**, 1385–1391.

Thompson, J.G., Partridge, R.J., Houghton, F.D., Cox, C.I. and Leese, H.J. (1996) Oxygen uptake and carbohydrate metabolism by *in vitro* derived bovine embryos. *J. Reprod. Fertil.*, **106**, 299–306.

Tiffin, G.J., Rieger, D., Betteridge, K.J., Yadav, B.R. and King, W.A. (1991) Glucose and glutamine metabolism in pre-attachment cattle embryos in relation to sex and stage of development. *J. Reprod. Fertil.*, **93**, 125–132.

Tsunoda, Y., Tokunaga, T. and Sugie, T. (1985) Altered sex ratio of live young after transfer of fast and slow developing mouse embryos. *Gamete Res.*, **12**, 301–304.

Van Inzen, W.G., van Stekelenburg-Hamers, A.E.P., Weima, S.M., Kruip, T.A.M., Bevers, M.M. and Mummery, C.L. (1995) Culture of bovine embryos to the blastocyst stage using buffalo rate liver (BRL) cells. *Theriogenology*, **43**, 723–738.

Van Winkle, L.J. (1988) Amino acid transport in developing animal oocytes and early conceptuses, *Biochim. Biophys. Acta*, **947**, 173–208.

Van Winkle, L.J., Haghighat, N. and Campione, A.L. (1990) Glycine protects preimplantation mouse conceptuses from a detrimental effect on development of the inorganic ions in oviductal fluid. *J. Exp. Zool.*, **253**, 215–219.

Walker, S.K., Heard, T.M. and Seamark, R.F. (1992) *In vitro* culture of sheep embryos without co-culture: success and perspectives. *Theriogenology*, **37**, 111–126.

Walker, S.K., Hill, J.L., Kleemann, D.O. and Nancarrow, C.D. (1996) Development of ovine embryos in synthetic oviduct fluid containing amino acids at oviductal fluid concentration. *Biol. Reprod.*, **55**, 703–708.

Watson, A.J., Hogan, A., Hahnel, A., Wiemer, K.E. and Schultz, G.A. (1992) Expression of growth factor ligand and receptor genes in the preimplantation bovine embryo. *Mol. Reprod. Dev.*, **31**, 87–95.

Watson, A.J., Watson, P.H., Arcellana-Panlilio, M., Warnes, D., Walker, S.K., Schultz, G.A., Armstrong, D.T. and Seamark, R.F. (1994) A growth factor map for ovine preimplantation development. *Biol. Reprod.*, **50**, 725–733.

Wenner, C.E. and Tomei, L.D. (1981) Phenotypic expression of malignant transformation and its relationship to energy metabolism. In *The Transformed Cell*, edited by I.L. Cameron and T.B. Pool, pp. 163–188, New York: Academic Press.

West, J.D. (1982) X chromosome expression during mouse embryogenesis. In *Genetic Control of Gamete Production and Function*, edited by P.G. Crosignani, B.L. Rubin and M. Fraccaro, pp. 49–91. London: Academic Press.

Whitten, W.K. (1956) Culture of tubal mouse ova. *Nature*, **177**, 96–97.

Whitten, W.K. (1957) Culture of tubal ova. *Nature*, **179**, 1081–1082.

Whitten, W.K. and Biggers, J.D. (1968) Complete development *in vitro* of the preimplantation stages of the mouse embryo in a simple chemically defined medium. *J. Reprod. Fertil.*, **17**, 399–401.

Whittingham, D.G. (1966) A critical phase in the cultivation of mouse ova *in vitro*. *J. Cell Biol.*, **31**, 123A.

Whittingham, D.G. and Biggers, J.D. (1967) Fallopian tube and early cleavage in the mouse embryo. *Nature*, **213**, 942–943.

Wiemer, K.E., Watson, A.J., Polanski, V., McKena, A.I., Fick, G.H. and Schultz, G.A. (1991) Effects of maturation and co-culture treatments on the development capacity of early bovine embryos. *Molec. Reprod. Dev.*, **30**, 330–338.

Wiley, L.M., Yamami, S. and Van Muyden, D. (1986) Effect of potassium concentration, type of protein supplement, and embryo density on mouse preimplantation development *in vitro*. *Fertil. Steril.*, **45**, 111–119.

Willadsen, S.M. (1979) A method for culture of micromanipulated sheep embryos and its use to produce monozygotic twins. *Nature*, **277**, 298–300.

Williams, T.J. (1986) A technique for sexing mouse embryos by a visual colorimetric assay of the X-linked enzyme glucose 6-phosphate dehydrogenase. *Theriogenology*, **25**, 733–739.

Wilson, J.M., Zalesky, D.D., Looney, C.R., Bondioli, K.R. and Magness, R.R. (1992) Hormone secretion by preimplantation embryos in a dynamic *in vitro* culture system. *Biol. Reprod.*, **46**, 295–300.

Wright, R.W. Jr. and Bondioli, K.R. (1981) Aspects of *in vitro* fertilization and embryo culture in domestic animals. *J. Anim. Sci.*, **53**, 702–729.

Xu, K.P., Yadav, B.R., King, W.A. and Betteridge, K.J. (1992) Sex-related differences in developmental rates of bovine embryos produced and cultured *in vitro*. *Molec. Reprod. Devel.*, **31**, 249–252.

Yadav, B.R., King, W.A. and Betteridge, K.J. (1993) Relationships between the completion of the cleavage and the chromosomal complement, sex, and developmental rates of bovine embryos generated *in vitro*. *Mol. Reprod. Dev.*, **36**, 434–439.

Zhang, L., Jiang, S., Wozniak, P.J., Yang, X. and Godke, R.A. (1995) Cumulus cell function during bovine oocyte maturation, fertilization, and embryo development *in vitro*. *Mol. Reprod. Dev.*, **40**, 338–344.

Zuelke, K.A. and Brackett, B.G. (1992) Effects of luteinizing hormone on glucose metabolism in cumulus enclosed bovine oocytes matured *in vitro*. *Endocrinology*, **131**, 2690–2696.

Zuelke, K.A. and Brackett, B.G. (1993) Increased glutamine metabolism in bovine cumulus cell enclosed and denuded oocytes after *in vitro* maturation with luteinizing hormone. *Biol. Reprod.*, **48**, 815–820.

2. NUCLEAR TRANSFER

KEITH H.S. CAMPBELL* and IAN WILMUT

Roslin Institute (Edinburgh), Roslin, Midlothian EH25 9PS, UK

There are two potential roles for nuclear transfer in animal breeding. First, the production of multiple copies of elite embryos by reconstruction using embryonic blastomeres. Secondly, nuclear transfer from cultured cell populations may be used for the production of genetically modified progenitor animals, either for the introduction of genetic change into nucleus herds, or for increasing the rate of dissemination of genetic modification into the population as a whole. The purpose of this review is to discuss some of the factors that affect the development of reconstructed embryos and the means by which nuclear transfer can be used to achieve these goals.

KEY WORDS: nuclear transfer; cell cycle; embryo development; nuclear reprogramming; genetic modification.

INTRODUCTION

Embryo reconstruction by nuclear transfer involves the transfer of a single nucleus to an unfertilised oocyte or one cell zygote from which the genetic material has been removed. In farm animals the use of unfertilised oocytes arrested at metaphase of the second meiotic division (MII) as recipient cells has become the method of choice. The donor cell used for reconstruction is dependent upon the application of the technology, for embryo multiplication blastomeres from selected embryos are used as nuclear donors (First, 1991). More recently live offspring in sheep were produced using cells cultured *in vitro* as nuclear donors (Campbell *et al.*, 1996b). This approach will prove extremely useful in the field of genetic manipulation. The development of embryos reconstructed by nuclear transfer is dependent on many factors. These include cell cycle effects of both donor and recipient cells, the methods of activation and culture, the stage of development or differentiated state of the donor nucleus. Recently it has been suggested that the chromatin state of the donor nucleus at the time of transfer may be a function of cell cycle phase and directly affect the efficiency of nuclear transfer.

METHOD OF EMBRYO RECONSTRUCTION

Historically two types of recipient cell have mainly been used for nuclear transfer, pronuclear zygotes and oocytes arrested at metaphase of the second meiotic division. More recently the use of two cell stage mouse embryos has been

* Corresponding author. Present address: PPL Therapeutics, Roslin, Midlothian EH25 9PP UK. Tel.: 0131-440-4777. Fax: 0131-440-4888. E-mail: Campbell@pplros.demon.co.uk.

reported (Tsunoda *et al.*, 1987). In farm animal species no development has been reported when using pronuclear zygotes as recipients, except when pronuclei are exchanged between zygotes (e.g. in cattle, Robl *et al.*, 1987; pig, Prather *et al.*, 1989) and oocytes arrested at MII have become the recipient of choice.

Sources of Recipient Oocytes

MII oocytes for use as recipient cells in embryo reconstruction can be obtained following *in vitro* maturation of oocytes recovered at slaughter in cattle (Barnes *et al.*, 1993), sheep (Pugh *et al.*, 1991) and pig (Hirao *et al.*, 1994). Alternatively MII oocytes can be obtained by maturation of oocytes collected by *in vivo* aspiration (ovum pickup, OPU) in cattle (for review see Bols *et al.*, 1994), maturation *in vivo* and collection by flushing from the oviduct after ovulation (all species) (e.g. sheep, Campbell *et al.*, 1994a) or possibly by careful timing and aspiration of follicles following oocyte maturation, prior to ovulation.

Enucleation of Recipient Oocytes

The term enucleation is used to describe the removal of the genetic material from the recipient cell. Oocytes arrested at MII do not contain a nucleus, the chromatin is condensed as chromosomes which are arranged on the spindle. Treatment of oocytes with the microtubule inhibitor Cytochalasin B imparts an elasticity to the plasma membrane and by using a small glass pipette (15–20 µm diameter) a membrane enclosed portion of cytoplasm can be removed. The metaphase plate is not visible under the light microscope, however it is located below the 1st polar body which can be used as a guide. Enucleation is confirmed by staining the karyoplast with a DNA specific fluorochrome such as Hoescht 3332 either following aspiration (Westhusin *et al.*, 1990) or during the aspiration procedure as is used routinely in our laboratory (Campbell *et al.*, 1993b) (see Figure 2.1).

Embryo Reconstruction

Following enucleation the genetic material from the donor cell (karyoplast) must be introduced into the enucleated oocyte (cytoplast). In general this has been achieved by fusion of the two cells although more recently direct injection techniques have been reported (Collas and Barnes, 1994; Ritchie and Campbell, 1995). Cell fusion is induced by a number of agents including Sendai virus (Graham, 1969), polyethylene glycol (PEG) i.e. (Kanka *et al.*, 1991) or application of a DC electric current (Willadsen, 1986). In farm animal species electro-fusion is the most commonly used method, although Sendai virus is efficient in the mouse, its effects are variable in other species such as sheep (Willadsen, 1986). The use of PEG requires its fast and efficient removal after fusion due to its toxicity.

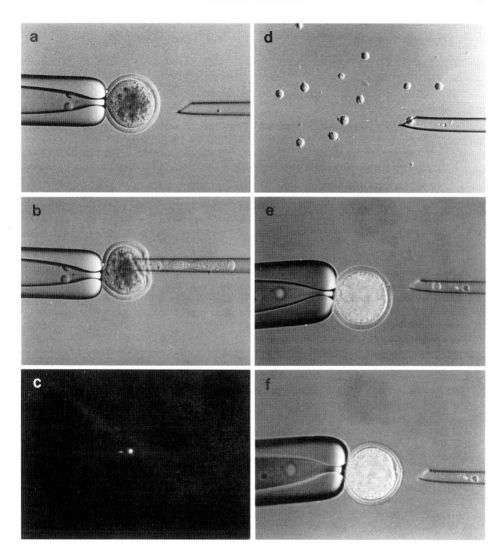

Figure 2.1 This series of figures shows the method of embryo reconstruction employed for the production of cloned sheep from a cultured cell line (Campbell *et al.*, 1996b) (magnification × 400). (a) MII oocyte attached to holding pipette prior to enucleation. (b) Removal of a karyoplast (containing the chromosomes) from below the 1st polar body. (c) Checking the enucleation procedure, the aspirated karyoplast is illuminated by UV light, fluorescence of the polar body (*right*) and metaphase spindle (*left*) confirms enucleation. (d–f) A donor cell is aspirated into the pipette and placed into contact with the enucleated oocyte via the previously made hole in the zona pellucida.

ACTIVATION OF THE RECONSTRUCTED EMBRYOS

Following introduction of the donor genetic material the reconstructed embryo has to begin development. At fertilisation, sperm penetration initiates a cascade of events which result in the onset of development. Many studies have shown that fertilisation initiates a series of calcium peaks. These appear to be sufficient and necessary for development, although the timing and duration vary between species e.g. mouse (Cuthbertson and Cobbold, 1985; Vitullo and Ozil, 1992), cow (Collas et al., 1993). Without sperm, treatments must be applied which can mimic these events and induce development. During recent years many treatments have been reported which cause oocyte activation and induce development, although comparative studies of these treatments have not been reported. Such treatments have included electrical stimulation using either a single DC pulse e.g. pig (Prochazka et al., 1992), cattle (Kono et al., 1989) (for review see Robl et al., 1992) or multiple electrical stimuli coinciding with the reported calcium peaks following fertilisation i.e. rabbit (Ozil, 1990), cattle (Collas et al., 1993). Chemical treatments have included phorbol ester e.g. mouse (Cuthbertson and Cobbold, 1985), calcium ionophores such as A23187 (Ware et al., 1989; Aoyagi, 1992), ionomycin in cattle (Susko Parrish et al., 1994), components of 2nd messenger systems e.g. IP3 (inositol tris-phosphate), in mouse (Jones et al., 1995), cattle (for review see White and Yue, 1996), ethanol (i.e. cattle, Nagai, 1987), strontium chloride (i.e. mouse, O'Neill, Rolfe and Kaufman, 1991). The rate and frequency of oocyte activation are dependent upon the age of the oocyte following the onset of maturation. As oocyte age increases, activation can occur spontaneously as a result of changes in temperature, or other manipulations and in addition pronuclear formation occurs more rapidly e.g. cattle (Ware et al., 1989; Presicce and Yang, 1994). In contrast activation of 'young' oocytes has proved more difficult, in cattle (Pressice and Yang, 1994) and pigs (Nussbaum and Prather, 1995) treatment of young MII oocytes with an activation stimulus combined with inhibitors of protein synthesis (i.e. cycloheximide or puromycin) can overcome this block. More recently, soluble sperm factors have been extracted which can induce activation following injection into mouse oocytes (Parrington et al., 1996); for review see Swann (1996).

The role of activation in subsequent development is slowly being elucidated. Calcium oscillations continue throughout the 1st cell cycle in the mouse and are associated with mitotic division (Kono et al., 1996; Jones et al., 1995). Activation of mouse oocytes with strontium chloride and continued exposure until after the first cleavage division has been shown to increase the size of measurable calcium oscillations at first mitosis to that observed in fertilised zygotes (Jones et al., 1995; Kono et al., 1996). In addition, cell number at the blastocyst stage has also been reported to increase (Jones et al., 1996) suggesting that the efficiency of activation may have far reaching developmental effects.

CULTURE OF RECONSTRUCTED EMBRYOS

Following reconstruction the embryo must be cultured to a stage at which it can be transferred to a synchronised recipient animal for development to term, generally at the morula or blastocyst stage. Two options are available, culture *in vitro* or culture *in vivo*. Many systems exist for the culture of embryos *in vitro* and research in this area has resulted in an increase in the frequency and the quality of development (for review see Campbell and Wilmut, 1994b). Traditionally reconstructed embryos from cattle and sheep have been cultured in the ligated oviduct of a temporary recipient ewe (Willadsen, 1986). Due to the hole made in the zona pellucida during manipulation this requires the encapsulation of each embryo in agar. The function of the agar chip is twofold, it holds the embryo in the zona pellucida, and it prevents attack by macrophages within the oviduct.

NUCLEAR–CYTOPLASMIC INTERACTIONS IN RECONSTRUCTED EMBRYOS

The successful development of reconstituted embryos is dependent upon a large range of factors. In fertilised zygotes early events are controlled by maternally inherited RNA's and proteins, until the zygotic nucleus assumes control. In reconstituted embryos both the cytoplasm and the transferred nucleus must be able to recapitulate these events. Changes in nuclear structure, chromatin structure and gene activity have been reported and these will be discussed in relation to the differentiated state of the donor nucleus.

Nuclear Events During the First Cell Cycle

Interactions between cytoplasmic factors within the cytoplast and the cell cycle stage of the donor nucleus at the time of fusion are crucial to the avoidance of DNA damage and the maintenance of correct ploidy (for review see Campbell *et al.*, 1996a). Early development is characterised by a series of reduction divisions and no net growth occurs. The major events of the first cell cycle concern only the nucleus involving DNA replication during which the genetic material is duplicated, followed by mitosis and cleavage when the duplicated material is equally segregated to the two daughter cells. The onset of both meiotic and mitotic divisions is controlled by a cytoplasmic activity termed MPF (maturation/mitosis/meiosis promoting factor). MII oocytes arrest at metaphase of the 2nd meiotic division and contain high levels of MPF activity. Upon fertilisation or activation MPF activity declines to basal levels until the G2-phase of the cycle when increasing MPF activity induces entry to 1st mitosis. When nuclei are fused to MII oocytes, MPF activity induces the transferred nucleus to enter a mitotic division precociously and this is characterised by nuclear envelope breakdown (NEBD) and chromatin condensation. The effects of this premature entry to mitosis, or premature chromosome condensation (PCC) as it has been termed, on the transferred nucleus are dependent upon its cell cycle phase. Nuclei in S-phase undergo large amounts of DNA damage, whereas nuclei that are pre (2C) or post (4C) S-phase form single or double chromatids respectively and appear to avoid DNA damage. NEBD also results in DNA synthesis occurring in all nuclei, regardless of their cell cycle stage, thus only diploid nuclei will avoid DNA damage and retain correct ploidy. In contrast if embryos are reconstructed following the decline of MPF activity no NEBD or PCC occurs, DNA synthesis is controlled by the cell cycle stage of the donor nucleus and correct ploidy is maintained (for review see Campbell *et al.*, 1996a; summarised in Table 2.1).

The occurrence of NEBD and PCC may not be related solely to the activity of MPF. In cattle oocytes MPF activity, when measured biochemically, declines within 2–3 hours following activation (Campbell *et al.*, 1993a,b; Collas *et al.*, 1993). However, in embryos reconstructed at different times following activation and examined one hour after application of the fusion pulse, NEBD of the transferred nucleus is observed for approximately 9 hours following activation (Campbell *et al.*, 1993b). This discrepancy may be the result of further cytoplasmic factor/s, such as MAP kinase. This cytoplasmic kinase becomes activated early during the 1st cell cycle of murine zygotes and its presence is incompatible with pronuclear formation (for review see Whittaker, 1996).

Nuclear/Chromatin Changes as Evidence of 'Reprogramming'

The only true measure of 'reprogramming' of the reconstituted embryo is normal development to term. Early development is controlled by maternally inherited RNA and proteins and little or no transcription is detectable from the zygotic nucleus. At a particular stage of development, which is species dependent (see Table 2.2), a switch to zygotic genome control occurs and this is characterised by a large increase in detectable transcription (for review see Telford *et al.*, 1990).

Table 2.1   The effects of different cell cycle combinations of donor and recipient cells on the chromatin and ploidy of reconstructed embryos during the 1st cell cycle. In the mouse the formation of a second polar body from the donor chromatin alters these effects (for review see Campbell *et al.*, 1996a).

Cell cycle stage of recipient	MPF Activity	Ploidy/cell cycle stage of donor	Effect on nucleus	Effect on chromatin	DNA synthesis	Ploidy of daughter cells
MII	High	2C (G0/G1)	NEBD	SC's	+	2C
MII	High	4C (G2)	NEBD	DC's	+	4C
MII	High	2–4C (S)	NEBD	Pulverised	+	?2–4C
G1/S	Low	2C (G0/G1)	NO NEBD		+	2C
G1/S	Low	4C (G2)	NO NEBD		−	2C
G1/S	Low	2–4C (S)	NO NEBD		+	2C

SC's = single chromatids, DC's = double chromatids, 2C = diploid, 4C = tetraploid, ?2–4C = unknown ploidy.

Table 2.2 A comparison between the stage of development at which transcription from the embryonic genome begins and the most advanced stage of development from which nuclei transferred to enucleated oocytes have been able to support development to adulthood. Data on nuclear transfer from Illmensee and Hoppe, 1981; Collas and Robl, 1991; Collas and Barnes, 1994; Campbell *et al.*, 1996b; Wilmut *et al.*, 1997; Gurdon, 1962a,b. Data on transcription from Bolton *et al.*, 1984; Van Blerkom and Manes, 1974; King *et al.*, 1985, 1988; Camous *et al.*, 1986 Calarco and McClaren, 1976; Newport and Kirschner, 1982.

Species	Mouse	Rabbit	Cow	Sheep	Xenopus
Onset of transcription	2 cell	4 cell	8–16 cell	8–16 cell	4000 cells
Nuclear totipotency	Morula ICM	32 cell	ICM	Cultured differentiated cell populations derived from: (1) Embryo (2) Foetus (3) Adult mammary gland	Tadpole intestinal epithelium

The zygotic nucleus must then control development in a spatial and temporal manner and result in the formation of specific differentiated cell types. Nuclear transfer was originally proposed as a method for the study of differentiation (Spemann, 1938). Successful development in the frog from differentiated tadpole intestinal epithelial cells resulted in the concept of 'nuclear equivalence': all nuclei contain all of the information required for development and differentiation is achieved by differential gene expression (Gurdon, 1962a,b, 1974). The mechanisms responsible for differential gene expression are, however, poorly understood. It is thought that genomic imprinting mediated by DNA methylation is associated with differential gene expression (Levine *et al.*, 1992) and alterations in methylation/imprinting are associated with developmental abnormalities (for reviews see Reik *et al.*, 1990; Schultz *et al.*, 1992). For successful development the transferred nucleus must therefore firstly abolish transcription and then re-establish the temporal spatial and quantitative patterns of gene expression associated with normal development.

In reconstituted embryos there is an apparent correlation between the developmental or differentiated stage of the donor cell and the ability of the nucleus and chromatin to return to the zygotic state and control development. In the mouse (Howlett *et al.*, 1987) and rabbit (Kanka *et al.*, 1996) inhibition of transcription and establishment of zygotic gene expression profiles have been reported when transferring transcriptionally active blastomere nuclei, suggesting 'reprogramming'. In cattle the reports are less clear, continued transcription was reported following transfer of blastomere nuclei from 16–40 cell embryos to enucleated preactivated oocytes but rapid inhibition was seen when these nuclei were transferred to MII oocytes (Smith *et al.*, 1996). By studying nucleolar morphology King *et al.* (1996) reported that transcription in nuclear transfer embryos reduced over the first few cleavage divisions. In our laboratory inhibition of transcription is observed after transfer of fibroblast nuclei however, this is dependent not only upon the cell cycle phase of the recipient cytoplasm but also that of the donor nucleus at the time of transfer (Iwasaki and Campbell unpublished data). Studies on gene expression in reconstituted cattle embryos have shown altered levels of transcripts from a number of genes including bFGF, TGFα, IGF-II and IGF-I receptor which were up regulated and IGF-I which was down regulated (Westhusin *et al.*, 1995). It is interesting that reports in the mouse suggest that these genes are potentially imprinted (for review see Beechey and Cattanach, 1994). Immuno-cytochemical studies have demonstrated a number of changes in the transferred nucleus (for review see Stricker *et al.*, 1989). These include accumulation of B type lamins in cattle and pigs (Prather *et al.*, 1989) and mouse (Prather *et al.*, 1991) (B type lamins are associated with embryonic blastomeres and undifferentiated cells (Galli *et al.*, 1994)). Changes in snRNP's have been observed (Prather and Rickords, 1992), and in cattle, the removal of somatic Histone H2 and its replacement with the embryonic form (Smith *et al.*, 1995) and the stage specific expression of a protein as defined by the monoclonal antibody TEC-03 (Van Stekelenberg-Hamers *et al.*, 1994) have been reported. Whether these changes are indicative of, or are involved in, nuclear remodelling and chromatin reprogramming is unclear.

CELL CYCLE CO-ORDINATION AND DEVELOPMENT

As detailed earlier, inappropriate choice of donor and recipient cell cycle stages can result in chromosomal damage and aneuploidy during the 1st cell cycle. Two approaches can be used to avoid these problems. Firstly, diploid nuclei can be transferred to MII oocytes and, secondly, G0/G1, S and G2-phase nuclei can be transferred after the decline of cytoplasmic activities which induce NEBD (for review see Campbell *et al.*, 1996a). The former of these approaches requires the synchronisation or selection of nuclear donors that are in specific phases of the cell cycle. In addition to chromosomal damage and aneuploidy induced by inappropriate cell cycle combinations, the cell cycle stage of both donor and recipient cells can interact via other mechanisms to affect development.

Embryonic Blastomeres as Nuclear Donors

In early embryos, at any one time, the majority of nuclei are in S-phase. Although synchronisation of embryonic blastomeres has been successful in the mouse (Otaegui *et al.*, 1994) similar methods have proved unreliable in farm animal species in our hands. The use of pre-activated oocytes as cytoplast recipients for unsynchronised blastomeres results in a significant increase in the frequency of development to the blastocyst stage in both sheep (Campbell *et al.*, 1994b) and cattle (Stice *et al.*, 1994). As an alternative to pre-activation, treatment of MI enucleated cattle oocytes with 6-dimethyl amino purine results in the oocyte arresting in an unactivated state with low levels of MPF (Susko Parrish et al., 1994). This situation mimics the use of pre-activated oocytes as cytoplast recipients in that the transferred nuclei do not undergo NEBD and upon subsequent activation DNA replication is controlled by the cell cycle phase of the donor nucleus thus maintaining ploidy.

The ability to synchronise the blastomeres of early murine embryos has allowed more detailed studies of cytoplast/karyoplast cell cycle combinations. Recent reports in the mouse have demonstrated the use of mitotically arrested cells as donors of genetic material (Kwon and Kono, 1996). Briefly blastomeres from nocodazole treated embryos arrested in mitosis are transferred to enucleated MII oocytes. Extrusion of a polar body is inhibited by treatment with cytochalasin B and this results in the formation of two (pro) nuclei. Each of these nuclei is then transferred individually to an enucleated one cell embryo. Using this method these authors produced 6 identical pups from a single 4 cell embryo. Development has also been obtained from 20 cell embryos (personal communication). In a further study Otaegui and co-workers (1996) suggest that during the late G2 and early G1 phase of the donor cell cycle the chromatin is better able to re-direct development. Together these two studies suggest that during late G2, M and early G1 a permissive state exists which allows nuclear reprogramming. One possible explanation for these observations is that during these cell cycle phases, certain factors are released from the chromatin, thus allowing access of oocyte derived factors. This hypothesis is supported by two lines of evidence. Firstly, during mitosis transcription factors become displaced from the chromatin (Schermoen and O'Farrell, 1991; Martinez-Balbas et al., 1995) and, secondly, recent evidence that live offspring can be produced from cultured, differentiated cell lines induced to exit the growth cycle and enter a state of quiescence (see below).

Other Cell Populations

One of the aims of developmental biologists and biotechnologists is to produce offspring from cell populations that can be maintained in culture. For nuclear transfer the availability of a cultured cell line would facilitate cell cycle synchronisation of the donor nucleus and allow optimisation of cell cycle co-ordination in the reconstituted embryo. In the frog, development to term was obtained following the transplantation of intestinal epithelial cell nuclei (Gurdon, 1962a,b). In mammals a number of cell types including embryonic stem (ES) cells in the mouse and primordial germ cells have been proposed as being totipotent (for review see Wilmut, Campbell and O'Neill, 1992), however, as yet development to term has not been demonstrated by nuclear transplantation for cattle PGC's (Moens et al., 1996) or for murine ES cells (Modlinski et al., 1996). Recently, however, we have reported development to term of ovine embryos reconstructed using an embryo derived, epithelial like cell population as nuclear donors (Campbell et al., 1996b). In these experiments the cells were arrested in a G0 or quiescent state by the reduction of serum levels in the growth medium. Quiescent cells exit the growth cycle during the G1-phase and arrest with a diploid DNA content. The differentiated nature of the donor cells used in these studies (as suggested by morphology and expression of the differentiation associated antigens A-type nuclear lamins, vimentin and cytokeratins) prompted speculation that this property may not be limited to embryo derived cell lines and development from adult somatic populations may be a possibility (Solter, 1996).

To extend our observations and address this possibility three new cell populations were derived from (1) the embryonic disc of a day-9 embryo, (2) an eviscerated day-26 foetus and (3) the mammary gland of a 6 year old ewe in the last trimester of pregnancy. All three cell populations were induced to enter quiescence and then used as nuclear donors for embryo reconstruction by transfer to enucleated metaphase II oocytes, as previously described (Campbell et al., 1996b). Live offspring were obtained from all three cell populations (Wilmut et al., 1997) confirming the previous speculation that differentiated cells may be used as nuclear donors.

The role of quiescent donor nuclei in the success of these studies may be related to a number of factors. Firstly a stable population of diploid cells allows the co-ordination of donor and recipient cell cycle. Secondly, when cells enter quiescence a number of changes occur; these include a reduction in transcription, a reduction in translation, active degradation of mRNA and chromatin condensation (Whitfield et al., 1985). These changes may render both the cytoplasm and the chromatin more compatible with the cytoplast and facilitate a greater reprogramming of the donor chromatin by maternally derived cytoplasmic factors as discussed in the previous section. The role of quiescence in changing chromatin structure and the ability of donor nuclei to re-control development after nuclear transfer requires further studies.

In summary a period of 'permissiveness' appears to exist during late G2, M, early G1 and G0 stages of the donor cell cycle. During this period the chromatin appears more able to be modified to re-control embryonic and foetal development of reconstructed embryos.

THE USE OF NUCLEAR TRANSFER IN GENETIC MODIFICATION

The role of nuclear transfer in agriculture and biotechnology can be roughly divided into two areas: firstly multiplication of selected genotypes/phenotypes can be achieved by cloning from selected embryos/animals, secondly the role of nuclear transfer in the production of genetically modified animals as progenitors for traditional breeding programmes.

The ability to produce live offspring from cultured cell populations may herald a new era in genetic modification of farm animal species. Previously genetic modification was restricted to the addition of genetic material by injection into pronuclear zygotes. This technique has a number of disadvantages (for review see Campbell and Wilmut, 1997); firstly the efficiency is low, secondly, integration of the added DNA occurs at random during the early cell cycles. This causes a

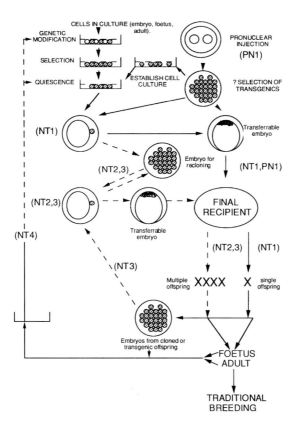

Figure 2.2 Potential roles for nuclear transfer in genetic modification and breeding of farm animal species. Two methods of producing genetically modified offspring are included. Firstly, the genetic modification of a cultured cell population and the production of embryos by nuclear transfer (NT1) and secondly the production of transgenic embryos by pronuclear injection. The potential fates of embryos produced by each method are denoted by the arrows. A single embryo produced by nuclear transfer from a cultured cell can be transferred directly to a final recipient resulting in a single offspring, or submitted to a second or more round/s (NT2) of multiplication resulting in multiple offspring. A single embryo produced by pronuclear injection could, with the development of reliable technology, be screened for transgenesis and transferred to a final recipient resulting in a single offspring or recloned by one (NT1) or more (NT2) rounds of nuclear transfer producing multiple offspring. Offspring produced by these methods could be used in traditional breeding programmes, alternatively embryos produced from these offspring could be cloned by nuclear transfer (NT3) in order to increase the number of modified animals and accelerate the rate of dissemination of the desired characteristic into the population. When using cultured cells multiple offspring may be produced by a single round of nuclear transfer, however, the use of recloning may increase the frequency of development. Selected transgenic embryos or foetuses or adults produced by pronuclear injection may also be used for the production of a cell line which may then be used to produce multiple embryos (dotted arrows indicate re-cloning steps). Transgenic embryos, foetuses or adults produced by these methods may similarly be used to establish cell lines which may be used for additional genetic modification or for multiplication procedures (NT4).

number of problems. Firstly random integration results in the production of variably expressing off-spring and for a particular gene modification a number of offspring would be required to obtain one that expressed the gene in the correct tissue and at the level required. Secondly the timing of integration results in the production of mosaic animals in which only some of the cells in the embryo and consequently the animal produced carry the modification. Therefore the gene may not be expressed in the correct tissue and transmission of the gene through the germline may not occur. The availability of cultured cells has a number of advantages, this allows genetic modification and selection of the cells before embryo reconstruction, the nature of the modifications that can be performed are greatly increased allowing gene knockouts, gene additions, precise modification of control regions to control expression levels and selective modification of gene products.

In addition to increasing the precision of genetic modification nuclear transfer increases the rate at which genetic modification can be made in a population. Sexing of embryos or cell lines allows modification of both male and female lines for breeding to homozygosity, alternatively this may be achieved by using double knockout techniques. The production of multiple copies of selected animals will accelerate the rate at which animal derived products may be tested and brought into commercial use. Figure 2.2 outlines some of the potential roles of nuclear transfer in animal production and breeding.

REFERENCES

Aoyagi, Y. (1992) Artificial activation of bovine oocytes matured *in vitro* by electric shock or exposure to ionophore A23187. *Theriogenology*, **37**, 188–180.

Barnes, F., Endebrock, M., Looney, C., Powell, R., Westhusin, M. and Bondioli, K. (1993) Embryo cloning in cattle: the use of *in vitro* matured oocytes. *Journal of Reproduction and Fertility*, **97**, 317–320.

Beechey, C.V. and Cattanach, B.M. (1994) Genetic imprinting map. *Mouse Genome*, **92**, 108–110.

Bols, P.E.J., Soom, A., Kruif, A., Van Soom, A. and De Kruif, A. (1994) Ovum pick-up in the cow, a review Ovum pick-up (OPU) bij het rund. *Vlaams Diergeneeskundig Tijdschrift*, **63**, 101–108.

Bolton, V.N., Oades, P.J. and Johnson, M.H. (1984) The relationship between cleavage, DNA replication and gene expression in the mouse two-cell embryo. *Journal of Embryology and Experimental Morphology*, **190**, 139–256.

Calarco, P.G. and McClaren, A. (1976) Ultrastructural observations of primplantation stages of sheep. *Journal of Embryology and Experimental Morphology*, **36**, 609–622.

Camous, S., Kopechny, V. and Flechon, J.E. (1986) Autoradiographic detection of the earliest stage of [^{3}H]-uridine incorporation into the cow embryo. *Biology of the Cell*, **58**, 195–200.

Campbell, K.H.S., Ritchie, W.A. and Wilmut, I. (1993a) Disappearance of maturation promoting factor and the formation of pronuclei in electrically activated *in-vitro* matured bovine oocytes. *Theriogenology*, **39**, 199–190.

Campbell, K.H.S., Ritchie, W.A. and Wilmut, I. (1993b) Nuclear–cytoplasmic interactions during the first cell cycle of nuclear transfer reconstructed bovine embryos: Implications for deoxyribonucleic acid replication and development. *Biology of Reproduction*, **49**, 933–942.

Campbell, K.H.S., Loi, P., Cappai, P. and Wilmut, I. (1994a) Improved development to blastocyst of ovine nuclear transfer embryos reconstructed during the presumptive S-phase of enucleated activated oocytes. *Biology of Reproduction*, **50**, 1385–1393.

Campbell, K. and Wilmut, I. (1994b) Recent advances on *in vitro* culture and cloning of ungulate embryos. *Proceedings 5th World Congress on Genetics Applied to Livestock Production*, **20**, 180–187.

Campbell, K.H.S., McWhir, J., Ritchie, W. and Wilmut, I. (1995) Production of live lambs following nuclear transfer of cultured embryonic disc cells. *Theriogenology*, **43**, 181.

Campbell, K.H.S., Loi, P., Otaegui, P.J. and Wilmut, I. (1996a) Cell cycle co-ordination in embryo cloning by nuclear transfer. *Reviews of Reproduction*, **1**, 40–46.

Campbell, K.H.S., McWhir, J., Ritchie, W.A. and Wilmut, I. (1996b) Sheep cloned by nuclear transfer from a cultured cell line. *Nature London*, **380**, 64–66.

Campbell, K.H.S. and Wilmut, I. (1997) Totipotency or multipotentiality of cultured cells: Applications and progress. *Theriogenology*, **47**, 63–72.

Collas, P. and Robl, J.M. (1991) Factors affecting the efficiency of nuclear transplantation in the rabbit embryo. *Biology of Reproduction*, **43**, 877–884.

Collas, P., Fissore, R., Robl, J.M., Sullivan, E.J. and Barnes, F.L. (1993) Electrically induced calcium elevation, activation, and parthenogenetic development of bovine oocytes. *Molecular Reproduction and Development*, **34**, 212–223.

Collas, P., Sullivan, E.J. and Barnes, F.L. (1993) Histone H1 kinase activity in bovine oocytes following calcium stimulation. *Molecular Reproduction and Development*, **34**, 224–231.

Collas, P. and Barnes, F.L. (1994) Nuclear transplantation by microinjection of inner cell mass and granulosa cell nuclei. *Molecular Reproduction and Development*, **38**, 264–267.

Cuthbertson, K.S.R. and Cobbold, P.H. (1985) Phorbol ester and sperm activates mouse oocytes by inducing sustained oscillations in cell Ca^{2+}. *Nature*, **316**, 541–542.

First, N.L. (1991) Manipulation techniques with potential use in animal agriculture. *Preimplantation Genetics: Proceedings First International Symposium 14–19 September 1990*, Chicago, Illinois, 49–61.

Galli, C., Lazzari, G., Flechon, J.E. and Moor, R.M. (1994) Embryonic stem cells in farm animals. *Zygote*, **2**, 385–389.

Graham, C.F. (1969) The fusion of cells with one- and two-cell mouse embryos. *Wistar Institute. Symposium. Monograph*, **9**, 19–33.

Gurdon, J.B. (1962a) The developmental capacity of nuclei taken from intestinal epithelium cells of feeding tadpoles. *Journal of Embryology and Experimental Morphology*, **10**, 622–640.

Gurdon, J.B. (1962b) Adult frogs from the nuclei of single somatic cells. *Developmental Biology*, **4**, 256–273.

Gurdon, J.B. (1974) *The Control of Gene Expression in Animal Development*, Oxford: Clarendon Press.

Hirao, Y., Nagai, T., Kubo, M., Miyano, T., Miyake, M. and Kato, S. (1994) *In vitro* growth and maturation of pig oocytes. *Journal of Reproduction and Fertility*, **100**, 333–339.

Howlett, S.K., Barton, S.C. and Surani, M.A. (1987) Nuclear cytoplasmic interactions following nuclear transplantation in mouse embryos. *Development*, **101**, 915–923.

Illmensee, K. and Hoppe, P.C. (1981) Nuclear transplantation in Mus musculus: development potential of nuclei from preimplantation embryos. *Cell*, **23**, 9–18.

Jones, K.T., Carroll, J., Merriman J.A., Whittingham, D.G. and Kono, T. (1995) Repetitive sperm-induced Ca^{2+} transients in mouse oocytes are cell cycle dependent. *Development*, **132**, 915–923.

Jones, K.T., Carroll, J. and Whittingham, D.G. (1995) Ionomycin, thapsigargin, ryanodine, and sperm induced Ca^{2+} release increase during meiotic maturation of mouse oocytes. *Journal of Biological Chemistry*, **270**, 6671–6677.

Jones, K.T., Bos-Mikich, A. and Whittingham, D.G. (1996) Ca^{2+} oscillations during exit from meiosis and first mitotic division influence inner cell mass and trophectoderm number in mouse blastocysts. *Journal of Reproduction and Fertility*, **17**, 5 (Abstract).

Kanka, J., Hozak, P., Heyman, Y., Chesne, P., Degrolard, J., Renard, J.P. *et al.* (1996) Transcriptional activity and nucleolar ultrastructure of embryonic rabbit nuclei after transplantation to enucleated oocytes. *Molecular Reproduction and Development*, **43**, 135–144.

Kanka, J., Fulka, J. Jr., Fulka, J. and Petr, J. (1991) Nuclear transplantation in bovine embryo: Fine structural and autoradiographic studies. *Molecular Reproduction and Development*, **29**, 110–116.

King, W.A., Nair, A. and Betteridge, K.J. (1985) The nucleolus organizer regions of early bovine embryos. *Journal of Dairy Science*, **68** (suppl.), 249–240.

King, W.A., Shepherd, D.L., Plante, L., Lavoir, M.-C., Looney, C.R. and Barnes, F.L. (1996) Nucleolar architecture over the first few cleavage divisions in bovine nuclear transfer embryos. *Molecular Reproduction and Development*, **44**, 499–506.

Kono, T., Jones, K.T., Bos Mikich, A., Whittingham, D.G. and Carroll, J. (1996) A cell cycle-associated change in Ca^{2+} releasing activity leads to the generation of Ca^{2+} transients in mouse embryos during the first mitotic division. *Journal of Cell Biology*, **132**, 915–923.

Kono, T., Iwasaki, S. and Nakahara, T. (1989) Parthenogenetic activation by electric stimulus of bovine oocytes matured *in vitro* . *Theriogenology*, **33**, 569–576.

Kwon, O.Y. and Kono, T. (1996) Production of sextuplet mice by transferring metaphase nuclei from 4-cell embryos. *Proceedings of the National Academy of Sciences of the United States of America*, **93**, 13010–13013.

Levine, A., Cantoni, G.L. and Razin, A. (1992) Methylation in the preinitiation domain suppresses gene transcription by an indirect mechanism. *Proceedings of the National Academy of Sciences of the United States of America*, **89**, 10119–10123.

Martinez-Balbas, M.A., Dey, A., Rabindran, S.K., Ozato, K. and Wu, C. (1995) Displacement of sequence specific transcription factors from mitotic chromatin. *Cell*, **83**(1), 29–38.

Modlinski, J.A., Reed, M.A., Wagner, T.E. and Karasiewicz, J. (1996) Embryonic Stem Cells: developmental capabilities and their possible use in mammalian embryo cloning. In *Animal Reproduction: Research and Practice*, edited by Stone, G.M. and Evans, G., pp. 437–446. Elsevier.

Moens, A., Chesne, P., Delhaise, F., Delval, F., Ectors, F., Dessy, F., Renard, J.P. and Heyman, Y. (1996) Assessment of nuclear totipotency of fetal bovine diploid germ cells by nuclear transfer. *Theriogenology*, **46**, 871–880.

Nagai, T. (1987) Parthenogenetic activation of cattle follicular oocytes *in vitro* with ethanol. *Gamete Research*, **16**, 243–249.

Newport, J. and Kirschner, M. (1982) A major transition in early xenopus embryos: II. Control of the onset of transcription. *Cell*, **30**, 687–696.

Nussbaum, D.J. and Prather, R.S. (1995) Differential effects of protein synthesis inhibitors on porcine oocyte activation. *Molecular Reproduction and Development*, **41**, 70–75.

O'Neill, G.T., Rolfe, L.R. and Kaufman, M.H. (1991) Developmental potential and chromosome constitution of strontium-induced mouse parthenogenones. *Molecular Reproduction and Development*, **30**, 214–219.

Otaegui, P.J., O'Neill, G.T., Campbell, K.H.S., and Wilmut, I. (1994) Transfer of nuclei from 8-cell stage mouse embryos following use of nocodazole to control the cell cycle. *Molecular Reproduction and Development*, **39**, 147–152.

Otaegui, P.J., Campbell, K.H.S., Ansell, J., Waddington, D. and Wilmut, I. (1996) The influence of cell cycle stage of donor blastomere and recipient cytoplast on development of mouse embryos reconstructed by nuclear transfer, (manuscript in preparation).

Ozil, J.P. (1990) The Parthenogenetic development of rabbit oocytes after repetitive pulsatile electrical stimulation. *Development*, **109**, 117–127.

Parrington, J., Swann, K., Shevchenko, V.I., Sesay, A.K. and Lai, F.A. (1996). Calcium oscillations in mammalian eggs triggered by a soluble sperm protein. *Nature London*, **379**, 364–368.

Prather, R.S., Sims, M.M. and First, N.L. (1989) Nuclear transplantation in early pig embryos. *Biology of Reproduction*, **41**, 414–418.

Prather, R.S., Sims, M.M., Maul, G.G., First, N.L. and Schatten, G. (1989) Nuclear lamin antigens are developmentally regulated during porcine and bovine embryogenesis. *Biology of Reproduction*, **40**, 123–132.

Prather, R.S., Kubiak, J., Maul, G.G., First, N.L. and Schatten, G. (1991) The expression of nuclear lamin A and C epitopes is regulated by the developmental stage of the cytoplasm in mouse oocytes or embryos. *Journal of Experimental Zoology*, **257**, 110–114.

Prather, R.S. and Rickords. L.F. (1992) Developmental regulation of an snRNP core protein epitope during pig embryogenesis and after nuclear transfer for cloning. *Molecular Reproduction and Development*, **33**, 119–123.

Presicce, G.A. and Yang, X. (1994) Nuclear dynamics of parthenogenesis of bovine oocytes matured *in vitro* for 20 and 40 hours and activated with combined ethanol and cycloheximide treatment. *Molecular Reproduction and Development*, **37**, 61–68.

Prochazka, R., Kanka, J., Sutovsky, P., Fulka, J. and Motlik, J. (1992) Development of pronuclei in pig oocytes activated by a single electric pulse. *Journal of Reproduction and Fertility*, **96**, 725–734.

Pugh, P.A., Fukui, Y., Tervit, H.R. and Thompson, J.G. (1991) Developmental ability of *in vitro* matured sheep oocytes collected during the nonbreeding season and fertilized *in vitro* with frozen ram semen. *Theriogenology*, **36**, 771–778.

Reik, W., Howlett, S.K. and Surani, M.A. (1990) Imprinting by DNA methylation: from transgenes to endogenous gene sequences. *Development*, Supplement, 99–106.

Ritchie, W.A. and Campbell, K.H.S. (1995) Intracytoplasmic nuclear injection as an alternative to cell fusion for the production of bovine embryos by nuclear transfer. *Journal of Reproduction and Fertility*, **15**, 60 (Abstract).

Robl, J.M., Prather, R., Barnes, F., Eyestone, W., Northey, D., Gilligan, B. *et al.* (1987) Nuclear transplantation in bovine embryos. *Journal of Animal Science*, **64**, 642–647.

Robl, J.M., Fissore, R., Collas, P. and Duby, R.T. (1992) Cell fusion and oocyte activation. In *Symposium on Cloning Mammals by Nuclear Transplantation*, edited by Seidel, G.E.J., pp. 24–27. Colorado: Colorado State University.

Schermoen, A.W. and O'Farrell, P.H. (1991) Progression of the cell cycle through mitosis leads to abortion of nascent transcripts. *Cell*, **67**, 303–310.

Schultz, G.A., Hogan, A., Watson, A.J., Smith, R.M. and Heyner, S. (1992) Insulin, insulin-like growth factors and glucose transporters: temporal patterns of gene expression in early murine and bovine embryos. *Symposium on growth factors in early embryonic development, University of Sydney, Australia, 3 October 1991. Reproduction, Fertility and Development*, **4**, 361–371.

Smith, S.D., Soloy, E., Kanka, J., Holm, P. and Callesen, H. (1996) Influence of recipient cytoplasm stage on transcription in bovine nucleus transplant embryos. *Molecular Reproduction and Development*, **45**, 444–450.

Smith, L.C., Meirelles, F.V., Bustin, M. and Clarke, H.J. (1995) Assembly of somatic histone H1 onto chromatin during bovine early embryogenesis. *Journal of Experimental Zoology*, **273**, 317–326.

Solter, D. (1996) Lambing by nuclear transfer. *Nature*, **380**, 24–25.

Spemann, H. (1938) *Embryonic development and induction*, pp. 210–211. New York: Hafner Publishing Company.

Stice, S.L., Keefer, C.L. and Matthews, L. (1994) Bovine nuclear transfer embryos: Oocyte activation prior to blastomere fusion. *Molecular Reproduction and Development*, **38**, 61–68.

Stricker, S., Prather, R., Simerly, C., Schatten, H. and Schatten, G. (1989) Nuclear Architectural Changes during Fertilization and Development. In *The Cell Biology of Fertilization*, edited by Schatten, H. and Schatten, G., pp. 225–250. Orlando: Academic Press.

Susko Parrish, J.L., Leibfried Rutledge, M.L., Northey, D.L., Schutzkus, V. and First, N.L. (1994) Inhibition of protein kinases after an induced calcium transient causes transition of bovine oocytes to embryonic cycles without meiotic completion. *Developmental Biology*, **166**, 729–739.

Swann, K. (1996) Soluble sperm factors and Ca^{2+} release in eggs at fertilization. *Reviews of Reproduction*, **1**, 33–39.

Telford, N., Watson, Andrew J. and Schultz, Gilbert A. (1990) Transition from maternal to embryonic control in early mammalian development: A comparison of several species. *Molecular Reproduction and Development*, **26**, 90–100.

Tsunoda, Y., Yasui, T., Shioda, Y., Nakamura, K., Uchida, T. and Sugie, T. (1987) Full-term development of mouse blastomere nuclei transplanted into enucleated two-cell embryos. *Journal of Experimental Zoology*, **242**, 147–140.

Vitullo, A.D. and Ozil, J.P. (1992) Repetitive calcium stimuli drive meiotic resumption and pronuclear development during mouse oocyte activation. *Developmental Biology*, **151**, 128–136.

Van Blerkom, J. and Manes, C. (1974) Development of preimplantation rabbit embryos *in vivo* and *in vitro* II. A comparison of qualitative aspects of protein synthesis. *Developmental Biology*, **40**, 40–51.

Van Stekelenberg-Hamers, A.E.P., Rebel, H.G., Van Inzen, W.G., Deloos, F.M., Drost, M., Mummery, C.L., Weima, S.M. and Trounson, A.O. (1994) Stage specific appearance of the mouse antigen TEC-3 in normal and nuclear transfer bovine embryos: Re-expression after nuclear transfer. *Molecular Reproduction and Development*, **37**, 27–33.

Wall, R.J. (1996) Transgenic livestock: Progress and prospects for the future. *Theriogenology*, **45**, 57–68.

Ware, C.B., Barnes, F.L., Maiki Laurila, M. and First, N.L. (1989) Age dependence of bovine oocyte activation. *Gamete Research*, **22**, 265–275.

Westhusin, M.E., Arcellana-Panilio, M., Harvey, M., Jones, K. and Schultz, G.A. (1995) Gene expression in cloned bovine embryos. In *Application of Molecular Biology to Reproduction. IETS Satellite Symposium*.

Westhusin, M.E., Levanduski, M.J., Scarborough, R., Looney, C.R. and Bondioli, K.R. (1990) Utilization of fluorescent staining to identify enucleated demi-oocytes for utilization in bovine nuclear transfer. *Biology of Reproduction (suppl.)*, **42**, 176–170.

White, K.L. and Yue, C. (1996) Intracellular receptors and agents that induce activation in bovine oocytes. *Theriogenology*, **45**, 91–100.

Whitfield, J.F., Boynton, A.L., Rixon, A.L. and Youdale, T. (1985) The control of cell proliferation by calcium, Ca^{2+}-calmodulin and cyclic AMP. In *Control of Animal Cell Proliferation. Volume 1*, edited by Boynton, A.L. and Leffert, H.L., pp. 331–365. London: Academic Press Inc.

Whittaker, M. (1996) Control of meiotic arrest. *Reviews of Reproduction*, **1**, 127–135.

Willadsen, S.M. (1986) Nuclear transplantation in sheep embryos. *Nature*, **320**, 63–65.

Wilmut, I., Campbell, K.H.S. and O'Neill, G.T. (1992) Sources of totipotent nuclei including embryonic stem cells. In *Symposium on Cloning Mammals by Nuclear Transfer*, edited by Seidel, G.E.J., pp. 8–16. Colorado: Colorado State University.

Wilmut, I., Schnieke, A., McWhir, J., Kind, A. and Campbell, K.H.S. (1997) Viable offspring derived from fetal and adult mammalian cells. *Nature*, **385**, 810–813.

3. OPPORTUNITIES AND CHALLENGES IN DOMESTIC ANIMAL EMBRYONIC STEM CELL RESEARCH

STEVEN L. STICE*

Advanced Cell Technology, Paige Laboratory, University of Massachusetts, Amherst, MA 01003, USA

Research applications using mouse ES cell technologies continue to expand, and are encouraging researchers to attempt to produce similar cell lines in domestic animal species. However, unlike the mouse, domestic animal ES cells with germ-line transmission capabilities remains an elusive goal. Debates continue on which *in vitro* environment and genetic factors are responsible for the differences observed among species. At the core of this debate is the question, should domestic animal ES be identical to mouse ES cells in respect to morphological and differentiation characteristics? Additional informative differentiation markers should help answer this question, ultimately leading to more successful ES studies in farm species. The presence and absence of molecular markers such as Oct-4, REX-1 and H-19 are well characterized in mice development. They may also be informative in farm animal embryonic development and ES cell studies. Preliminary studies using informative molecular differentiation markers will ease decisions on which putative ES cell lines to test for *in vivo* pluri- and totipotency. Useful *in vitro* data is particularly important in farm species given the huge time and resource commitments needed in well replicated *in vivo* potency studies. As additional cell lines are developed, research on how best to genetically engineer these cells is required to produce transgenic livestock through ES cell technology in the future.

KEY WORDS: embryonic stem cells; markers; chimera; nuclear transfer; domestic animal.

MOUSE AND DOMESTIC ANIMAL ES CELLS

The ultimate goal of most laboratories conducting domestic animal embryonic stem (ES) cell research is to produce a cell line that can contribute to the germ-line of resulting offspring. Mouse ES cell technologies have progressed rapidly since germ-line transmission was first demonstrated (Bradley *et al.*, 1984). These advances include important new methods of propagating, characterizing and genetically modifying mouse ES cells. Conversely, the production of domestic animal ES cells line has been a more formidable task. Despite the problems, farm animal ES cell research continues because of the huge potential these cells have in advancing animal biotechnology efforts. Germ-line transmittable domestic animal ES cell uses range from improved production livestock to advancing our understanding of early embryonic development. Future biomedical uses include producing transgenic animals for cell and organ replacement therapies and as "bioreactors" to manufacture proteins of interest. Introducing foreign DNA into ES cells will result in germ-line transmission of specific gene targeting events.

*Tel.: (413) 545-2427. Fax: (413) 545-6326. E-mail: stice@vasci.umass.edu.

This capability will have a tremendous impact on the production of transgenic farm animals. In the end, ES cells enable researchers to make specific genomic modifications, a clear advancement over the pronuclear microinjection approach (see Chapter 4.1 this volume).

The wide gaps in accomplishments between mouse ES cells and domestic animal ES cells research, warrants new approaches toward isolating and propagating domestic animal ES cells. Results from previous attempts to produce germline ES cells through chimera approaches have fallen short (pig, Piedrahita *et al.*, 1990; Gerfen and Wheeler, 1995; Anderson *et al.*, 1994). Possible reasons for these results are numerous. Of course the most obvious one being that cultured cells have differentiated during propagation and thus can no longer contribute to all cell types in the developing fetus. However, determination of *in vitro* differentiation in these cells is problematic, due to a lack of specific domestic animal ES cell markers.

Therefore, most if not all domestic animal ES cell studies have attempted to compare putative domestic ES cells to mouse ES cells. Most studies use morphological, mouse ES cell markers and *in vitro* and *in vivo* differentiation characteristics to evaluate a particular cell line (see review by Stice and Strelchenko, 1996). One problem that arises in making morphological comparisons is that domestic ES cells may differ from mouse ES cells. This idea stems from the fact that early embryonic development differs between mice and domestic animals (see review by Betteridge and Flechon, 1988). The mouse embryo develops as an egg cylinder whereas the farm species forms an embryonic disk. These differences also question how informative mouse ES cells will be in domestic animal ES cell studies. In addition, it is unclear whether gene expression during early developmental stages is comparable among species. Surprisingly, comprehensive molecular developmental marker studies on both domestic animal embryonic development and on the putative ES cells derived from these cells are lacking. This is particularly true for molecular markers. An improved understanding of molecular events in early domestic embryonic development would obviously be useful in germ-line ES cells isolation experiments.

Markers for Embryonic Stem Cell

Recently, researchers have suggested the use of mouse embryonic and ES cell markers in studies attempting to derive domestic animal ES cell lines (Flechon, 1995). Some of these cells markers include alkaline phosphatase (AP) activity, cytokeratin 8 + 18, lamins A/C, and SSEA-1 epitope. These cell markers are informative in mouse ES cell studies and may also be also useful in isolating domestic animal ES cells. Differences in marker characteristics among putative ES cell lines are often more informative than morphological descriptions. Markers can also be helpful in defining spatial and temporal changes that occur in any cultured pluri- or totipotent cell line. However, the use of a single marker or even a set of markers to determine the potency of cell lines cannot replace *in vivo* differentiation studies. In the end, appropriate animal studies (chimera and/or nuclear transfer) must be done to decide whether a cell line should be considered an ES cell line (Flechon, 1995). Animal studies are expensive and time consuming. Given these circumstances, not all putative ES cell lines can be tested *in vivo*. Therefore, it is imperative to develop a set of *in vitro* markers that accurately reflect the differentiated state and/or potency of putative ES cell lines.

Alkaline phosphatase activity is often associated with undifferentiated mouse ES cells and primordial germ cells (Pease *et al.*, 1990). Mouse ES cells lose AP activity upon differentiation *in vitro*. The inner cell mass (ICM) and the trophoblast of pig, sheep and cattle embryos are AP positive (Talbot *et al.*, 1993, Talbot *et al.*, 1995). In these studies, cells derived from the ICM lost AP activity after *in vitro* propagation. However, AP activity is also present in various embryonic tissues. The mouse embryonic AP gene is expressed until the blastocyst stage, but a nonspecific AP gene is expressed through later embryonic stages (Hahnel *et al.*, 1990). Careful interpretation of AP results must be made considering the fact that there are multiple AP genes. Nonspecific expression AP genes or loss of expression in domestic species may prove misleading sometimes. In our laboratory, embryonic cell lines that were originally AP negative, differentiated *in vitro* into various AP positive cells (Figure 3.1). Some of these cells are morphologically similar to neurons (Talbot *et al.*, 1993). Putative bovine ES cells lacking AP activity (Strelchenko *et al.*, 1995) when used in nuclear transfer procedures directed embryonic development through organogenesis (Stice *et al.*, 1996). In addition, AP gene expression differs among species. Mouse AP activity is found in germ cells but not in the gonad somatic cells. However, AP activity is found in both the germ and somatic cells of the developing bovine gonad (Lavior *et al.*, 1994). Therefore, AP activity in domestic species may not be as informative in domestic animals as it is in the mouse (Van Stekelenburg-Hamers *et al.*, 1995).

Other cell markers have been less thoroughly studied, but they may also have short comings when used to screen domestic animal putative ES cells. ES cell characterization studies often use cytokeratin 18, because it is found in the trophectoderm but not in the mouse ICM (Emerson, 1988). After probing porcine putative ES cells for cytokeratin 18, negative cell lines were used to attempt to produce chimeric offspring (Piedrahita *et al.*, 1990). However, these putative ES cells did not produce chimeric offspring. More recently, nuclear transfer experiment using a cytokeratin 18 positive embryonic disc derived cell line resulted in the birth of live lambs (Campbell *et al.*, 1996). Therefore, an absence of cytokeratin does not independently suggest that a particular cell line will contribute to chimeric offspring, nor does its presence indicate a loss of totipotency. As for SSEA-1, this mouse ICM epitope is not found on bovine ICM cells or cells derived from the ICM (Van Stekelenburg-Hamers *et al.*, 1995). However, SSEA markers were present in pluripotent rat (Iannaccone *et al.*, 1994) and primate (Thomson *et al.*, 1995) embryonic cell lines. These mixed results questions the usefulness of this marker in screening putative ES cell lines derived from domestic animal embryos. Antibody labeling of lamins A/C gradually decreases in porcine embryos at the four-cell stage and was absent through the blastocyst stage (Prather *et al.*, 1989). Unfortunately, both the ICM and the

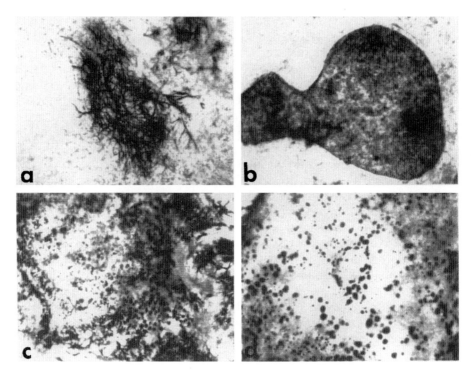

Figure 3.1 Alkaline phosphate staining of putative porcine ES cells undergoing *in vitro* differentiation: (a) neuronal-like cells (100×), (b) large cells which form dome-like structures (100×), (c) neuronal-like mixed with large unattached individual cells (100×) (d) large unattached cells (100×).

trophectoderm are negative for lamins A/C. Therefore, this marker does not distinguish differences between two different types of cells in the early embryos. Therefore, embryonic cell markers that are specifically associated with the differentiation of the ICM may be more informative than most of the markers used thus far.

Developmentally regulated murine gene expression has been extensively analyzed in murine ES cells and various murine early embryonic cell types (for a review see Pederson, 1994). Many of these genes vary considerably in expression patterns during early embryonic development and in undifferentiated and differentiated ES cells. There are many candidate marker genes, but three genes of particular interest, REX-1, Oct-4 and H19 are described below. Each has its own independent expression pattern during early embryonic development (Figure 3.2). Expression of these genes is different for the ICM vs. trophectoderm, primitive ectoderm vs. primitive endoderm and differentiated vs. undifferentiated ES cells (Figure 3.2). There are many examples of how these markers can be used. One study determined how differentiation of mouse ES cells into

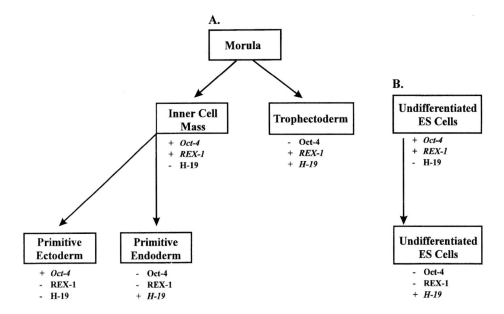

Figure 3.2 REX-1, Oct-4 and H19 are differentially expressed in (A) mouse embryonic tissue and (B) mouse ES cells.

primitive endoderm and ectoderm was affected by LIF (Shen and Leder, 1992). Similar differentiation studies might be done with putative domestic animal ES cells using these three genes.

REX-1 is a positive marker for ICM cells but is lost as these cells differentiate into primitive ectoderm; however, Oct-4 is present in both the ICM and the primitive ectoderm. REX-1 (for reduced expression) cDNA (1,745 nucleotides) was isolated by differential screening of a mouse F9 stem cell cDNA library (Hosler *et al.*, 1989). DNA sequence analysis suggests that REX-1 encodes for a regulatory protein. It was found that steady mRNA levels were seven-fold lower in retinoic acid induced differentiated F9 cells than undifferentiated F9 cells. Similarly, using Northern analysis, REX-1 is high in mouse ES cells and reduced in differentiated ES cells (Roger *et al.*, 1991). Using *in situ* hybridization in this same study, REX-1 was found in the ICM and polar trophoblast of day 4.5 embryos. After two days it was still present in some trophoblast derived tissue but much reduced in the primitive ectoderm. Oct-3 (Okamoto *et al.*, 1990) and Oct-4 (Rosner *et al.*, 1990) was later found to be one in the same and will be called Oct-4 in this manuscript. Oct-4 is found in both the ICM and embryonic ectoderm but absent in the trophoblast or the primitive endoderm (Scholer *et al.*, 1990). Oct-4 is also in germ cells and undifferentiated stem cells but is lost as ES cells begin to differentiate. Both Oct-4 and REX-1 genes may play a role in maintaining the pluripotency of embryonic cells.

In contrast to REX-1 and Oct-4, H19 is a positive marker for differentiation. H19 is not present in undifferentiated mouse ES cells but is present after differentiation (Poirier *et al.*, 1991). At the time of implantation this mRNA is active in extra-embryonic cell types. Again using *in situ* hybridization, H19 was not found in the ICM or primitive ectoderm. H19 was found in day 4.5 trophoblast and later in the ectoplacental cone, trophoblastic giant cells, extra-embryonic endoderm and ectoderm. H19 was also found in various tissues of the mid gestation embryo and adult tissues. Rapid induction of H19 mRNA in differentiating mouse ES cells makes it a candidate marker for differentiated domestic animal ES cells. It may also be useful in defining cell types in developing embryos.

Although it is unclear whether all murine markers will be as informative in domestic animals, differential expression found with at least some of these markers will be beneficial. At first appearance it may seem redundant to use a battery of markers. Rather, the overlap in tissue expression patterns leads to additional information that each marker by itself cannot provide. For example, although REX-1 and Oct-4 are present in the ICM, only Oct-4 is present in the murine primitive ectoderm. There are certainly other genetic markers that may be as useful as these three genes. In addition, differential display techniques (Liang and Pardee, 1992) and cDNA subtraction libraries may produce new markers specific for livestock species. In the end, gene expression studies may provide new markers that correlate well with differentiation events in early domestic animal embryos and putative ES cells.

Testing Putative Embryonic Stem Cells for Totipotency

Mouse ES cells were shown to be totipotent when chimera studies produced stable ES germ-line chimeric offspring (Bradley *et al.*, 1984). This opened the possibility of making transgenic animals using genetically modified ES cells. Unfortunately, germ-line chimeric animals have not been reported in any species other than the mouse. Farm animal species are at a great disadvantage in this regard. These types of experiments require several months to conduct in mice. However, in farm animals, especially cattle, this process may require several years. In particular, ES cell chimera experiments have the inherent disadvantage of requiring two generations of animals to definitively demonstrate germ-line transmission. The cost of feeding and maintaining, any number of farm animals over several years is high. Often hundreds of animals are used to serve as embryo donors and recipients, especially if testing more than one putative ES cell line. This especially holds true in non-litter bearing species. Sheep and goats present yet another obstacle since they are seasonal breeders. Unless additional animal management procedures are used, experiments in these species are conducted only during certain times of the year. All these factors have contributed to the limited number of studies examining the totipotency of putative domestic animal ES cells.

Chimeras

Despite the constraints of chimera studies in livestock species, researchers have made some progress. In rabbits (Giles *et al.*, 1993) and short term cultured ICM cells (five days, rabbit) injected into recipient embryos resulted in offspring. Similar studies in the pig proved that a freshly isolated ICM could contribute to a chimeric offspring (Anderson *et al.*, 1994). However, cells cultured for longer periods did not produce chimeric offspring in these studies. These are in agreement with other studies (Piedrahita *et al.*, 1990; Gerfen and Wheeler, 1995). There is reported evidence of chimeric pigs derived from a putative ES cell line, but as yet the germ-line contribution of these embryonic cells has not been demonstrated (see review by Wheeler, 1994). Similarly, rat embryonic cell lines produced coat color chimeras, but not germ-line chimeras (Iannaccone *et al.*, 1994). Therefore, further refinements in non-mouse ES cell propagation techniques may be needed before producing germ-line ES cell chimeric animals.

Chimera studies using primordial germ (PG) cells or fetal germ (FG) cells have produced some encouraging results. In mice, only PG cells induced to dedifferentiate into cell lines similar to mouse ES cells were useful in producing chimeric offspring (Stewart *et al.*, 1994). However, in the rabbit, freshly isolated FG cells did contribute to the gonad of near term fetuses (Moens *et al.*, 1996). Cultured cattle PG cells maintained Oct-4 activity (Cherney and Merier, 1994), and propagated pig PG cells were AP positive and expressed SSEA-1 (Shim, *et al.*, 1997). This appears to be a promising area of research for the future.

Nuclear Transfer

Major advances have been made in using nuclear transfer (cloning) to test the totipotency of a particular embryonic cell line. This is an area in which farm species seem to have an advantage over the mouse. Chapter 2 of this book discusses nuclear transfer experiments in farm animals. Embryonic cell lines derived from cattle (Stice *et al.*, 1996) and sheep (Campbell, 1996) embryos having morphological and marker characteristics differing from those observed in mouse ES cells were used in nuclear transfer studies. The bovine embryonic cell lines are epithelial-like and AP negative (Strelchenko, *et al.*, 1995; Stice *et al.*, 1996). The sheep cell lines were also epithelial and positive for both cytokeratin and lamin A/C (Campbell *et al.*, 1996). The bovine nuclear transfer embryos developed through organogenesis while similar sheep embryos developed to offspring. In another study, bovine cultured ICM cells grown in suspension were reported to have totipotent properties, since these cells produced nuclear transfer calves (Sims and First, 1994). Also, bovine embryonic cell line derived nuclear transfer embryos were aggregated with *in vitro* fertilized embryos a chimeric fetus reached the second trimester (Stice *et al.*, 1996).

The successful nuclear transfer studies raise some intriguing questions about the potency of cultured embryonic cells and current *in vitro* markers used to indirectly indicate pluri- and totipotency. Why do cells that have marker characteristics associated with differentiated cells direct fetal development and sometimes result in offspring? A plausible explanation is that the nuclear transfer procedure itself induces nuclear reprogramming in these differentiated nuclei. If so, these cell lines may not be useful in traditional germ-line chimera experiments. Depending on the results of additional nuclear transfer studies, the need to isolate murine-like ES cells in domestic animal species may become less important. Producing nuclear transfer embryos has some clear advantages over chimera systems. A nuclear transfer system eliminates the recovery and use of host embryos. However, probably the most importance advantage nuclear transfer has is the elimination of a generation of chimeric animals. Using the nuclear transfer procedure, transgenic animals may be produced directly from transfected cell lines. However, in the pig, embryo nuclear transfer studies have not been as successful as those in sheep and cattle. Therefore, germ-line porcine offspring may still be generated through chimera approaches. No matter whether chimera or nuclear transfer procedures are used, domestic animal specific marker(s) are still needed. Markers will still be useful in tracking differences between cell lines and the potency or differentiation of individual cell lines.

TRANSGENIC LIVESTOCK USING EMBRYONIC STEM CELL TECHNOLOGY

Although nuclear transfer and chimera studies are encouraging, it is premature to suggest that producing a gene targeted animal is feasible using any totipotent cell line. In order for this to happen, the cell lines should have certain characteristics in common with mouse ES cells. First, mouse ES cells undergo clonal propagation. These cells maintain their totipotent characteristics even when passaged as single cells or low cell density for short periods. This is important because homologous recombination selection strategies use clonal culture techniques. Cell colonies that are clonally derived, can then be screened for recombination events. Gene targeting events occur in only 1×10^{-4} to 1×10^{-8} using standard electroporation techniques. Only a few individual cells will survive selection procedures and form a new colony (for a review of procedures see Ramirez-Solis et al., 1993).

Presently, clonal propagation of putative domestic animal ES cells has not been reported. A number of techniques have been used to disaggregate domestic embryonic cell lines including mechanical (Stice et al., 1996), enzymatic including trypsin (Piedrahita et al., 1990) collagenase and trypsin (Strojek et al., 1990; Talbot et al., 1993) or pronase (Stice et al., 1996). Often these techniques can disaggregate these cells into small clumps and single cells. However, it is unknown whether various cell lines can be clonally propagated, since there is no available information on plating efficiencies using these various techniques. Also, electroporation procedures require single cell suspensions. The electrical pulse that induces pores in the ES cells membrane for DNA entry into the cells might also induce unwanted cell fusion and/or poor transfection rates if ES cell doublets or clumps are used. Therefore, transfection and selection procedures currently used to produce transgenic mouse ES cells present additional requirements and stresses on a domestic animal cell lines.

In addition to clonal propagation, research is needed in the area of transgenic ES cell selection procedures. Selectable genes such as neomycin transferase are commonly used in mouse gene targeting DNA constructs. Mouse ES cells are selected over time in medium containing G418. Resistant transgenic colonies can be screened further for the desired gene targeting event using a wide variety of techniques (see review by Melton, 1994). Little research has been done with domestic species in this area. Cell survival rates may vary considerably after porcine embryonic cell lines are exposed to G418 selection medium (Rund *et al.*, 1994). Additional differences between mouse ES cells and putative domestic animal ES cell lines, such as longer cell doubling time, may require innovative cell selection methods. Lastly, the ability of various cell lines to express reporter genes or genes of interest remains undetermined. New expression vectors designed for unique cell lines may be needed. Depending on the totipotent cell type developed, these experiments may or may not be as formidable as the studies done to test the potency of the cells. However, when germ-line domestic animals are available, these areas will attract more focused attention.

REFERENCES

Anderson, G.B., Choi, S.J. and BonDurant, R.H. (1994) Survival of porcine inner cell masses in culture and after injection into blastocysts. *Theriogen.*, **42**, 204–212.

Betteridge, K.J. and Flechon, J.E. (1988) The anatomy and physiology of pre-attachment bovine embryos. *Theriogen.*, **29**, 155–186.

Bradley, A., Evans, M., Kaufman, M.H. and Robertson E. (1984) Embryo-derived stem cells: A tool for elucidating the developmental genetics of the mouse. *Nature (London)*, **309**, 255–256.

Campbell, K.H.S., McWhir, J., Ritchie, W.A. and Wilmut, I. (1996) Sheep cloned by nuclear transfer from a cultured cell line. *Nature*, **380**, 64–66.

Cherney, R.A. and Merier, J. (1994) Evidence for pluripotency of bovine primordial germ cell-derived cell lines maintained in long-term culture. *Theriogen.*, **41**, 175 (Abstr.).

Emerson, J.A. (1988) Disruption of the cytokeratin filament network in the preimplantation mouse embryo. *Development*, **104**, 219–234.

Flechon, J.E. (1995) Request for a consensus on the definition of putative embryonic cells. *Mol. Reprod. Dev.*, **41**, 274.

Gerfen, R.W. and Wheeler, M.B. (1995) Isolation of embryonic cell-lines from porcine blastocysts. *Anim. Biotech.*, **6**, 1–14.

Giles, J.R., Yang, X., Mark, W. and Foote, R.H. (1993) Pluripotency of cultured rabbit inner cell mass cells detected by isozyme analysis and eye pigmentation of fetuses following injection into blastocysts or morulae. *Mol. Reprod. Dev.*, **36**, 130–138.

Hahnel, A.C., Rappolee, D.A., Millan, J.L., Manes, T., Ziomek, C.A., Theodosiou, N.G. *et al.* (1990) Two alkaline phosphatase genes are expressed during early development in the mouse. *Development*, **110**, 555–564.

Hosler, B.A., Larosa, G.J., Grippo, J.F. and Gudas, L.J. (1989) Expression of REX-1, a gene containing zinc finger motifs, is rapidly reduced by retinoic acid in F9 teratocarcinoma cells. *Mol. Cell. Biol.* **9**, 5623–5629.

Iannaccone, P.M., Taborn, G.U., Garton, R.L., Caplice, M.D. and Brenin, D.R. (1994) Pluripotent embryonic stem cells from the rat are capable of producing chimeras. *Dev. Biol.*, **163**, 288–292.

Lavior, M.C., Basrur, P.K. and Betteridge, K.J. (1994) Isolation of germ cells from fetal bovine ovaries. *Mol. Reprod. Dev.*, **37**, 413–424.

Liang, P. and Pardee, A.B. (1992) Differential display of eukaryotic messenger RNA by means of the polymerase chain reaction. *Science*, **257**, 967–971.

Melton, D.W. (1994) Gene trageting. *BioEssays*, **16**, 633–638.

Moens, A., Betteridge, K.J., Brunet, A. and Renard, J.P. (1996) Low levels of chimerism in rabbit fetuses produced from preimplantation embryos microinjected with fetal gonadal cells. *Mol. Reprod. Dev.*, **43**, 38–46.

Okamoto, K., Okazawa, H., Okuda, A., Sakai, M., Muramatsu, M. and Hamada, H. (1990) A novel octamer binding transcription factor is differentially expressed in mouse embryonic cells. *Cell*, **60**, 461–472.

Pederson, R. (1994) Studies of *in vitro* differentiation with embryonic stem cells. *Reprod. Fert. Dev.*, **6**, 543–552.

Pease, S., Braghetta, P., Gearing, D., Grail, D. and Williams, R.L. (1990) Isolation of embryonic stem (ES) cells in media supplemented with recombinant leukemia inhibitory factor (LIF). *Dev. Biol.*, **141**, 344–352.

Piedrahita, J.A., Anderson, G.B. and BonDurant, R.H. (1990) On the isolation of embryonic stem cells: Comparative behavior of murine, porcine and ovine embryos. *Theriogen.*, **34**, 865–877.

Poirier, F., Chan, C.T.J., Timmons, P.M., Robertson, E.J., Evans, M.J. and Rigby, P.W.J. (1991) The murine H19 gene is activated during embryonic stem cell differentiation *in vitro* and at the time of implantation in the developing embryo. *Development*, **113**, 1105–1114.

Prather, R.S., Sims, M.M., Maul, G.G., First, N.L. and Schatten G. (1989) Nuclear lamin antigen are developmentally regulated during porcine and bovine embryogenesis. *Biol. Reprod.*, **40**, 123–132.

Ramirez-Solis, R., Davis, A.C. and Bradley, A. (1993) Gene targeting in embryonic stem cells. In *Guide to Techniques in Mouse Development: Meth. Enzym.*, edited by P.M. Wasserman and M.L. DePamphilis **225**, 855–877, San Diego: Academic Press Inc.

Roger, M.B., Hosler, B.A. and Gudas, L.J. (1991) Specific expression of a retinoic acid-regulated, zinc-finger gene, Rex-1, in preimplantation embryos, trophoblast and spermatocytes. *Development*, **113**, 815–824.

Rosner, M.H., Vigano, M.A., Ozato, K., Timmons, P.M., Poirier, F., Rigby, P.W. *et al.* (1990) A POU-domain transcription factor in early stem cell and germ cells of the mammalian embryo. *Nature (London)* **345**, 686–692.

Rund, A., Grum, L.R., Bleck, G.T., Leach, T.E. and Wheeler, M.B. (1994) Comparison of murine ES cell and porcine ES-like cell sensitivity to antibiotic G418. *Biol. Reprod.*, **50**, suppl. 1, 125, (Abstr).

Sims, M. and First, N.L. (1994) Production of calves by nuclear transfer of nuclei from cultured inner cell mass cells. *Proc. Natl. Acad. Sci. USA*, **91**, 6143–6147.

Scholer, H.R., Dressler, G.R., Balling, R., Rohdewohld, H. and Gruss, P. Oct-4: a germline-specific transcription factor mapping to the mouse t-complex. *EMBO*, **9**, 2185–2195.

Shen, M.M. and Leder, P. (1992) Leukemia inhibitory factor is expressed by the preimplantation uterus and selectively blocks primitive ectoderm formation *in vitro*. *Proc. Natl. Acad. Sci. USA*, **89**, 8240–8244.

Shim, H., Gutierrez-Adan, A. Chen, L.R., BonDurant, R.H. and Anderson, G.B. (1997) Isolation of pluripotent stem cells from culture primordial germ cells. *Therio.*, **47**, 245 (Abstr.).

Stewart, C.L., Gadi, I. and Bhatt, H. (1994) Stem cells from primordial germ cells can reenter the germ line. *Dev. Biol.*, **161**, 626–628.

Stice, S.L. and Strelchenko, N.S. (1996) Domestic animal embryonic stem cells: progress towards germ-line contribution. *Biotechnology's Role in the Genetic Improvement of Farm Animals* edited by R.H. Miller, V.G. Pursel and H.D. Norman. *American Soc. Animal Sci.* 189–201.

Stice, S.L., Strelchenko, N.S., Keefer, C.L. and Matthews, L. (1996) Pluripotent bovine embryonic cell lines direct development following nuclear transfer. *Biol. Reprod.*, **54**, 100–110.

Strelchenko, N., Miltipova, M. and Stice, S. (1995) Further characterization of bovine pluripotent stem cells. *Theriogen.*, **43**, 327 (Abstr.).

Strojek, R.M., Reed, M.A., Hoover, J.L. and Wagner, T.E. (1990) A method for cultivating morphologically undifferentiated embryonic stem cells from porcine blastocysts. *Theriogen.*, **33**, 901–913.

Talbot, N.C., Rexroad, C.E., Pursel, V.G. and Powell, A.M. (1993) Alkaline phosphatase staining of pig and sheep epiblast cells in culture. *Mol. Reprod. and Dev.*, **36**, 139–147.

Talbot, N.C., Powell, A.M. and Rexroad, C.E. (1995) *In vitro* pluripotency of epiblasts derived from bovine blastocysts. *Mol. Reprod. Dev.*, **42**, 35–52.

Thomson, J.A., Kalishman, J., Golos, T.G., During, M., Harris, C.P., Becker, R.A. and Hern J.P. (1995) Isolation of a primate embryonic stem cell line. *Proc. Natl. Acad. Sci. USA*, **92**, 7844–7848.

Van Stekelenburg-Hamers, A.E.P., Van Achterberg, T.A.E., Reble, H.G., Flechon, J.E., Campbell, K.H.S., Weima, S.M. *et al.* (1995) Isolation and characterization of permanent cell lines from inner cell mass cells of bovine blastocysts. *Mol. Reprod. Dev.*, **40**, 444–454.

Wheeler, M.B. (1994) Development and validation of swine embryonic stem cells — a review. *Reprod. Fert. Dev.*, **6**, 563–568.

Part 2
MAPPING THE GENOME

4. MAPPING GENES UNDERLYING PRODUCTION TRAITS IN LIVESTOCK

MICHEL GEORGES*

Department of Genetics, Faculty of Veterinary Medicine, University of Liège (B43), 20 Boulevard de Colonster, 4000-Liège, Belgium

With the advent of recombinant DNA, it is now possible to identify the genes that underly the genetic variation of production traits observed in livestock species. Identifying these genes is expected to allow for more efficient marker aided breeding programs and to yield novel insights in to the physiology of the corresponding traits. The most popular approach consists in an initial genetic localisation of the corresponding genes using linkage strategies, followed by positional cloning of the corresponding genes based on their known map location. In this chapter, the general principles of linkage analysis are reviewed with special emphasis on linkage analysis for quantitative trait loci (QTL). Developments in marker technology that have allowed for the generation of whole genome marker maps in livestock species in recent years are discussed, as well as new areas of research aiming at more efficient genotyping methods. Alternative mapping strategies such as bulk segregant analysis, representational difference analysis, identity-by-descent mapping and genome mismatch scanning are briefly described with their specific applications. Finally, we provide an overview of recent mapping experiments in which the described methods have been applied succesfully to livestock production traits.

INTRODUCTION

Domestication rhymes with gene manipulation. Indeed by selecting animals exhibiting desired properties, early agriculturalists were already sorting amongst alleles, albeit unwittingly. More recently, by modelling an individual's phenotype as the sum of an environmental and genotypic component, quantitative genetic theory has allowed for a considerable increase in genetic response. Although it is recognized that for most production traits the genotypic component likely reflects the joint contribution of multiple "polygenes", their actual identity and precise mode of action remains unknown.

With the advent of recombinant DNA it has become feasible — at least in principle — to dissect this "black box" into its individual Mendelian components. This prospect has received a lot of attention, not only because an understanding of the molecular architecture of complex heritable traits is of fundamental interest, but also because it might contribute to the improvement of breeding designs.

Today, the preferred strategy for identifying the genes that account for the genetic variation of a trait of interest as observed either within or between populations, is referred to as "positional candidate cloning" (Collins, 1995). In a first stage, this approach requires the chromosomal localisation of the pursued genes

*Tel.: 32-4-366.41.51. Fax: 32-4-366.41.22. E-mail: michel@stat.fmv.ulg.ac.be.

using linkage analysis or related strategies, followed by the actual identification of the causal gene and sequence variants amongst the "candidate" genes known from transcript maps to be located in the corresponding chromosomal area. While comprehensive transcript maps will not become available for domestic species in the near future, the remarkable conservation of synteny observed between mammals will allow animal geneticists to benefit from the human transcript map, which will soon be complete.

The success of the positional candidate cloning approach amongst animal geneticist is not only due to recent methodological breakthroughs — catalyzed by the Human Genome Initiative — that have rendered this strategy so effective, but also to the perspective that mapping data alone could lead to more effective Marker Assisted Selection (MAS) in the near future.

The purpose of this chapter is to review principles and recent developments underlying the first step in the positional candidate approach towards cloning production genes in livestock, that is the genetic localisation. After a review of the principles underlying linkage analysis, especially as it applies to quantitative traits, we will describe recent advances in marker technology that allowed for efficient linkage mapping in mammalian systems. Emerging alternative mapping strategies are briefly described, followed by an overview of successful implementations of the described methods in livestock.

This chapter will be followed by a chapter by Leif Andersson devoted to the second step, that is cloning the gene based on its map position.

LINKAGE ANALYSIS

General Principles: Two-Point Linkage Analysis

Assuming a pair of loci, a double heterozygous parent can transmit four types of gametes. Two of these reconstitute the genotype of the grandparental gametes and are therefore referred to as "parentals". A reassortment of grandparental alleles generates the two other gametic types referred to as "recombinants". Unambiguously recognizing the parental or recombinant gametic state therefore requires knowledge of the grandparental gametes or parental "phase".

The proportion of parental versus recombinant gametes informs us about the relative location of the loci analyzed. Indeed, we know from Mendel's second law that two loci on different chromosomes will assort independently, i.e. parental and recombinant gametes will be represented in equal proportions. On the contrary, for loci located on the same chromosome, production of a recombinant gamete requires crossing-over between the two loci. The occurrence of this event is more unlikely the closer the two loci are. As a consequence, the proportion of recombinant gametes drops with increasing proximity of the two loci.

The recombination rate, however, is only informing us accurately about genetic distance for relatively small distances. Due to multiple cross-overs, recombination rate saturates at 50% above a certain limit (an even number of cross-overs between a pair of loci will produce apparently non-recombinant parental gametes). The relationship between the recombination rate observed for a pair of loci and the actual genetic distance is referred to as a mapping function. Several mapping functions are known, accounting or not for the non-independence of multiple cross-overs in a given interval or "interference". Kosambi's mapping function is the most commonly used one for mammalian genomes (Ott, 1991).

To study the relative location of a pair of loci one could directly genotype sperm cells or oocytes and count gametic types. With the advent of the Polymerase Chain Reaction (PCR), this has become possible for DNA markers and has been used to some extend to construct DNA marker maps of specific chromosomal areas (e.g. Arnheim *et al.*, 1990; Lewin *et al.*, 1992). Usually, however, offspring are being generated, and the gametic genotype inferred from the offspring's genotype, accounting for the contribution of the mate. For loci traced via the segregation of a phenotype not expressed at the gametic stage, this approach is obviously the only practical one.

Performing a linkage study with a given marker therefore requires not only a heterozygous parent, but sufficient information to trace its segregation in the offspring. The informativeness of a marker is a function of the number of alleles, their population frequency and their dominance/recessive relationships. The informativeness of a marker is commonly measured by its "Polymorphism Information Content" (Botstein *et al.*, 1980).

A variety of statistical tests have been applied to test for significant deviations from independent assortment of a pair of loci (Ott, 1991). The most commonly used one is a sequential maximum likelihood (ML) procedure referred to as the lodscore test (Morton, 1955). The lodscore corresponds to the $\log_{10}$ of a likelihood ratio: likelihood of the genotypic data under the alternative hypothesis (H_1) of linkage between the two loci at a given recombination rate ($\theta \neq 0.5$), divided by the likelihood of the genotypic data under the null hypothesis (H_0) of independent assortment of both loci ($\theta = 0.5$). The value of θ maximizing the likelihood of the data is determined and the H_0 hypothesis is rejected in favour of linkage at the corresponding recombination rate if the lodscore is superior to 3. This high threshold (associated Type I error rate or probability to reject H_0 when it is right, of 5%) is needed because of the low prior probability of linkage ($\approx 1/50$) for a typical mammalian genome. Linkage at the corresponding θ can be excluded when lodscores inferior to -2 are obtained, while the lodscore is considered inconclusive for intermediate lodscores values ($-2 <$ lodscore < 3) requiring additional data.

Manual computation of lodscores is feasible for relatively small and simple pedigrees. In order to extract all the information in more complex situations (phase unknown, missing genotypic data, inbreeding and marriage loops, etc., ...), however, the calculations become quite tedious and lodscores are more conveniently computed using computer programs. Probably the most popular one of these are the LINKAGE package (Lathrop and Lalouel, 1984) and the faster FASTLINK (Cottingham *et al.*, 1993) and VITESSE (O'Connell and Weeks, 1995) programs, exploiting the Elston–Stewart algorithm (Elston and Stewart, 1971). Two-point lodscore tables (i.e. lodscore for a range of $0 < \theta < 0.5$) can be computed with the MLINK option, while ML two-point lodscores with associated θ are directly obtained with the LODSCORE option.

Multipoint Linkage Analysis: Map Construction and Location Scores

Although two-point methods enable the identification of groups of linked loci, determining the most likely order and recombination rates between adjacent markers using two-point results is not always obvious. More reliable ordering is obtained by including several, if not all, linked markers jointly in the likelihood calculations. Traditionally, three-point crosses were used to establish gene order, exploiting the low frequency of the double-recombinant class whose identification establishes the order. Today, the likelihood of the genotypic data is calculated for the different possible marker orders. For each order, the recombination rates between adjacent markers that maximize the likelihood under the corresponding order are determined with maximization routines. The order and associated recombination rates maximizing the likelihood are traditionally accepted as the correct order if the odds versus alternative orders is > 1000. Such calculations can be performed with for instance the ILINK option of the LINKAGE package (Lathrop and Lalouel, 1984).

Amongst other factors, the recombination rate between two loci is known to be affected by sex, being usually reduced in the heterogametic sex (Ott, 1991). Male- and female-specific recombination rates are therefore sometimes estimated independently.

As the number of markers increases, the multipoint likelihood calculations can become very time-consuming as the number of possible orders increases dramatically. Exploring all possible orders therefore becomes unfeasible, and alternative strategies are required to identify the most likely one. A commonly used strategy consists of a step-wise procedure where markers are progressively added to a growing map, the most informative markers being considered first. The position of the new marker is determined by sliding its hypothetical location through the previously positioned markers which are held in a fixed order (reviewed in Buetow, 1994).

It should be noted that multipoint linkage analysis is very sensitive to genotyping errors. Genotyping errors can be detected to some extend by the abnormal distribution of recombinational events they generate. Tests for heterogeneity in the pairwise recombination fractions across the family material (e.g. Lathrop et al., 1988), as well as changes in recombination patterns associated with the introduction of loci within the map, are particularly useful to validate the genotyping data. The latter are conveniently identified with, for instance, the CHROMPIC option of the CRIMAP package, another popular set of linkage analysis programs (P. Green, unpublished).

Typically, marker maps are constructed using material from shared reference families which have been selected to be optimal for map construction using the linkage analysis procedures described above. Within the human gene mapping community, two large family panels have been established: the CEPH and Venezuelan pedigrees (reviewed in Buetow, 1994). Similar strategies have been adopted by the animal genetics community, and reference pedigrees are being shared for the construction of marker maps in most domestic species (e.g. Hetzel, 1993). The linkage maps which are generated can then be assigned to specific chromosomes using somatic cell hybrids and fluorescent *in situ* hybridisation (FISH mapping), which also allows for an accurate monitoring of progress in total genome coverage.

The resulting, high quality reference marker maps can then be used *as is* to position any gene underlying an economically important trait, as long as one has access to appropriate segregating pedigrees for the trait of interest. The hypothetical position of the gene to be mapped is moved through the reference map held fixed and evidence in favour of the location of the gene at a given position in the map is expressed as a lod score or location score curve which can conveniently be generated using for instance the LINKMAP option of the LINKAGE programs (Lathrop *et al.*, 1984). Figure 4.1 shows such a lod score curve obtained for the bovine *mh* gene (causing double-muscling) segregating in the Belgian Blue population, with respect to a marker map constructed on the IBRP reference families (International Bovine Reference Panel; Hetzel, 1993).

Mapping Genes Underlying Complex Traits

Many phenotypic traits known from epidemiological studies to be genetically determined, do not, however, follow simple Mendelian transmission, i.e. dominant or

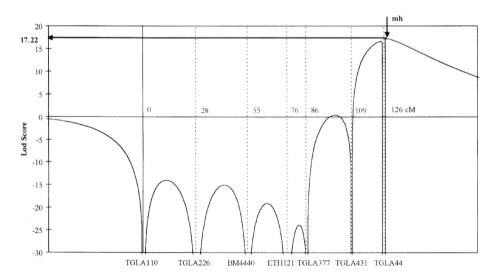

Figure 4.1   Lod score curve obtained with the LINKMAP option of the LINKAGE program for the *mh* gene causing double-muscling in cattle with respect to a bovine chromosome 2 marker map.

recessive/autosomal or sex linked. Classification into distinct phenotypes is still possible for some of these traits (e.g. affected for a genetic disorder or not), whereas for others the phenotypes are said to be quantitative and are distributed on a continuous scale. Evidence for the role of genes in the observed familial clustering is typically measured as a *relative risk* (probability that a relative of an "affected" person exhibits the phenotype compared to the frequency of the phenotype in the general population) for the first set of complex traits, and by their *heritability* (genetic variance component as a proportion of the total phenotypic variance) for the second group.

The origin of the observed complexities are multiple but — as pointed out by Lander and Schork (1994) — all result in the breakdown of the simple correspondence between genotype and phenotype, either because the same genotype can result in different phenotypes, or different genotypes can result in the same phenotype. More specifically, one can distinguish (i) non-genetic causes of complexity: environmental and random effects, and (ii) genetic causes of complexity: locus heterogeneity, oligogenic and polygenic modes of inheritance, and even non-Mendelian inheritance mechanisms (cytoplasmic inheritance, parental imprinting, etc.).

In some circumstances, the genes underlying discrete traits can still be located using the "parametric" linkage strategies that were described above, as long as one includes the appropriate *penetrance functions*. Simply stated, penetrance functions allow for discrepancies between genotype and phenotype to be due to "something else" other than recombination. They are a way of acknowledging the shortcomings of the applied genetic model. Mapping methods applied to complex traits, however, most often reduce to so-called model-free or non-parametric approaches. For discrete traits, individuals are sorted by phenotype and one looks for a non-random distribution of specific chromosome segments in the resulting groups. The most common of these strategies in human genetics are the sib-pair and affected-pedigree-member analyses (reviewed in Lander and Schork, 1994; Weeks and Lathrop, 1994). For continuously distributed traits, the approach usually consists of sorting the individuals by genotype as inferred from marker data and looking for differences in the distribution (mean and/or variance) of the quantitative phenotype. An example of such a strategy that has been used in human populations consists in regressing the squared difference in a trait between two relatives on the proportion of alleles shared identical-by-descent at a given locus (Haseman and Elston, 1972). The choice of method applied in animal genetics is primarily determined by the choice of experimental design.

Choice of Experimental Design to Map QTL in Livestock Species

The vast majority of traits dealt with by animal breeders are complex traits of the second type, i.e. continuously distributed quantitative traits. Typical examples include milk yield and composition (protein and fat) in dairy cattle, growth and carcass characteristics in beef cattle, pigs and poultry, etc. The experiments designed to identify the genes underlying these traits, referred to as Quantitative Trait Loci or QTL, are primarily of two kinds.

(i) Experimental Crosses

In this first approach, one attempts to identify the genes contributing to the differences observed for a trait of interest between two strains, breeds or even subspecies. Well-known examples of this strategy are the experiments aimed at mapping genes underlying the multitude of phenotypic differences observed between wild boar and domestic pig as a result of thousands of years of domestication (Andersson et al., 1994), or the efforts to map the genes accounting for the differences in fertility between Chinese and European pig breeds.

To map the corresponding genes, an experimental cross is set up by mating the selected, divergent parental lines, and using the resulting F_1 individuals to generate a large segregating F_2 or backcross population. A number of statistical methods are available for the detection of QTL in such crosses using the collected marker genotypes and phenotypes of interest. The most commonly used methods share a multipoint approach (often referred to as interval mapping) in which the position of a hypothetical QTL is moved through a fixed marker map. Evidence in favour of the presence of the QTL is computed for each position using either maximum likelihood methods (e.g. Lander and Botstein, 1989), multiple regression (e.g. Haley and Knott, 1992; Martinez and Curnow, 1992; Haley et al., 1994) or non-parametric rank-based tests (Kruglyak and Lander, 1995).

This approach offers several advantages. It is reasonable to assume that phenotypically highly divergent strains will have fixed or nearly fixed highly divergent QTL alleles. Most if not all F_1 animals will, therefore, be heterozygous for the same QTL alleles (genetic homogeneity), expected to generate relatively important QTL allele substitution effects in the F_2 or backcross generations. Likewise, F_1 individuals resulting from a cross between divergent parental lines have an increased likelihood of being heterozygous at the marker loci, thus increasing the marker information content. Finally, crosses such as these being usually performed under properly controlled environmental conditions, non-genetic noise will be concomitantly reduced.

The experimental cross approach has, however, some disadvantages as well. Setting up such crosses in livestock species is an expensive and time-consuming endeavour. Moreover, most ongoing breeding programs in livestock species target the genetic variation that exists within elite commercial strains. It has yet to be demonstrated that the loci explaining differences between highly divergent lines are also contributing to the within-strain variation present in commercial populations.

The prospect of using Marker Assisted Introgression to move favourable QTL alleles between strains might, however, alter this view in the future (Hospital et al., 1992).

(ii) Outbred Pedigrees

The objective of the second type of design is to map the QTL that are underlying the genetic variance observed for a trait of interest in a commercial population. As previously mentioned, these genes are the molecular substrate of most ongoing breeding programs, and their identification is therefore expected to directly allow for more efficient "Marker Asssisted Selection" or MAS schemes (see Chapter 6 in this volume). The most widespread examples of such experimental designs in livestock production, are the multitude of projects attempting to map genes affecting milk production traits in dairy cattle populations.

Such experiments may seem very ambitious at first glance as they lack all the advantageous features listed for the experimental cross design. Elite populations are subjected to intense selection pressure which is expected to rapidly fix or nearly fix alleles with large effects, leaving only modest allele substitution effects to be mapped. Marker heterozygosity and therefore information content will generally be lower in such outbred populations whose population structure usually leads to a reduced effective population size and, therefore, genetic polymorphism. Moreover, different sets of QTL loci and QTL alleles are likely to segregate in different families, exacerbating the genetic complexity (locus and allelic heterogeneity) of the studied phenotype in such outbred populations. Finally, phenotypic information collected under field conditions is often of variable quality. Fortunately, animal geneticist have the advantage over their colleagues studying complex traits in the human, that much larger sibships are readily available, reflecting the prolificity of most domestic species. The extensive use of artificial insemination (AI) in cattle, for instance, results in pedigrees comprising hundreds if not thousands of paternal half-sibs, which are the basis of most ongoing QTL mapping efforts.

The statistical methods presently used to detect QTL in such paternal half-sib designs are in essence very similar to those used in experimental crosses. Animals are sorted by paternal QTL genotype based on flanking marker genotypes, and the resulting multipoint likelihoods are used to estimate the effects of the hypothetical QTL alleles on the trait of interest using maximum likelihood procedures (e.g. Georges *et al.*, 1995), multiple regression (Knott *et al.*, 1994) or non-parametric rank-based strategies (Coppieters *et al.*, 1998b). Analyses are either performed within (Georges *et al.*, 1995) or across (Knott *et al.*, 1994; Coppieters *et al.*, 1998b) family. To optimally extract a maximum of information from the available data set, particularly by accounting for all known relationships between individuals composing the available pedigree material, remains an area of intense research, relying on state-of-the-art statistical procedures (e.g. Uimari *et al.*, 1996; Van Arendonk *et al.*, personal communication).

Strategies to Increase the Power of QTL Mapping

While 10 to 20 informative individuals might be sufficient to confidently map a single gene trait by linkage analysis, mapping genes underlying complex traits requires considerably larger experiments to reveal what is expected to be a relatively modest contribution of individual loci or QTL to the overall trait variance. Experimental cross designs typically count hundreds of offspring, while outbred designs may require thousands. Considerable attention has therefore been given to maximize the power of QTL mapping experiments in order to limit their size whenever possible. Some of the most commonly used strategies are:

(i) Selective Genotyping

For continuously distributed traits, the amount of information contributed by an individual is affected by its phenotypic value. Indeed, the QTL genotype is best inferred for individuals exhibiting extreme phenotypes. By selecting individuals whose phenotype deviates by one or two standard deviations from the mean, the required sample can be reduced by respectively 60% and 80% without loss of power (e.g. Lander and Botstein, 1989; Darvasi and Soller, 1994).

Note that truncation selection, which may affect samples in some circumstances, may — when not accounted for — either decrease the power to detect QTL if it affects the entire sample (Mackinnon and Georges, 1992), or increase this power when it affects part of the sample (Coppieters *et al.*, 1998a).

(ii) Progeny-Testing

For traits with low heritability, breeding values estimated from phenotypic values of descendants, may be used instead of the actual individual's phenotype. A well-known example of this strategy is the so-called grand-daughter design to map QTL affecting milk production in dairy cattle (Weller *et al.*, 1990). The pedigree material used in this design — which is readily available in commercial dairy cattle populations — is composed of paternal half-brother pedigrees generated by artificial insemination. The sires and their sons are the only individuals to be marker-genotyped, while the phenotypes used for QTL mapping are the son's breeding values estimated from their respective milking daughters. Most sons having of the order of 100 daughters, the heritability of the breeding value estimates reaches 80% versus the 30% heritability of the actual phenotype. This approach leads to a nearly fourfold reduction in required sample size (Weller *et al.*, 1990; Georges *et al.*, 1995).

(iii) Simultaneous Search

While the purpose of progeny-testing is to reduce the environmental noise, the aim of simultaneous search is to reduce the noise due to other segregating loci when attempting to map a given causal gene. For discrete traits, computer programs are available to perform an analysis under a model implying two independent causal loci that can be modeled to act in any number of ways (Schork *et al.*, 1993). For continuously distributed traits, regression based programs are available to test for the presence of two QTL on the same chromosome (Haley and Knott, 1992). Composite interval mapping (Zeng, 1994) or MQM (Multiple QTL Model) mapping (Jansen, 1994) are alternative methods allowing to account for genetic variance associated with other markers, when performing QTL interval mapping.

Choice of an Appropriate Significance Threshold

A lodscore threshold of three has traditionally been used to declare linkage between two loci. This stringent threshold (1000 : 1 likelihood ratio) is considered to correspond to a Type I error (see above) of approximately 5% based on Baysian arguments assuming a prior probability of linkage between two randomly selected loci of the order of 1/50.

The rigourous choice of an appropriate significance threshold has recently been the matter of much debate in the context of complex trait analysis (e.g. Lander and Kruglyak, 1995). Key issues are choice of null hypothesis, distribution of the used statistic under the chosen null hypothesis, appropriate correction for multiple testing due to whole-genome scan approaches and analyses of multiple phenotypes. While elegant analytical approaches have been described to address some of these issues (e.g. Lander and Botstein, 1989), pragmatic simulation based approaches are now routinely applied. One commonly used strategy consists in randomly permutating the phenotypes amongst individuals to determine the distribution of the statistic used when phenotype and genotype are effectively disconnected (Churchill and Doerge, 1994). Multipoint analysis methods allow for the determination of chromosome-wise significance thresholds which can then be adjusted using Bonferroni corrections to account for the analysis of multiple chromosomes and, if necessary, multiple traits (e.g. Spelman et al., 1996). These approaches, however, require several tens or hundreds of thousands of permutations, and are therefore only applicable with very fast analysis algorithms.

Mapping Resolution

The mapping resolution that can be reached by linkage strategies is limited by (i) the density of the available marker map in the region of interest, and (ii) the number and distribution of cross-over events flanking the gene of interest in the available pedigree material. Boehnke (1994) examined the distribution of the distance between nearest flanking cross-overs, which would fix the upper limit of the resolution power that could be achieved when mapping a simple Mendelian trait. He demonstrated that as many as 400 informative meioses are required to have a 90% chance to define a 1 cM chromosome segment containing the gene of interest, a resolution compatible with positional candidate gene approach.

The situation is even more problematic for complex traits as individual cross-over events cannot be unambiguously identified. Resolution therefore becomes statistical, yielding support intervals of the order of several tens of cM in most QTL mapping experiments. Fine-mapping QTL therefore remains a major intellectual challenge. It is likely to involve specific breeding combined with progeny-testing whenever experimental crosses can be generated, and identity-by-descent or related mapping methods (see hereafter) in outbred populations (Georges and Andersson, 1996).

MARKER TECHNOLOGY AND MARKER MAPS

Microsatellite Marker Maps

While the theoretical foundations of linkage mapping were laid in the beginning of this century, the actual implementation of this approach in mammals was hampered by the paucity of suitable genetic markers. The description of the first RFLPs in man triggered the realization that these might serve as an abundant source of genetic markers and form the basis of whole-genome marker maps (Botstein *et al.*, 1980). It is however the description of the Polymerase Chain Reaction (PCR) in combination with the discovery of microsatellites as an abundant source of evenly distributed highly polymorphic markers (Weber and May, 1989; Litt and Luty, 1989), that has boosted the construction of DNA marker maps in a wide range of mammalian species in the last five years.

Microsatellites are sequences characterized by the tandem repetition of short motifs, from one to four base pairs in length, which is why they are also referred to as Short Tandem Repeats (STR). A wide range of motifs can be found; however, in mammals the $(CA)_n$ family of microsatellites is by far the most abundant (Beckman and Weber, 1992). In man, it is estimated that a variable $(CA)_n$ repeat occurs approximately every 40 to 50 kb, with highly variable repeats occurring every 300 to 500 kb. Their function, if any, is essentially unknown. A subset of short tandem repeats is associated with the 3' end of retroposons and retrotranscripts (e.g. Economou *et al.*, 1990). Alternating purine:pyrimidine sequences are known to adopt Z-DNA or triple helix configuration (e.g. Baran *et al.*, 1991) which might be indicative of a regulatory role. While not the rule, a subset of microsatellites is characterized by remarkable interspecies conservation pointing to some possible functionality as well (e.g. Moore *et al.*, 1991).

As other satellite sequences (maxi- and minisatellites), microsatellites are highly polymorphic due to allelic differences in the number of repeats, heterozygosities above 75% being common in outbred populations. This high level of polymorphism finds its origin in a mutation rate of the order of 10^{-4}. The actual mechanism underlying mutational events remains essentially unknown. Interestingly, microsatellites exhibit increased instability in some (MIN+) forms of hereditary nonpolyposis colon cancer (HNPCC), subsequently shown to involve mutations in mutator genes (MSH2, MLH1, PMS1 and PMS2), homologous to the *E. Coli* MutHLS error correction components (Fishel *et al.*, 1993).

Microsatellite polymorphism can be conveniently revealed after PCR amplification using flanking primers, and electrophoretic size separation of the amplification product. The size of the amplification product reflects the number of repeats and therefore the allelic identity. Technological improvements of different kinds, including the possibility to perform PCR amplification in microtiter format with the aid of robotic stations, the possibility to perform multiplex genotyping, combined or not with multiplex PCR amplification (Ziegle *et al.*, 1994), and developments towards automated data-capture now allow for throughputs of the order of 500–1000 genotypes per person per day (e.g. Hall *et al.*, 1996; Ghosh *et al.*, 1997).

Since the first description of microsatellite markers in man, individual as well as internationally coordinated efforts have lead to the generation of a number of microsatellite-based linkage maps in the different livestock species (reviewed in Beattie, 1994; Georges and Andersson, 1996). At this point, the available maps count of the order of 1100 markers for cattle and pig (C. Beattie, personal communication), 700 for sheep (A.M. Crawford, personal communication) and 450 for poultry (M.A.M. Groenen, personal communication). These maps provide very adequate genome coverage, especially for cattle and pig where the average between marker interval is now of the order of 2.5–5 cM.

Sequence conservation has proven to be sufficiently high between cattle and sheep to allow for approximately 50% of primer sequences developed in one species to work in the other (Moore et al., 1991). This percentage is considerably higher than what has been observed for the mouse and rat which are thought to be evolutionary as closely related. As expected this cross-species use of microsatellite markers has proven inefficient for more distantly related domestic species despite the occasional demonstration of remarkable conservation of microsatellite position (e.g. Moore et al., 1991).

Fluorescence in situ hybridization (FISH) mapping has allowed to anchor and orient most of the linkage groups to specific chromosomes in cattle and pig. In poultry, establishing connections between the linkage and cytogenetic maps is complicated by non identifiable minichromosomes which might represent as much as 30% of the genome.

These mapping data are being compiled in a number of databases conveniently accessed via the internet.

Future Developments

There is no doubt that it is the discovery of microsatellites that has allowed for the rejuvenation of mammalian genetics in recent years and that these markers will continue to be invaluable genetic tools for several years to come. Microsatellites are by no means perfect, however, and scientists are already looking for improved marker technology. The main drawbacks of microsatellites are the need for an electrophoretic size separation of the PCR products and the associated difficulties to efficiently automate data-capture. These drawbacks impose considerable limits on throughput and therefore cost-effectiveness of microsatellite-based genotyping.

Contemplating the need for very high throughput genotyping in order to address the molecular architecture of complex traits in outbred populations (e.g. Risch and Merikangas, 1996; Lander, 1996), a number of teams have therefore expressed a renewed interest in point mutations as a source of genetic markers. Indeed, the potential advantage of point mutations over microsatellites is the possibility to develop all-or-none, binary detection systems, that are much more conveniently automated. The reduced PIC of individual point mutations, when compared to polyallelic satellite-based markers, is compensated for by a modest increase in the density of markers (2–3 fold). Strategies that are explored for high-throughput genotyping of point mutations are multiple and include the Oligonucleotide Ligation Assay (OLA) (e.g. Nickerson et al., 1990), the Ligase Chain Reaction (LCR) (e.g. Barany, 1991), nucleotide incorporation assays (e.g. Sheperd et al., 1991), "Taqman" assays (e.g. Livak et al., 1995; Heid et al., 1996) and reverse dot-blot (e.g. Kawasaki et al., 1993). The emerging DNA chip technology is likely the most promising route to dramatically increase throughput of reverse dot-blot and is a matter of intense research and development (e.g. Southern, 1996; Chee *et al.*, 1996).

It is estimated that a polymorphic nucleotide is encountered at least every 1000 base pairs in man, therefore providing a virtually unlimited source of potential polymorphic sites. While the frequency of point mutations is likely to be slightly lower in most domestic species, the number of available polymorphisms should be enormous in animal species as well. There is, however, a need for the development of methods that will allow for the quick identification of large numbers of polymorphic sites.

Single Stranded Conformation Polymorphism (SSCP) and Denaturing Gradient Gel Electrophoresis (DGGE) — among other mutation scanning techniques (reviewed in Cotton, 1997) — allow for the detection of the majority of polymorphic sites characterizing a specific DNA fragment. SSCP (Orita *et al.*, 1989) exploits the differential migration of single stranded DNA molecules differing by as little as one base pair, due to the adoption of distinct conformations in native gels. DGGE (e.g. Myers *et al.*, 1988) is based on the differential melting pattern and therefore migration of sequence variants in denaturing gels. Both methods are typically used in conjunction with PCR and therefore require prior sequence information of the corresponding DNA fragment.

RAPDs (Williams *et al.*, 1990) and AFLPs (Vos *et al.*, 1995), on the contrary, allow for the simultaneous detection of tens of polymorphic DNA fragments due to mutations in arbitrary primer recognition sites (RAPD) and restriction sites (AFLP) respectively. To generate RAPDs, random tenmers are typically used as primers to PCR amplify a sample of genomic fragments flanked by inverted repetitions of the respective tenmer which are close enough to allow for efficient amplification of the bounded DNA segment. Out of the 10–20 or so fragments that are typically amplified from a mammalian genome, a small subset will often be polymorphic due to mutations in the respective primer recognition site. In the AFLP technology, adapters are ligated to genomic DNA fragments generated with specific pairs of restriction enzymes, allowing for their subsequent PCR amplification. PCR fragments bounded by two different restriction sites are specifically visualized, yielding complex patterns comprising hundreds of fragments. As for RAPDs, a subset of these will often be polymorphic usually due to point mutations in the corresponding restriction sites. The AFLP technology allows for the simultaneous detection of tens of genetic markers. Particularly in plant genetics, RAPDs and AFLPs have been used as a source of genetic markers for the construction of linkage maps. In addition to the reduced PIC of the mostly recessive point mutations, both systems suffer also from the need for an electrophoretic separation. RAPDs and AFLPs are likely therefore to be superseeded by alternative detection systems. Especially when used in conjunction with SSCP and DGGE, however, both technologies could be used for the identification of large numbers of point mutation, which could then be adapted to more efficient detection systems, such as DNA chips.

The use of Representational Difference Analysis (RDA — see hereafter; Lisitsyn *et al.*, 1993a) has also been suggested for the detection of random DNA sequence polymorphisms differentiating two DNA samples, but has not found widespread application so far.

Despite the considerable investments in the development and use of microsatellite markers, animal geneticists need to be prepared to accompany human, and mouse geneticists in their ongoing technological revolution.

ALTERNATIVE MAPPING STRATEGIES

DNA Pooling/Bulk Segregant Analysis

As previously mentioned, linkage between a causative locus and a genetic marker will manifest itself by a reciprocal segregation distortion of the marker locus in off-spring sorted by phenotype. This segregation distortion is typically measured from the compilation of individual genotypes. Most genotyping methods, however, are not only qualitative — allowing for a distinction between allelic forms — but can be optimized to become quantitative as well — therefore allowing to measure differences in allelic frequencies between samples. Rather than genotype individuals separately, one can attempt to genotype DNA pools composed of equimolar mixtures of DNA from individuals sorted by phenotype, and directly look for reciprocal shifts in allele frequencies: a procedure referred to as bulk segregant analysis (Michelmore *et al.*, 1991). This approach dramatically reduces the number of samples to be analyzed, and therefore has the potential to considerably accelerate and reduce the costs of the initial whole-genome scan (reviewed in Sheffield *et al.*, 1995). The method can be adapted to continuously distributed traits if combined with selective genotyping, i.e. by comparing marker allele frequencies in DNA pools from the tails of the phenotypic distribution (e.g. Plotsky *et al.*, 1990).

Genetically Directed Representational Difference Analysis or GDRDA

Bulk Segregant Analysis still requires the use of a battery of genetic markers dispersed across the whole genome. By contrast, Representational Difference Analysis or RDA allows the investigator to directly identify DNA sequences differing between two samples, with no prior requirement for genetic markers (Lisitsyn *et al.*, 1993a). The principles underlying RDA are schematized in Figure 4.2. Assume that one wants to isolate DNA sequences present in DNA sample A that are absent in sample B. All common sequences are substracted from sample A used as "tester" by hybridisation to an excess of sample B DNA used as "driver". Homoduplex A:A molecules, preferentially formed between DNA sequences not present in sample B, are then selected by a homoduplex-specific PCR amplification. Successive rounds of substractive hybridisation and PCR selection of tester:tester homoduplex DNA leads to a remarkable enrichment allowing for the isolation of a unique sequence distinguishing the two DNA samples.

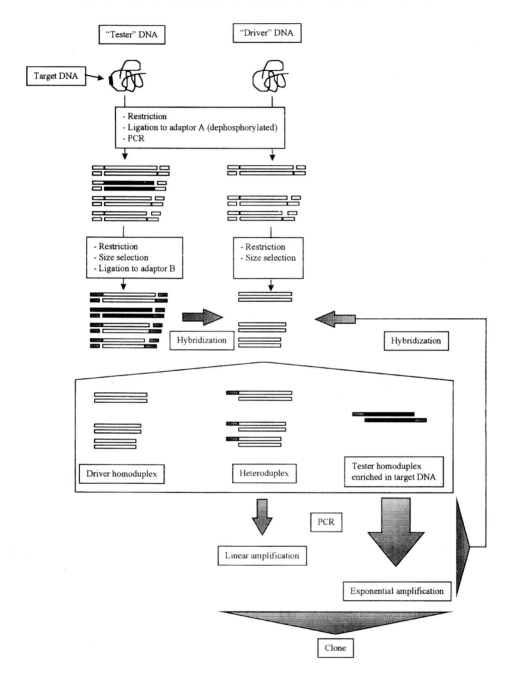

Figure 4.2   Principles of Representational Difference Analysis (RDA) for the detection of DNA sequences differing between two genomes.

A key step in the RDA procedure is the prior reduction of the complexity of the genomes to be compared by restriction digestion and preferential PCR amplification of the resulting smaller restriction fragments, resulting in tester and driver "amplicons". DNA sequence polymorphisms affecting the corresponding restriction sites and distinguishing the DNA samples to be analyzed might result in differences between tester and driver amplicons, therefore allowing for the identification of RFLPs by RDA.

For most genetically determined phenotypes it is usually difficult to identify samples that differ only in the DNA sequences causing the phenotype or DNA sequences flanking this causative locus. Congenic strains, obtained by introgressing a mutant locus from a donor strain into a recipient strain by repeated backcrossing, are amongst the few examples where RDA can be directly applied to isolate the causative locus using congenic and recipient DNA as tester and driver respectively. To overcome this limitation, however, RDA can be applied on carefully designed DNA pools, reducing the DNA sequence differences to the causative locus: an approach dubbed Genetically Directed Representational Difference or GDRDA (Lisitsyn et $al.$, 1993b). An example of such approach — successfully applied to the nude and staggerer loci in mice — uses pooled DNA from affected F_2's as driver and DNA from the unaffected parental line as tester. Indeed, for any randomly selected locus, the unaffected parental genome will represent on average halve of the F_2 DNA. Provided sufficient F_2 individuals contribute to the driver DNA to accomodate the stochastic fluctuations around this value of one half, this will allow for an efficient substractive hybridisation of the entire unaffected parental genome, with the exception of the region(s) flanking the causative gene(s) for which unaffected sequence variants would not be represented in the driver pool.

Association Studies and IBD-Mapping

Classical linkage analysis exploits the non-random allelic association observed for linked loci amongst sibs. For closely linked genes, this linkage disequilibrium will endure over several generations and can therefore be observed amongst more distantly related individuals.

In its simplest form, one hypothesises that individuals sampled from a given population based on a common phenotype, will share a unique (assuming genetic homogeneity) or a limited number (assuming genetic heterogeneity) of identical-by-descent (IBD) causal mutations tracing back to one or a limited number of common ancestors. Linked marker alleles associated with the causal mutation(s) in the founder(s) cosegregate with the causal mutation in subsequent generations, and are therefore expected to be enriched amongst "affected" descendents when compared to non-affected controls. The degree of "residual" allelic association observed at a given time will be a function of the number of generations to the common founder and the recombination rate between marker and disease locus. The efficacy of detecting enrichment of a given marker allele amongst affected descendents is greatly affected by the population frequency of the considered allele. Indeed, if the marker allele has a high frequency in the general population, the IBD signal will be confounded by a large proportion of alleles that are identical-by-state rather than by-descent. This limitation can be alleviated by considering multiple linked markers jointly as haplotypes. The low population frequency of any multi–site haplotype concomitantly enhances the IBD signal, resulting in so-called IBD-mapping (e.g. Houwen *et al.*, 1995; Charlier *et al.*, 1996b; Dunner *et al.*, 1997). Figure 4.3 summarizes the principles of IBD and linkage disequilibrium mapping.

Genome Mismatch Scanning (GMS)

Efficient IBD mapping requires high density marker maps. Genome Mismatch Scanning (GMS) is an elegant method developed to directly isolate relatively large chromosome segments shared identical-by-descent by two or more individuals, without the need for a high density marker map (Nelson *et al.*, 1993; Brown, 1994). After digestion with a restriction enzyme generating fragments of the order of several Kb, the DNA of two individuals is differentiated by methylating only one of them using a restriction methylase. The differentiated DNAs are then hybridized and the heteroduplexes isolated by virtue of their hemimethylated status. While IBD heteroduplexes are expected to be identical over their entire length, most heteroduplexes will show mismatches at a rate reflecting the nucleotide diversity of the population from which the individuals were sampled (of the order of 1/500 bases in most human populations). The *Ecoli* MutHLS mismatch repair enzyme system can then be used to eliminate the non-IBD heteroduplexes. The complex pool of DNA fragments isolated by this procedure, representing regions of identity-by-descent between the two samples, can then be labelled and mapped using a variety of approaches, including hybridisation to ordered microarrays of DNAs representing the entire genome. Figure 4.4 is illustrating the principles of GMS.

EXAMPLES OF SUCCESSFUL LINKAGE MAPPING OF PRODUCTION TRAITS IN LIVESTOCK

Comprehensive marker maps becoming available in most livestock species, systematic genome scans are increasingly being undertaken in order to locate genes of interest by linkage analysis. Table 4.1 reports single gene traits that were succesfully mapped in livestock species using this strategy. While most of these efforts used a conventional linkage analysis approach, mapping the *syndactyly* locus used an IBD mapping approach (Charlier *et al.*, 1996b), while the *dominant white* locus in poultry was mapped by bulk segregant analysis (Ruyter-Spira *et al.*, 1997).

In addition to these studies of monogenic traits, a number of whole genome scans have been undertaken to map QTL affecting a variety of quantitative production traits (Haley, 1995). The first of these attempts in pigs (Andersson *et al.*,

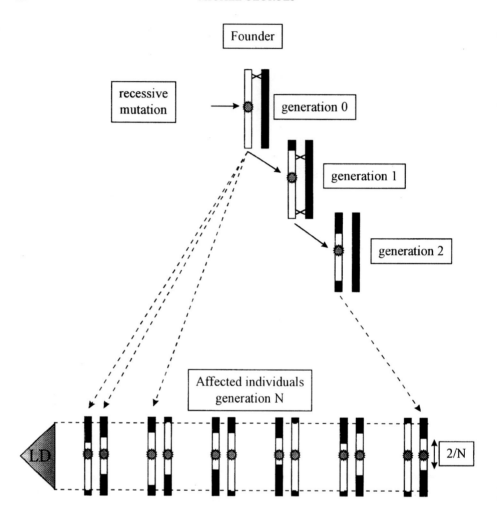

LD: gradient of linkage disequilibrium due to increased frequency of IBD chromosome segment shared by affected individuals.

Figure 4.3 Principles of linkage disequilibrium and IBD mapping of a recessive trait in genetic isolates. Assume a founder (generation 0) carrying a recessive mutation on one of its chromosomes (asterisk on shaded box). In a genetically isolated population, chromosomes from affected individuals sampled at generation "n" are assumed to trace back to the founder chromosome. In these individuals, the causal mutation is therefore expected to be flanked by identical-by-descent chromosome segments originating in the founder.

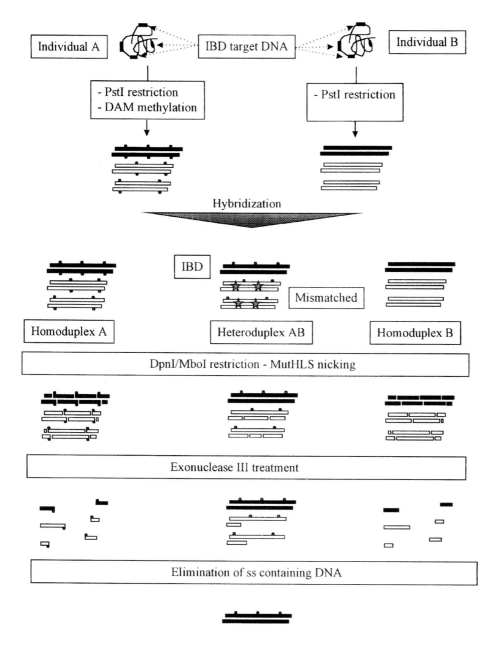

Figure 4.4   Principles underlying Genome Mismatch Scanning (GMS) for the detection of identical-by-descent chromosome segments shared by two individuals.

Table 4.1 Single gene traits mapped in livestock species.

Species	Locus	Trait	Position	Gene	Reference
Pig	MH	Malignant hyperthemia	6	CRC	Fuji et al., 1991
	I	Dominant white coat color	8	KIT	Johansson et al., 1992; Johansson Moller et al., 1996
	E	Extension coat color locus	6	?	Mariani et al., 1996
	Rn	Muscle glycogen content	15	?	Milan et al., 1995, 1996; Mariani et al., 1996
	ECK88ab, acR	Intestinal receptor for E.coli K88ab, ac fimbriae	13	?	Guérin et al., 1993; Edfors-Lija et al., 1995
	ECF107R	Intestinal receptor for E.coli F107 fimbriae	6	?	Voegeli et al., 1994
	CPS	Campus tremor syndrome	7	?	Tammen, I. and Harlizius, B., personal communication
Cattle	PDME	Weaver	4	?	Georges et al., 1993a
	Polled	Presence/Absence of horns	1	?	Georges et al., 1993b
	Roan	Roan coat color locus	5	?	Charlier et al., 1996a
	MH	Double muscling	2	?	Charlier et al., 1995
	E	Extension coat color locus	18	MC1R	Klungland et al., 1995
	Sy	Syndactyly	15	?	Charlier et al., 1996b
Sheep	FecB	Booroola fecundity gene	6	?	Montgomery et al., 1994
	CLPG	Callipyge muscular hypertrophy	18	?	Cockett et al., 1994, 1996
Goat	Polled	Presence/Absence of horns	1	?	Vaiman et al., 1996
Horse	E	Extension coat color locus	LGII	MC1R	Johansson et al., 1994; Marklund, L., Johansson Moller, M., Sandberg, K. and Andersson, L., personal communication
Poultry	DW	Dominant white	LG22	?	Ruyter-Spira, C.P., van der Poel, J.J., Groenen, M.A.M., personal communication
	SLD	Sex linked dwarfism	Z	GHR	Huang et al., 1993; Duriez et al., 1993

1994) and cattle (Georges *et al.*, 1995), have convincingly demonstrated that QTL can indeed be mapped using both experimental cross and outbred designs.

The first study (Andersson *et al.*, 1994) identified very strong effects on pig chromosome 4 accounting for a large part of the difference between wild boar and domestic pig in growth rate, fatness and length of the small intestine. The second study (Georges *et al.*, 1995) exploited the grand-daughter design to map genes affecting milk production traits in elite Holstein Friesian dairy cattle. A total of 1,518 sires, with progeny tests based on the milking performances of >150,000 daughters jointly, was genotyped for 159 autosomal microsatellites bracketing 1645 cM or approximately two thirds of the genome. Using a maximum likelihood multilocus procedure accounting for variance heterogeneity of the phenotypes, five chromosome regions were identified that gave very strong evidence for the presence of QTL controlling milk production: chromosomes 1, 6, 9, 10 and 20.

Several similar studies are presently being performed around the world and will likely yield a rich crop of QTL relevant for livestock production in the very near future. Initial QTL localisations will have to be followed by fine-mapping and positional cloning efforts to provide animal breeders with the tools required to harvest the benefits of QTL mapping efforts via Marker Assisted Selection.

REFERENCES

Andersson, L., Haley, C.S., Ellegren, H., Knott, S.A., Johansson, M., Andersson, K., Andersson-Eklund, L., Edfors-Lilja, I., Fredholm, M., Hansson, I., Håkansson, J. and Lundström, K. (1994) Genetic mapping of quantitative trait loci for growth and fatness in pigs. *Science* **263**, 1771–1774.

Arnheim, N., Li, H. and Cui, X. (1990) PCR analysis of DNA sequences in single cells: single sperm mapping and genetic disease diagnosis. *Genomics* **8**, 415–419.

Baran, N., Lapidot, A. and Manor, H. (1991) Formation of DNA triplexes accounts for arrest of DNA synthesis at d(TC)n and d(GA)n tracts. *Proc. Natl. Acad. Sc. USA* **88**, 507–511.

Barany, F. (1991) Genetic disease detection and DNA amplification using cloned thermostable ligase. *Proc. Natl. Acad. Sc. USA* **88**, 189–193.

Beattie, C. (1994) Livestock genome maps. *Trends in Genetics* **10**(9), 334–338.

Beckman, J.S. and Weber, J.L. (1992) Survey of human and rat microsatellites. *Genomics* **12**, 627–631.

Boehnke, M. (1994) Limits of resolution of linkage studies: implications for the positional cloning of disease genes. *Am. J. Hum. Genet.* **55**, 379–390.

Botstein, D., White, R.L., Skolnick, M. and Davis, R.W. (1980) Construction of a genetic linkage map in man using restriction fragment length polymorphisms. *Am. J. Hum. Genet.* **32**, 314–331.

Brown, P.O. (1994) Genome scanning methods. *Current Opinions in Genetics and Development* **4**, 366–373.

Buetow, K.H. (1994) Construction of reference genetic maps. In *Current Protocols in Human Genetics*, Volume I, Unit 1.5., John Wiley and Sons, Inc.

Charlier, C., Coppieters, W., Farnir, F., Grobet, L., Leroy, P., Michaux, C., Mni, M., Schwers, A., Vanmanshoven, P., Hanset, R. and Georges, M. (1995) The *mh* gene causing double-muscling in cattle maps to bovine chromosome 2. *Mammalian Genome* **6**, 788–792.

Charlier, C., Denys, B., Belanche, J.I., Coppieters, W., Grobet, L., Mni, M., Womack, J., Hanset, R. and Georges, M. (1996a) Microsatellite mapping of a major determinant of *White Heifer Disease*: the bovine *roan* locus. *Mammalian Genome* **7**, 138–142.

Charlier, C., Farnir, F., Berzi, P., Vanmanshoven, P., Brouwers, B. and Georges, M. (1996b) Identity-by-descent mapping of recessive traits in livestock: application to map the bovine syndactyly locus to chromosome 15. *Genome Research* **6**, 580–589.

Chee, M., Yang, R., Hubbell, E., Berno, A., Huang, X.C., Stern, D., Winkler, J., Lockhart, D.J., Morris, M.S. and Fodor, S.P.A. (1996) Accessing genetic information with high-density DNA arrays. *Science* **274**, 610–614.

Churchill, G.A. and Doerge, R.W. (1994) Empirical threshold values for quantitative trait mapping. *Genetics* **138**, 963–971.

Cockett, N.E., Jackson, S.P., Shay, T.D., Nielsen, D., Green, R.D. and Georges, M. (1994) Chromosomal localization of the callipyge gene in sheep (Ovis aries) using bovine DNA markers. *Proceedings of the National Academy of Sciences, USA* **91**, 3019–3023.

Cockett, N.E., Jackson, S.P., Shay, T.D., Farnir, F., Berghmans, S., Snowder, G., Nielsen, D. and Georges, M. (1996) Polar overdominance at the ovine callipyge locus. *Science* **273**, 236–238.

Collins, F.S. (1995) Positional cloning moves from perditional to traditional. *Nature Genetics* **9**, 347–350.

Coppieters, W., Mackinnon, M. and Georges, M. (1998a) A note on the effect of selection on linkage analysis for quantitative traits. *J. Heredity* (in press).

Coppieters, W., Kvasz, A., Arranz, J., Grisart, B., Farnir, F., Mackinnon, M. and Georges, M. (1998b) A rank-based non parametric method to map QTL in outbred half-sib pedigrees: application to milk production in a grand-daughter design (submitted for publication).

Cottingham, R.W., Idury, R.M. and Schäffer, A.A. (1993) Faster sequential genetic linkage computations. *Am. J. Hum. Genet.* **53**, 252–263.

Cotton, R.G.H. (1997) Slowly but surely towards better scanning for mutations. *Trends in Genetics* **13**(2), 43–46.

Darvasi, A. and Soller, M. (1992) Selective genotyping for determination of linkage between a marker locus and a quantitatve trait locus. *Theor. Appl. Genet.* **85**, 353–359.

Dunner, S., Charlier, C., Farnir, F., Brouwers, B., Canon, J. and Georges, M. (1997) Towards interbreed IBD fine mapping of the mh locus: double-muscling in the Asturiana de los Valles breed involves the same locus as in the Belgian Blue cattle breed. *Mammalian Genome* **8**, 430–435.

Duriez, B., Sobrier, M.-L., Duquesnoy, P., Tixier-Boichard, M., Decuypere, E., Coquerelle, G., Zeman, M., Goossens, M. and Amselem, S. (1993) A naturally occuring growth hormone receptor mutation: *in vivo* and *in vitro* evidence for the functional importance of the WS motif common to all members of the cytokine receptor superfamily. *Molecular Endocrinology* **7**, 806–814.

Edfors-Lilja, I., Gustafsson, U., Duval-Iflah, Y., Ellegren, H., Johansson, M., Juneja, R.K., Marklund, L. and Andersson, L. (1995) The porcine intestinal receptor for Escherichia coli K88ab, K88ac: regional localization on chromosome 13 and influence on IgG response to the K88 antigen. *Animal Genetics* **26**, 237–242.

Economou, E.P., Bergen, A., Warren, A.C. and Antonorakis, S.E. (1990) The polydeoxyadenylate tract of Alu repetitive elements is polymorphic in the human genome. *Proc. Natl. Acad. Sc. USA* **87**, 2951–2954.

Elston, R.C. and Stewart, J. (1971) A general model for the genetic analysis of pedigree data. *Hum. Hered.* **21**, 523–542.

Fishel, R., Lescoe, M.K., Rao, M.R.S., Copeland, N.G., Jenkins, N.A., Garber, J., Kane, M. and Kolodner, R. (1993) *Cell* **75**, 1027–1038.

Fuji, J., Otsu, K., Zorzato, F., Deleon, S., Khanna, V.K., Weiler, J.E., O'Brien, P.J. and MacLennan, D.H. (1991) Identification of a mutation in the porcine ryanodine receptor associated with malignant hyperthermia. *Science* **253**, 448–451.

Georges, M., Lathrop, M., Dietz, A.B., Lefort, A., Libert, F., Mishra, A., Nielsen, D., Sargeant, L.S., Steele, M.R., Zhao, X., Leipold, H. and Womack, J.E. (1993a) Microsatellite mapping of the gene causing *weaver* disease in cattle will allow the study of an associated QTL. *Proceedings of the National Academy of Sciences, USA* **90**, 1058–1062.

Georges, M., Drinkwater, R., Lefort, A., Libert, F., King, T., Mishra, A., Nielsen, D., Sargeant, L.S., Sorensen, A., Steele, M.R., Zhao, X., Womack, J.E. and Hetzel, J. (1993b) Microsatellite mapping of a gene affecting horn development in Bos taurus. *Nature Genetics* **4**, 206–210.

Georges, M., Nielsen, D., Mackinnon, M., Mishra, A., Okimoto, R., Pasquino, A.T., Sargeant, L.S., Sorensen, A., Steele, M.R., Zhao, X., Womack, J.E. and Hoeschele, I. (1995) Mapping quantitative trait loci controlling milk production by exploiting progeny testing. *Genetics* **139**, 907–920.

Georges, M. and Andersson, L. (1996) Livestock Genomics comes of age. *Genome Research* **6**, 907–921.

Ghosh, S. *et al.* (1997) Methods for precise sizing, automated binning of alleles, and reduction of error rates in large-scale genotyping using fluorescently labeled dinucleotide markers. *Genome Research* **7**, 165–178.

Guérin, G., Duval-Iflah, Y., Bonneau, M., Bertaud, M., Guillaume, P. and Ollivier, L. (1993) Evidence for linkage between K88ab, K88ac intestinal receptor to Escherichia coli and transferrin loci in pigs. *Animal Genetics* **24**, 393–396.

Haley, C.S. and Knott, S. (1992) A simple regression method for mapping quantitative trait loci in line crosses using flanking markers. *Heredity* **69**, 315–324.

Haley, C.S., Knott, S.A. and Elsen, J.M. (1994) Mapping quantitatve trait loci in crosses between outbred lines using least squares. *Genetics* **136**, 1195–1207.

Haley, C.S. (1995) Livestock QTLs — bringing home the bacon? *Trends in Genetics* **11**(12), 488–492.

Hall, J.M., LeDuc, C.A., Watson, A.R. and Roter, A.H. (1996) An approach to high-throughput genotyping. *Genome Research* **6**, 781–790.

Haseman, J.K. and Elston, R.C. (1972) The investigation of linkage between a quantitatve trait and a marker locus. *Behav. Genet.* **2**, 3–19.

Heid, C.A., Stevens, J., Livak, K.J. and Williams, P.M. (1996) Real time quantitative PCR. *Genome Research* **6**, 986–994.

Hetzel, J., Brascamp, P., Leveziel, H., Lewin, H., Teale, A. and Womack, J. (1993) The International Bovine Reference Panel (IBRP). Report of the ISAG working party.

Hospital, F., Chevalet, C. and Mulsant, P. (1992) Using markers in gene introgression breeding programs. *Genetics* **132**, 1199–1210.

Houwen, R.H.J., Baharloo, S., Blankenship, K., Raeymaekers, P., Juyn, J., Sandkuijl, L.A. and Freimer, N.B. (1995) Genome screening by searching for shared segments: mapping a gene for benign recurrent intrahepatic cholestasis. *Nature Genetics* **8**, 380–386.

Huang, N., Cogburn, L.A., Agarwal, S.K., Marks, H.L. and Burnside, J. (1993) Overexpression of a truncated growth hormone receptor in the sex-linked dwarf chicken: evidence for a splice mutation. *Molecular Endocrinology* **7**, 1391–1398.

Jansen, R. (1994) Controlling the type I and II errors in mapping quantitative trait loci. *Genetics* **138**, 871–881.

Johansson, M., Ellegren, H., Marklund, L., Gustavsson, U., Ringmar-Cederberg, E., Andersson, K., Edfors-Lilja, I. and Andersson, L. (1992) The gene for dominant white color in the pig is closely linked to ALB and PDGFRA on chromosome 8. *Genomics* **14**, 965–969.

Johansson, M., Marklund, L., Sandberg, K. and Andersson, L. (1994) Cosegregation between the chestnut coat colour in horses and polymorphisms at the melanocyte stimulating hormone (MSH) receptor locus. *Anim. Genet.* **25** (suppl. 2), 35.

Johansson Moller, M., Chaudhary, R., Hellmén, E., Höyheim, B., Chowdhary, B. and Andersson, L. (1996) Pigs with the dominant white coat color phenotype carry a duplication of the KIT gene encoding the mast/stem cell growth factor receptor. *Mammalian Genome* **7**, 822–830.

Kawasaki, E., Saiki, R. and Erlich, H. (1993) Genetic analysis using polymerase chain reaction-amplified DNA and immobilized oligonucleotide probes: reverse dot-blot typing. *Methods Enzymol.* **218**, 369–381.

Klungland, H., Vage, D.I., Gomez-raya, L., Adalsteinsson, S. and Lien, S. (1995) The role of melanocyte-stimulating hormone (MSH) receptor in bovine coat color determination. *Mammalian Genome* **6**, 636–639.

Knott, S.A., Elsen, J.M. and Haley, C.S. (1994) Multiple marker mapping of quantitative trait loci in half-sib populations. *Proceedings 5th World Congress on Genetics Applied to Livestock Production* **21**, 33–36.

Kruglyak, L. and Lander, E.S. (1995) A nonparametric approach for mapping quantitative trait loci. *Genetics* **139**, 1421–1428.

Lander, E. (1996) The new genomics: global views of biology. *Science* **274**, 536–539.

Lander, E.S. and Botstein, D. (1989) Mapping mendelian factors underlying quantitative traits using RFLP linkage maps. *Genetics* **121**, 185–199.

Lander, E.S. and Schork, N.J. (1994) Genetic dissection of complex traits. *Science* **265**, 2037–2048.

Lander, E.S. and Kruglyak, L. (1995) Genetic dissection of complex traits: guidelines for interpreting and reporting linkage results. *Nat. Genet.* **11**, 241–247.

Lathrop, M. and Lalouel, J.-M. (1984) Easy calculations of lod scores and genetic risks on small computers. *Am. J. Hum. Genet.* **36**, 460–465.

Lathrop, G.M., Lalouel, J.-M., Julier, C. and Ott, J. (1984) Strategies for multilocus linkage analysis in humans. *Proc. Natl. Acad. Sci. USA* **81**, 3443–3446.

Lathrop, G.M., Nakamura, Y., Cartwright, P., O'Connell, P., Leppert, M., Jones, C., Tateishi, H., Bragg, T., Lalouel, J.-M. and White, R. (1988) A primary genetic map of markers for human chromosome 10. *Genomics* **2**, 157–164.

Lewin, H.A., Schmitt, K., Hubert, R., van Eijk, M.J.T. and Arnheim, N. (1992) Close linkage between bovine prolactin and Bola-DRB3 genes: genetic mapping in cattle by single sperm typing. *Genomics* **13**, 44–48.

Lisitsyn, N.A., Lisitsyn, N.M. and Wigler, M. (1993a) Cloning the differences between two complex genomes. *Science* **259**, 946–951.

Lisitsyn, N.A., Segre, J.A., Kusumi, K., Lisitsyn, N.M., Nadeau, J.H., Frankel, W.N., Wigler, M.H. and Lander, E.S. (1993b) Direct isolation of polymorphic markers linked to a trait by genetically directed representational difference analysis. *Nature Genetics* **6**, 57–63.

Litt, M. and Luty, J.A. (1989) A hypervariable microsatellite revealed by *in vitro* amplification of a dinucleotide repeat within the cardiac muscle actin gene. *Am. J. Hum. Genet.* **44**, 397–401.

Livak, K.J., Marmaro, J. and Todd, J.A. (1995) Towards fully automated genome-wide polymorphism screening. *Nature Genetics* **9**, 341–342.

Mackinnon, M. and Georges, M. (1992) The effect of selection on linkage analysis for quantitative traits. *Genetics* **132**, 1177–1185.

Mariani, P., Johansson, M., Høyheim, B., Marklund, L., Davies, W., Ellegren, H. and Andersson, L. (1996) The extension coat color locus and the loci for blood group O and tyrosine aminotransferase are on pig chromosome 6. *J. Heredity* **87**, 272–276.

Mariani, P., Lundstrom, K., Gustafsson, U., Enfalt, A.-C., Juneja, R.K. and Andersson, L. (1995) A major locus (Rn) affecting muscle glycogen content is located on pig chromosome 15. *Mammalian Genome* **7**, 52–54.

Martinez, O. and Curnow, R.N. (1992) Estimating the locations and the sizes of the effects of quantitative trait loci using flanking markers. *Theor. Appl. Genet.* **85**, 480–488.

Michelmore, R.W., Paran, I. and Kesseli, R.V. (1991) Identification of markers linked to disease-resistance genes by bulked segregant analysis: a rapid method to detect markers in specific genomic regions by using segregating populations. *Proc. Natl. Acad. Sci. USA* **88**, 9828–9832.

Milan, D., Le Roy, P., Woloszyn, N., Caritez, J.C., Elsen, J.M., Sellier, P. and Gellin, J. (1995) The RN locus for meat quality maps to pig chromosome 15. *Génétique Sélection Evolution* **27**, 195–199.

Milan, D., Woloszyn, N., Yerle, M., Leroy, P., Bonnet, M., Riquet, J., Lahbibmansais, Y., Caritez, J.C., Robic, A., Sellier, P., Elsen, J.M. and Gellin, J. (1996) Accurate Mapping of the Acid Meat RN Gene on Genetic and Physical Maps of Pig Chromosome 15. *Mammalian Genome* **7**, 47–51.

Moore, S.S., Sargeant, L., King, T.J., Mattick, J.S., Georges, M. and Hetzel, D.J.S. (1991) The conservation of dinucleotide microsatellites among mammalian genomes allows the use of heterologous PCR primer pairs in closely related species. *Genomics* **10**, 654–660.

Montgomery, G.W., Crawford, A.M., Penty, J.M., Dodds, K.G., Ede, A.J., Henry, H.M., Pierson, C.A., Lord, E.A., Galloway, S.M. and Schmack, A.E. *et al.* (1994) The ovine Booroola fecundity gene (FecB) is linked to markers from a region of human chromosome 4q. *Nature Genetics* **4**, 410–414.

Morton, N.E. (1955) Sequential tests for the detection of linkage. *Am. J. Hum. Genet.* **7**, 277–318.

Myers, R.M., Sheffield, V.C. and Cox, D.R. (1988) Detection of single base changes in DNA: ribonuclease cleavage and denaturing gradient gel electrophoresis, In *Genome Analysis: a practical approach*. Ed. K.E. Davies. IRL Press, pp. 95–139.

Nelson, S.F., McCusker, J.H., Sander, M.A., Kee, Y., Modrich, P. and Brown, P.O. (1993) Genome Mismatch Scanning: a new approach to genetic linkage mapping. *Nature Genetics* **4**, 11–18.

Nickerson, D.A., Kaiser, R., Lappin, S., Stewart, J., Hood, L. and Landegren, U. (1990) Automated DNA diagnostics using a ELISA-based oligonucleotide ligation essay. *Proc. Natl. Acad. Sci., USA* **87**, 8923–8927.

O'Connell, J.R. and Weeks, D.E. (1995) The VITESSE algorithm for rapid exact multilocus linkage analysis via genotype set-recoding and fuzzy inheritance. *Nat. Genet.* **11**, 402–408.

Orita, M., Suzuki, Y., Sekiya, T. and Hayashi, K. (1989) Rapid and sensitive detection of point mutations and DNA polymorphisms using the PCR. *Genomics* 874–879.

Ott, J. (1991) *Analysis of Human Genetic Linkage*. Johns Hopkins University Press, Baltimore.

Plotsky, Y., Cahaner, A., Haberfeld, A., Lavi, U. and Hillel, J. (1990) Analysis of genetic association between DNA fingerprint bands and quantitative traits using DNA mixes. *Proc. 4th World Congres GALP, Edinburgh 23–27 July 1990*, XIII,133–136.

Risch, N. and Merikangas, K. (1996) The future of genetic studies of complex human diseases. *Science* **273**, 1516–1517.

Rothshild, M., Jacobson, C., Vaske, D., Tuggle, C., Wang, L., Short, T., Eckardt, G., Sasaki, S., Vincent, A., McLaren, D., Southwood, O., van der Steen, H., Milehm, A. and Plastow, G. (1996) The estrogen receptor locus is associated with a major gene influencing litter size in pigs. *Proceedings of the National Academy of Sciences USA* **93**, 201–205.

Ruyter-Spira, C.P., van der Poel, J.J. and Groenen, M.A.M. (1997) Bulked segregant analysis using microsatellites: mapping of the dominant white locus in chicken, *Poultry Science* **76**, 386–391.

Sheffield, V.C., Nishimura, D.Y. and Stone, E.M. (1995) Novel approaches to linkage mapping. *Current Opinions in Genetics and Development* **5**(3), 335–341.

Shepherd, N.S., Pfrogner, B., Beaty, C., Livak, K. and Rafalski, A. (1991) A new technique for nucleic acid polymorphism analysis. Abstracts of papers presented at the 1991 meeting on Genome Mapping and Sequencing 1991. p. 188. Cold Spring Harbor Laboratory.

Schork, N.J., Boehnke, M., Terwilliger, J.D. and Ott, J. (1993) Two trait locus linkage analysis: a powerful strategy for mapping complex genetic traits. *Am. J. Hum. Genet.* **53**, 1127–1136.

Southern, E.M. (1996) DNA chips: analysing sequence by hybridization to oligonucleotides on a large scale. *Trends in Genetics* **12**(3), 110–115.

Spelman, R.J., Coppieters, W., van Arendonk, J.A.M. and Bovenhuis, H. (1996) Quantitatve Trait Loci analysis for five milk production traits on chromosome six in the dutch Holstein-Friesian population. *Genetics* **144**, 1799–1808.

Uimari, P., Thaller, G. and Hoeschele, I. (1996) The use of multiple markers in a Bayesian method for mapping quantitative trait loci. *Genetics* **143**, 1831–1842.

Vaiman, D., Koutita, O., Oustry, A., Elsen, J.M., Manfredi, E., Fellous, M. and Cribiu, E.P. (1996) Genetic mapping of the autosomal region involved in XX sex-reversal and horn development in goats. *Mammalian Genome* **7**, 133–137.

Voegeli, P., Fries, R., Leemann, G., Bertschinger, H.U. and Stranzinger, G. (1994) Genes for the AO inhibition (S-locus) are closely linked to the genes specifying receptors of F107 fimbriated Escherichia coli strains causing oedema disease and post-weaning diarrhoea in the pig. *Animal Genetics* **25** (Suppl 2), 66.

Vos, P., Hogers, R., Bleeker, M., Reijans, M., van de Lee, T., Hornes, M., Frijters, A., Pot, J., Peleman, J. and Kuiper, M. *et al.* (1995) AFLP: a new technique for DNA fingerprinting. *Nucleic Acids Res.* **23**, 4407–4414.

Weber, J.L. and May, P.E. (1989) Abundant class of human DNA polymorphisms which can be typed using the polymerase chain reaction. *Am. J. Hum. Genet.* **44**, 388–396.

Weeks, D. and Lathrop, G.M. (1994) Polygenic disease: methods for mapping complex disease traits. *Trends in Genetics* **11**(12), 513–519.

Weller, J.I., Kashi, Y. and Soller, M. (1990) Power of daughter and granddaughter designs for determining linkage between marker loci and quantitatve trait loci in dairy cattle. *J. Dairy Sc.* **73**, 2525–2537.

Williams, J.G., Kubelik, A.R., Livak, K.J., Rafalski, J.A. and Tingey, S.V. (1990) DNA polymorphisms amplified by arbitrary primers are useful as genetic markers. *Nucleic Acids Res.* **18**, 6531–6535.

Zeng, Z.B. (1994) Precision mapping of quantitatve trait loci. *Genetics* **136**, 1457–1468.

Ziegle, J.S., Su, Y., Corcoran, K.P., Nie, L., Mayrand, P.E., Hoff, L.B., McBride, L.J., Kronick, M.N. and Diehl, S.R. (1992) Application of automated DNA sizingtechnology for genotyping microsatellite loci. *Genomics* **14**, 1026–1031.

5. IDENTIFICATION AND CLONING OF TRAIT GENES

LEIF ANDERSSON *

Department of Animal Breeding and Genetics, Swedish University of Agricultural Sciences, Box 597, S-751 24 Uppsala, Sweden

Genome analysis makes it possible to clone a locus based on its phenotypic expression. The cloning of trait loci can roughly be divided into four strategies: functional cloning, candidate cloning, positional cloning and positional candidate cloning. Functional cloning implies that the cloning step is performed after the biochemical characterisation of the gene product. Candidate cloning is based on the identification of candidate genes for a given trait. The usefulness of this approach is dependent on the number of potential candidate genes. If this number is too large it may be more efficient to first map the trait locus to a chromosomal region and then ask the question whether there are any candidate genes already mapped to the same region. This strategy is called positional candidate cloning and is expected to be the major strategy in the future because of the rapid development of an almost complete human transcript map. Animal geneticists will be able to utilise this strategy by accessing the human transcript map by comparative gene mapping. Finally, in positional cloning the target gene is cloned on the basis of its map position and the function of the gene is revealed subsequently. The cloning of monogenic trait loci is a demanding undertaking but relatively straightforward when good pedigree material is available. The cloning of quantitative trait loci (QTLs) is much more problematic because the poor precision in QTL mapping and our vague ideas about the molecular nature of such loci.

KEY WORDS: cloning; livestock; phenotype; trait; QTL.

INTRODUCTION

The prospects for the genetic dissection of phenotypic traits is the driving force for gene mapping studies in livestock. Informative linkage maps, comprising 500–1000 genetic markers, have been established for all major farm animal species and they are already being exploited for mapping monogenic trait loci (for review see Georges and Andersson, 1996). Some convincing examples of the identification of quantitative trait loci (QTLs) have also been reported (Andersson *et al.*, 1994; Georges *et al.*, 1995). Information on the chromosomal localisation of a trait locus may be used in practical animal breeding by marker assisted selection (see Chapter 6 in this volume) but the mapping of a trait locus may also be the starting point for the cloning of the locus and the subsequent identification of the causative mutation.

The cloning of trait loci is justified from a scientific point of view since a central topic in current genome research is to understand the relationship between genotype and phenotype. It is anticipated that research on farm animals could make significant contributions to this area due to the long tradition of genetic

---
*Tel.: +46-184714904. Fax: +46-18504461. E-mail: leif.andersson@bmc.uu.se.

analysis of various phenotypic traits in breeding programs. This is particularly true for quantitative trait loci (QTLs). The cloning of QTLs would advance quantitative genetics theory and may open up new possibilities for the future use of transgenic technologies in animal improvement programs. The use of transgenesis in farm animals has been hampered by our ignorance concerning genes which control major phenotypic traits. The cloning of trait loci will also facilitate practical applications since a direct test for a causative mutation is more straightforward than a test based on linked markers and therefore more appealing to the breeding industry. This is well illustrated by the case for the mutation controlling malignant hyperthermia (MH) in pigs. Although several closely linked markers were known in the 1970s it was not until the causative mutation was identified (Fujii *et al.*, 1991) that large scale programs for reducing the incidence of MH were initiated in many countries.

So far only a limited number of mutations controlling phenotypic trait loci have been identified in farm animals. One of the most important ones from a practical point of view is the mutation controlling MH in pigs and the research resulting in the identification of this mutation will be used as an example throughout this chapter. This mutation is associated with the porcine stress syndrome (PSS) which involves the development of MH following stress or exposure to the anaesthetic gas halothane, and pale, soft and exudative (PSS) meat (see review by Archibald, 1991). Interestingly the *MH* mutation is also associated with a high lean content and it is very likely that selection for lean growth increased the incidence of this mutation in many breeds. The first report of the porcine stress syndrome came as early as 1953 (Ludvigsen, 1953) but at this time the genetic basis was unknown. Later it was found that a brief exposure to halothane could trigger the development of MH in susceptible pigs and that this was inherited as a simple recessive trait (Eikelenboom and Minkema, 1974). This allowed the mapping of the *MH* locus which in turn led to the identification of a missense mutation in the calcium release channel (CRC; also denoted the ryanodine receptor, RYR) which almost certainly is the causative mutation for MH (Fujii *et al.*, 1991). It has been proposed that this mutation is causing the effect on lean content (MacLennan and Philips, 1993) but it cannot be excluded that independent mutations in very closely linked genes explain the effect on leanness.

When discussing strategies for cloning trait genes it is important to distinguish between those traits controlled by a single gene (i.e. monogenic traits) and complex polygenic traits where the phenotype is controlled by an unknown number of genes and by environmental factors. The cloning of monogenic trait loci is today a fairly straightforward undertaking, although often very demanding, while the cloning of polygenic trait loci is much more problematic for several reasons. The possible strategies for cloning monogenic trait loci will therefore be described first and at the end of the chapter we will discuss the hurdles involved in cloning polygenic trait loci and how these may be managed.

STRATEGIES FOR CLONING GENES CONTROLLING MONOGENIC TRAITS

It is useful to recognise four major strategies for cloning trait loci: functional cloning, candidate cloning, positional cloning and positional candidate cloning. These are not mutually exclusive and a research group attempting to clone a trait locus will employ several in parallel.

Functional Cloning

Functional cloning is the classical way of cloning genes from cDNA or genomic libraries on the basis of previous biochemical characterisation of the gene product (see Old and Primrose, 1994). In the context of cloning trait loci, functional cloning implies screening for genetic variation at the protein level prior to molecular cloning. For instance, a straightforward way to clone a gene controlling a bleeding disorder is to carry out a biochemical investigation with the aim of revealing which of the well known coagulation factors is defective or missing. Information about the protein involved will subsequently be used to clone the gene. This may be accomplished for instance by screening a cDNA or genomic library with a heterologous probe (if the gene has been cloned in another species), an oligonucleotide probe designed on the basis of a partial amino acid sequence of the protein, or by screening a cDNA expression library with an antibody against the protein. Functional cloning may be very efficient if one has a good understanding of the biochemical pathway involved but its use is restricted to the limited set of gene products for which a biochemical assay is possible. The cloning of the *MH* mutation in pigs can at least partly be characterised as functional cloning since the identification of a mutation in the *CRC* gene was preceded by biochemical work showing that the tryptic digestion patterns of the gene product differed between pigs of different *MH* genotypes (Knudson *et al.*, 1990) showing the presence of a mutation.

Candidate Cloning

Candidate genes may be identified on the basis of their known function. For instance, the growth hormone gene is one (out of many) candidate genes for growth traits. A candidate gene may also be one controlling a strikingly similar phenotype (e.g. an inherited disorder) in another species. The candidate gene may be investigated by functional studies of the gene product (as described above) or by gene mapping, cloning and sequencing. The first step in the characterisation of a candidate gene is to find out whether it maps in the near vicinity of the trait locus. This may be accomplished with physical mapping (*in situ*-hybridisation or somatic cell mapping) or by linkage mapping. In the latter case one needs to develop a simple DNA polymorphism like a restriction fragment length polymorphism (RFLP) or single strand conformation polymorphism (SSCP) for the candidate gene. The presence of a single authentic recombinant (i.e. one which is not due to genotyping errors or incomplete penetrance, etc.) between the candidate and trait loci is sufficient to rule out the candidate gene.

There are already several examples of candidate cloning of mutations controlling monogenic traits in farm animals. For instance, the identification of the causative mutations for bovine leukocyte adhesion deficiency (BLAD; Shuster *et al.*, 1992) and for hyperkalaemic periodic paralysis (HYPP) in horses (Rudolph *et al.*, 1992) were based on the previous identification of mutations causing similar diseases in humans. Moreover, the finding of mutations in the melanocyte stimulating hormone receptor gene (*MC1R*) associated with coat colour variants in cattle (Klungland *et al.*, 1995) and in horses (Marklund *et al.*, 1996) followed the detection of mutations in the presumed homologous coat colour locus in mice (Robbins *et al.*, 1993).

Positional Cloning

Positional cloning is the strategy of choice when a trait locus has been mapped to a chromosomal region lacking obvious candidate genes. In contrast to functional cloning, the target gene is cloned on the basis of its map position while the function of the gene is revealed subsequent to cloning. Positional cloning is composed of four phases: (1) defining the chromosomal region in question as precisely as possible, (2) building a contig of genomic clones spanning the region, (3) screening for transcripts encoded within the defined segment and identification of candidate genes and (4) screening for causative mutations in candidate genes. Positional cloning is often a demanding task and the following resources are essential for a successful outcome: (1) a pedigree material including a large number of informative meioses, (2) a dense genetic map, (3) large insert libraries and (4) mRNA from the appropriate tissue isolated from both affected and nonaffected individuals. Furthermore, the research group or research consortium needs expertise in a wide range of molecular and cytogenetic techniques (cf. Sherrington *et al.*, 1995).

The chromosomal region which will be the target for positional cloning is defined by the two nearest flanking markers showing recombination to the trait locus. The rate limiting steps in positional cloning are the characterisation of candidate genes and screening for mutations. As a rule of thumb, 1 cM corresponds to about 1 Mbp in a mammalian genome and may harbour 20–30 genes; it must be strongly emphasised that these are average figures and the rate of recombination as well as gene density vary considerably in the genome. Consequently, it is essential to map a trait locus as precisely as possible. Boehnke (1994) has calculated the expected size of the distance between flanking markers conditional on the number of informative meioses and the map density. As illustrated in Figure 5.1, an acceptable size of the interval (on the order of the cM) is only achieved with a large number of informative meioses and a high marker density. Even with 200 informative meioses and an average marker distance of 2 cM the expected interval is 3 cM.

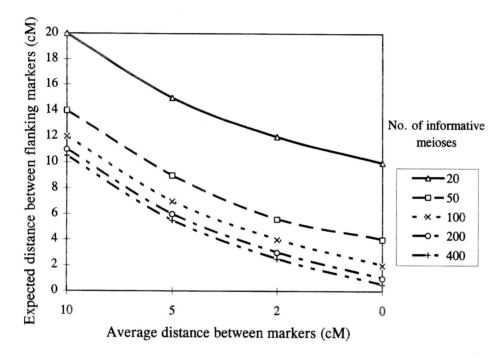

Figure 5.1 Expected distance between the two nearest flanking markers showing recombination to a trait locus as a function of the average distance between markers and the number of informative meioses. Based on data presented by Boehnke (1994).

The second phase involves construction of a physical map covering the region and building a contig of genomic clones from large insert libraries (**YAC, BAC, PAC** or **P1**). The critical issue in this work is to have access to large insert libraries with sufficient depth, i.e. containing manifold genome coverage, to ensure that the whole region is represented and that possible problems with chimerism can be resolved. The construction of long range restriction maps by pulsed field gel electrophoresis using genomic DNA from affected and unaffected individuals provides a reference for the contig map and may reveal chromosomal rearrangements (deletions, inversions, duplications) among affected individuals.

Once the physical map has been put in place, a number of alternative strategies are available for finding genes within the defined chromosomal region (see Monaco, 1994 for review). One of the first strategies to be used was so called zoo-blots in which genomic clones are used to probe Southern blots of genomic DNA from other species. Cross-hybridising fragments are likely to contain genes since primarily coding sequences are well conserved during evolution. Another strategy is to isolate genomic clones containing CpG islands which are often found in the 5'-end of house-keeping genes (Bird, 1986); CpG islands are fairly short stretches of DNA containing unmethylated CpG dinucleotides and the CG dinucleotide occurs here much more frequently than in the rest of the genome. A more direct approach is to use genomic clones as probes for screening cDNA libraries after suppression of repeated sequences in the probe. This works well for cosmid clones but less well for YAC clones for which the signal-to-noise ratio often becomes too low. Exon-trapping (Duyk *et al.*, 1990; Buckler *et al.*, 1991) is a novel method for finding genes present in genomic clones. By this method random genomic DNA fragments are inserted into an intron present in a mammalian expression vector. Subsequent to transfection, mRNA can be isolated and screened for the acquisition of one or more exons present in the genomic DNA fragment. The cloned exonic fragment can then be used to probe Northern blots and cDNA libraries. An advantage with this method is that it can be used to find genes without information in which tissue(s) or in which developmental stage(s) they are expressed. Finally, hybrid selection or direct selection (Lovett *et al.*, 1991; Parimoo *et al.*, 1991) involves solution hybridisation of target cDNA with a biotinylated genomic probe which could be a cosmid, BAC or even a whole YAC clone. cDNA hybridising to the genomic clone are enriched by avidin capture of the probe. The critical issue as regards the use of these methods is the extent of completeness for finding transcripts from the target region. Hattier *et al.* (1995) recently reported on the efficacy of hybrid selection. They isolated 931 clones from a 600-kb region harbouring the human *BRCA1* gene and found 118 nonoverlapping candidate expressed sequence tags (ESTs). They concluded that the region could be screened quickly without a huge investment of labour.

The first successful application of positional cloning was the identification of the gene causing Duchenne muscular dystrophy in humans (Hoffman *et al.*, 1987). This has been followed by a number of positionally cloned genes causing human diseases (Collins, 1995) or inherited disorders in mice (Copeland *et al.*, 1993). It is important to realise why positional cloning has been so successful in these two species. Firstly, excellent tools for genome analysis are available including dense genetic maps and large insert libraries. For instance, the most recently updated human linkage map contains 5264 microsatellite markers (Dib *et al.*, 1996) and most parts of the human genome are by now cloned in overlapping YAC clones (Chumakov *et al.*, 1995). In the mouse it is also possible to make large breeding experiments (1000 informative meioses or more) allowing precise mapping of trait loci. Secondly, many successful positional cloning experiments have been guided by chromosomal rearrangements (deletions, duplications, translocations or inversions) which have interrupted the coding sequence or altered gene expression. Thus, the cloning of the rearrangement breakpoint has been a convenient route towards the gene or its close vicinity. So far, few genes for which the phenotypic effect was due to a point mutation have been isolated by positional cloning (e.g. Zhang *et al.*, 1994; Sherrington *et al.*, 1995). Moreover, positional cloning experiments have primarily involved inherited disorders where a deleterious mutation has been expected. In such cases, the gene may be identified already in the screening process as one encoding a mRNA which are absent or showing an aberrant size in affected individuals. It will be more difficult to clone mutations causing variant forms of a gene product because normal mRNA expression is expected and it will be hard to distinguish the causative mutation from a linked polymorphism.

Prospects for Positional Cloning in Livestock

No gene controlling a trait locus in a farm animal has yet been positionally cloned. However, the strong research activity in livestock genomics including the development of large insert libraries (see Georges and Andersson, 1996, for review) holds promise that the first successful experiments are not far away. For instance, Eggen *et al.* (1996) reported construction of a YAC contig spanning the region harbouring the polled locus in cattle. The available marker maps in farm animals are sufficiently dense for mapping trait loci. But for most parts of the genome they are not dense enough for the precise mapping needed for positional cloning. This is illustrated by the recent mapping of the *RN* gene to pig chromosome 15 (Mariani *et al.*, 1996; Milan *et al.*, 1996); *RN* has a major influence on muscle glycogen content and meat quality. Despite that more than 1000 genetic markers are available in the pig (Rohrer *et al.*, 1996), the interval between flanking markers is about 10 cM. Thus, after mapping trait loci animal geneticists will be faced by the need to increase marker density in the region. There is a growing interest for targeted approaches to tackle this problem such as the isolation of genetic markers from chromosome- or region-specific genomic libraries constructed using flow-sorted chromosomes or microdissected chromosome segments.

   Another limiting factor for positional cloning in farm animals may be the number of informative meioses available as it may not be possible to increase the sample size due to the lack of suitable family material and the cost of producing experimental pedigrees. A solution to this dilemma can be to utilise the presence of linkage disequilibrium (LD) to define a narrow region containing the causative mutation as successfully applied for positional cloning of the gene causing diastrophic dysplasia in humans (Hästbacka *et al.*, 1994). The basis for LD-mapping is that individuals which have inherited a specific mutation from a common ancestor will share a chromosome segment which is identical by descent (IBD) and genetic polymorphisms within this region will show linkage disequilibrium. The expected physical size of the IBD segment is a function of the recombination rate in the interval and the number of independent meiotic events which the mutation has been transmitted from the common ancestor to the sample of descendants.

   Although positional cloning in livestock is possible, few labs will have the resources needed to carry out such an endeavour within a reasonable amount of time. However, animal geneticists will rarely use the positional cloning strategy solely but will aggressively exploit mapping information from other species when cloning trait genes (see next section).

Positional Candidate Cloning

A limitation with the candidate cloning approach is that for most traits there are many potential candidate genes and the characterisation of each of them in relation to the expression of a phenotype is demanding. An alternative is therefore to first map the trait locus and then look for candidate genes already assigned to that particular chromosomal region. This has been denoted positional candidate cloning which has already proven to be a very useful approach (see Copeland *et al.*, 1993) and will be the major future strategy for identifying trait genes in humans (Collins, 1995). The reason for this optimism is the rapid progress occurring within the human genome project which is expected to lead to an almost complete human transcript map in the near future. This will result from several large-scale cDNA sequencing projects. Also underway is development of ordered transcript maps by mapping the derived ESTs (expressed sequence tags) on radiation hybrid panels or YAC contigs (Hudson *et al.*, 1995). These initiatives will be complemented by the generation of the complete sequence of the human genome within the next 5–10 years. Together these resources will circumvent the need for positional cloning and the screening for potential candidate genes in a specific region will be made *in silico* using databases. This calls for the development of efficient means for accessing and cross-linking different databases.

Comparative Genomics Provides Opportunities for Positional Candidate Cloning in Livestock

A complete transcript map will not be available in the near future for any farm animal. However, animal geneticists will have the opportunity to exploit mapping information in humans and mice based on comparative gene mapping (see Chapter 7 of this volume). Coding sequences are often well conserved and it is possible to identify gene homologies even between distantly related species. This in combination with the remarkable conservation of vertebrate genome organisation make it possible to identify homologous chromosome segments between species. The regions of conserved synteny to the human genome have been established by comparative chromosome painting (Zoo-FISH) for cattle (Solinas-Toldo *et al.*, 1995; Chowdhary *et al.*, 1996), pig (Rettenberger *et al.*, 1995; Frönicke *et al.*, 1996) and horse (Raudsepp *et al.*, 1996). Although it is well established that intrachromosomal rearrangements may have occurred within regions of conserved synteny (e.g. Johansson *et al.*, 1995), colinearity to the human map is expected for large parts of farm animal genomes at least for those species within the mammalian class. Thus, after aligning an animal map with the human map based on the location of a set of homologous loci, it should be possible to access the human transcript map with great confidence. This opens up the possibility for positional candidate cloning based on comparative genomics. The human transcript map should also be a useful resource when there is a need to isolate genomic clones from a target region since human cDNA clones can be used to probe genomic libraries. This scenario makes a strong case for the development of high-resolution comparative maps for all major farm animals.

The identification of the mutation causing malignant hyperthermia (MH) in pigs (Fujii *et al.*, 1991) was the first example of positional candidate cloning of a trait gene in livestock. The *MH* locus was assigned to a linkage group on pig chromosome 6 (Davies *et al.*, 1988) and the major candidate gene encoding the calcium release channel (CRC) was subsequently mapped to the same region (Harbitz *et al.*, 1990). This prompted Fujii and coworkers to sequence the 15 000 bp *CRC* transcript from an affected and an unaffected pig which lead to the identification of a single missense mutation in the recessive allele.

Screening for Mutations in Candidate Genes

Once a putative causative gene has been identified using any of the four strategies described above there are several possible strategies for finding mutations. Northern blot analysis of mRNA from affected and non-affected individuals is an obvious approach for the initial characterisation of a candidate gene. This analysis may reveal differences in the level, or in the tissue distribution, of gene expression implying the presence of a regulatory mutation in the promoter or in another regulatory element. Moreover, a mRNA of aberrant size may be due to a deletion/insertion or a splice defect. Normal mRNA expression in affected individuals suggests that the mutation is a structural one and the next step is to screen for mutations using cDNA clones or RT-PCR products. There are several methods available which detect point mutations with varying efficiency (see Landegren, 1996) but in a search for a causative mutation most researchers would do the screening by sequence analysis. Sequence analysis of genomic DNA may be an attractive alternative to cDNA sequencing if the gene is not too large and/or it is difficult to isolate mRNA.

Finally, if a regulatory mutation is expected because of aberrant mRNA expression or if the coding sequence does not differ between affected and non-affected individuals it will be necessary to make the sequence comparison using genomic DNA. Once again this can be done by isolating clones from a genomic library or using PCR-based strategies depending upon how much sequence information is available from the target gene. A nightmare in this context is so called position effects which means that a mutation far away from the coding sequence may disregulate gene expression. There are several examples now where chromosomal alterations more than 100 kb from the gene apparently cause phenotypic effects (Bedell *et al.*, 1996). Therefore, it is wise to include traditional Southern blot analysis as well as Pulsed Field Gel Electrophoresis of genomic DNA in the screening for mutations since these methods may reveal chromosomal rearrangements.

A Causal Relationship between an Observed Mutation and the Phenotype Needs to Be Proven

When a putative mutation has been identified it is necessary to provide data supporting that the mutation causes the phenotypic effect. Genetic as well as functional evidence may be provided. For a monogenic trait with complete penetrance, all animals which are heterozygous and/or homozygous for the mutation (depending on whether the trait shows a dominant or recessive inheritance) should exhibit the phenotype in question. Moreover, individuals showing the phenotype but lacking the mutation may occur but they should then exhibit other mutations in the same gene.

Circumstantial evidence is provided if the expected effect of the mutation is consistent with the characteristics of the phenotype. This is the case if a nonsense mutation is identified and the phenotype is obviously due to the lack of gene expression. Strong indication for a causal relationship may also be provided if a missense mutation causes a substitution in a highly conserved and functionally important part of the molecule. However, even if there are striking indications of a causal relationship it is often difficult to exclude the possibility that the observed mutation is only very closely linked to the causative mutation and experimental work may be needed to provide conclusive evidence. This may be achieved by expressing the normal and variant form of the gene product *in vitro* and comparing their function. In many cases though, it will be necessary to study the phenotypic effect *in vivo* by producing transgenic animals carrying the specific mutation. This is well illustrated by the *MH* mutation in pigs. It may be possible to express the mutant and normal form of the Calcium Release Channel in muscle cell culture and show a functional difference but a transgenic model is needed to prove that this mutation causes malignant hyperthermia. Moreover, such a transgenic model would also be the only way to settle the long-standing question whether the association to leanness and meat quality traits is due to pleiotropic effects of the *MH* mutation or close linkage to other genes affecting these traits.

Prospects for Cloning Genes Controlling Polygenic Traits

Most traits of practical significance in animal breeding show a polygenic inheritance. This means that they are determined by an unknown number of genes together with environmental factors. A locus influencing a quantitative trait like milk yield or daily gain is generally referred to as a quantitative trait locus (QTL). The mapping and, if possible, cloning of QTLs is a major target in animal genome research. However, the cloning of QTLs will be a formidable task for two reasons: (1) the poor precision in QTL mapping and (2) the nature of causative mutations controlling quantitative traits. First we may ask the question "what is a QTL?". QTL simply denotes a chromosomal region controlling part of the genetic variation in a given quantitative trait. So, a QTL may reflect genetic variation in a single gene or the haplotype effect of several linked genes. With current technology, only QTLs with a large or at least moderate effect will be targets for cloning experiments.

The precision in the mapping of a QTL is much reduced compared with a monogenic trait locus as in the former case the phenotype is influenced by the environment as well as segregation at other loci. There is thus not a direct relationship between genotype and phenotype which prohibits a direct scoring of recombinants between the QTL and flanking markers. For instance, simulation studies showed that a QTL explaining 11% of the phenotypic variation in an F_2 population of 1000 animals and mapped using completely informative markers with a 10 cM spacing, would be mapped to an 8 cM interval (Knott and Haley, 1992). However, for a QTL with a major effect it is possible to deduce the genotype for an individual by progeny testing and by analysing flanking markers. This is illustrated in Figure 5.2 for a case where a QTL has been detected in a cross between two different lines A and B. A congenic line carrying the QTL allele from line A on a line B background can be produced over a few generations by using marker information to select informative recombinants for further breeding. This procedure will reveal whether the QTL is inherited as a distinct locus or is due to several linked loci which will break apart in subsequent generations. If it is inherited as a distinct locus this approach should make it possible to map the locus at the 1 cM resolution needed for cloning. The outlined strategy should be feasible for some farm animals like chicken and pig but would be very costly for others like cattle. However, in the case of dairy cattle, the extensive progeny testing schemes provide an opportunity to identify sires which are likely to have inherited a QTL allele from a common ancestor and use IBD mapping to define the QTL to a narrow region (Georges and Andersson, 1996).

Another approach to improve the precision of the localisation of the QTL is to refine the phenotype. Ideally the QTL should be transformed into a simple monogenic trait by genetic dissection of the polygenic trait. The key to such an achievement is that the QTL genotype can be predicted with high precision using flanking markers. It is thus possible to identify half- or full-sibs with different QTL genotypes which can be subjected to experimental work with the aim to reveal the action of the QTL. Once again we can use the *MH* mutation in pigs to illustrate this point. Sudden stress death, leanness and meat quality, which are all influenced by this mutation, have a complex genetic background making the cloning of the mutation difficult. A major breakthrough towards the identification of the *MH* mutation was therefore the observation that the development of malignant hyperthermia after exposure to halothane was inherited as a recessive trait with an almost complete penetrance.

The other major obstacle for cloning QTLs is our vague idea about the molecular nature of QTL mutations. Consider for instance a QTL allele increasing daily gain by 5% and let us assume that the effect is caused by a single mutation. It is very unlikely that this is due to a deleterious mutation which may be revealed by Northern blot analysis of candidate genes from the region. It is also highly unlikely that a chromosomal rearrangement will guide us towards the gene. Moreover, QTL alleles may well be due to regulatory mutations located far away from the coding sequence. Unfortunately, there is not much data available on this topic from experimental organisms which pave the way for animal geneticists towards their Holy Grail, the cloning of QTLs. It is clear that a major challenge in animal genetics will be to design strategies and experiments which can shed light on this central topic.

High resolution QTL mapping by selective back-crossing

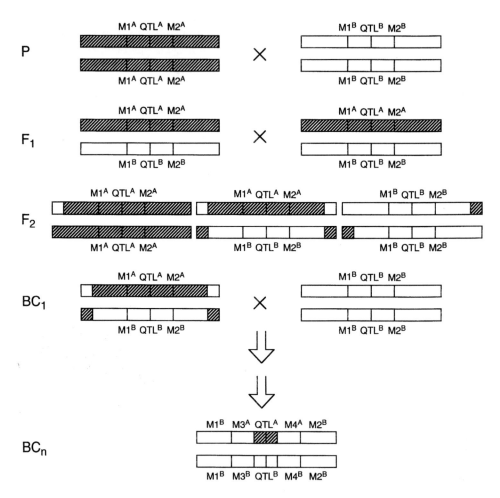

Figure 5.2 The principle of mapping a QTL fixed for different alleles in line A and B. The detection of the QTL by marker segregation analyses in the F_2 generation is followed by high-resolution QTL mapping by selective back-crossing. M1 to M4 represent marker loci 1 to 4.

ACKNOWLEDGEMENT

Sincere thanks are due to James Kijas and Lena Marklund for valuable help in preparing this manuscript.

REFERENCES

Andersson, L., Haley, C.S., Ellegren, H., Knott, S.A., Johansson, M., Andersson, K. *et al.* (1994) Genetic mapping of quantitative trait loci for growth and fatness in pigs. *Science*, **263**, 1771–1774.

Archibald, A.L. (1991) Inherited halothane-induced malignant hyperthermia in pigs. In *Breeding for Disease Resistance in Farm Animals*, edited by Owen, J.B., pp. 449–466. CAB International, UK.

Bird, A.P. (1986) CpG rich islands and the function of DNA methylation. *Nature*, **321**, 209–213.

Bedell, M.A., Jenkins, N.A. and Copeland, N.G. (1996) Good genes in bad neighbourhoods. *Nature Genetics*, **12**, 229–232.

Boehnke, M. (1994) Limits of resolution of genetic linkage studies: implications for the positional cloning of human disease genes. *Am. J. Hum. Genet.*, **55**, 379–390.

Buckler, A.J., Chang, D.D., Graw, S.L., Brook, D., Haber, D.A., Sharp, P.A. *et al.* (1991) Exon amplification: a strategy to isolate mammalian genes based on RNA splicing. *Proc. Natl. Acad. Sci. (USA)*, **88**, 4005–4009.

Chowdhary, B.P., Frönicke, L., Gustavsson, I. and Scherthan, H. (1996) Comparative analysis of the cattle and human genomes: detection of ZOO-FISH and gene mapping-based chromosomal homologies. *Mammalian Genome*, **7**, 297–302.

Chumakov, I.M., Rigault, P., LeGall, I., Bellanne-Chantelot, C., Billault, A. *et al.* (1995) A YAC contig of the human genome. *Nature*, **377**, 175–297.

Collins, F.S. (1995) Positional cloning moves from perditional to traditional. *Nature Genet.*, **9**, 347–350.

Copeland, N.G., Jenkins, N.A., Gilbert, D.J., Eppig, J.T., Maltais, L.J., Miller, J.C. *et al.* (1993) A genetic linkage map of the mouse: current applications and future prospects. *Science*, **235**, 1046–1049.

Davies, W., Harbitz, I., Fries, R., Stranzinger, G. and Hauge, J.G. (1988) Porcine malignant hyperthermia detection and chromosomal assignment using a linked probe. *Animal Genetics*, **19**, 203–212.

Dib, C., Fauré, S., Fizames, C., Samson, D., Drouot, N., Vignal, A. *et al.* (1996) A comprehensive genetic map of the human genome based on 5,264 microsatellites. *Nature*, **380**, 152–154.

Duyk, G.M., Kim, S.W., Myers, R.M. and Cox, D.R. (1990) Exon trapping: a genetic screen to identify candidate transcribed sequences in cloned mammalian DNA. *Proc. Natl. Acad. Sci. (USA)*, **87**, 8995–8999.

Eggen, A., Doud, L.K., Hayes, H., Murvke, B.T., Jurgella, G., Pfister-Genskow, M. *et al.* (1996) Construction of a YAC-contig in the vicinity of the polled locus in cattle. *Animal Genetics*, **27** (Suppl. 2), 58–59.

Eikelenboom, G. and Minkema, D. (1974) Prediction of pale, soft, exudative muscle with a nonlethal test for halothane induced porcine malignant hyperthermia. *Netherlands J. Vet. Sci.*, **99**, 421–426.

Frönicke, L., Chowdhary, B.P., Scherthan, H. and Gustavsson, I. (1996) A comparative map of the porcine and human genomes demonstrates ZOO-FISH and gene mapping-based chromosomal homologies. *Mammalian Genome*, **7**, 285–290.

Fujii, J., Otsu, K., Zorzato, F., de Leon, S., Khanna, V.K., Weiler, J. *et al.* (1991) Identification of a mutation in the porcine ryanodine receptor that is associated with malignant hyperthermia. *Science*, **253**, 448–451.

Georges, M. and Andersson, L. (1996) Livestock genomics comes of age. *Genome Research*, **6**, 907–921.

Georges, M., Nielsen, D., Mackinnon, M., Mishra, A., Okimoto, R., Pasquino, A.T. *et al.* (1995) Mapping quantitative trait loci controlling milk production in dairy cattle by exploiting progeny testing. *Genetics*, **139**, 907–920.

Harbitz, I., Chowdhary, B., Thomsen, P.D., Davies, W., Kaufmann, U., Kran, S. *et al.* (1990) Assignment of the porcine calcium release channel gene, a candidate for the malignant hyperthermia locus, to the 6p11–q21 segment of chromosome 6. *Genomics*, **8**, 243–248.

Hästbacka, J., de la Chapelle, A., Mahtani, M.M., Clines, G., Reevedaly, M.P., Daly, M. *et al.* (1994) The diastrophic dysplasia gene encodes a novel sulfate transporter — positional cloning by fine-structure linkage disequilibrium mapping. *Cell*, **78**, 1073–1087.

Hattier, T., Bell, R., Shaffer, D., Stone, S., Phelps, R.S., Tavtigian, S.V. *et al.* (1995) Monitoring the efficacy of hybrid selection during positional cloning: the search for BRCA1. *Mammalian Genome*, **6**, 873–879.

Hoffman, E.P., Brown, R.H. and Kunkel, L.M. (1987) Dystrophin: the protein product of the Duchenne muscular dystrophy locus. *Cell*, **51**, 919–928.

Hudson, T.J., Stein, L.D., Gerety, S.S., Ma, J., Castle, A.B., Silva, J. *et al.* (1995) An STS-based map of the human genome. *Science*, **270**, 1945–1954.

Johansson, M., Ellegren, H. and Andersson, L. (1995) Comparative mapping reveals extensive linkage conservation — but with gene order rearrangements — between the pig and human genomes. *Genomics*, **25**, 682–690.

Klungland, H., Våge, D.I., Gomez-Raya, L., Adalsteinsson, S. and Lien, S. (1995) The role of melanocyte-stimulating hormone (MSH) receptor in bovine coat color determination. *Mammalian Genome*, **6**, 636–639.

Knott, S.A. and Haley, C.S. (1992) Aspects of maximum likelihood methods for the mapping of quantitative trait loci in line crosses. *Genet. Res.*, **60**, 139–151.

Knudson, C.M., Mickelson, J.R., Louis, C.F. and Campbell, K.P. (1990) Distinct Immunopeptide maps of the sarcoplasmic-reticulum Ca^{2+} release channel in malignant hyperthermia. *J. Biol. Chem.*, **265**, 2421–2424.

Landegren, U. (Ed.) (1996) *Laboratory Protocols for Mutation Detection*. Oxford: Oxford University Press.

Lovett, M., Kere, J. and Hinton, L.M. (1991) Direct selection: a method for the isolation of cDNAs encoded by large genomic regions. *Proc. Natl. Acad. Sci. (USA)*, **88**, 9628–9633.

Ludvigsen, J. (1953) Muscular degeneration in hogs. In *15th International Veterinary Congress, Stockholm 1953*, pp. 251–263.

MacLennan, D.H. and Phillips, M.S. (1993) Malignant hyperthermia. *Science*, **256**, 789–794.

Mariani, P., Lundström, K., Gustafsson, U., Enfält, A.-C., Juneja, R.K. and Andersson, L. (1996) A major locus (*RN*) affecting muscle glycogen content is located on pig Chromosome 15. *Mammalian Genome*, **7**, 52–54.

Marklund, L., Johansson Moller, M., Sandberg, K. and Andersson, L. (1996) A missense mutation in the gene for the melanocyte-stimulating hormone receptor (*MC1R*) is associated with the chestnut coat colour in horses. *Mammalian Genome*, **7**, 895–899.

Milan, D., Woloszyn, N., Yerle, M., Le Roy, P., Bonnet, M., Riquet, J. *et al.* (1996) Accurate mapping of the acid meat RN gene on genetic and physical maps of pig chromosome 15. *Mammalian Genome*, **7**, 47–51.

Monaco, A.F. (1994) Isolation of genes from cloned DNA. *Currrent Opinion in Genetics and Development*, **4**, 360–365.

Old, R.W. and Primrose, S.B. (1994) *Principles of Gene Manipulation*, 5th edn. Oxford: Blackwell Scientific Publications.

Parimoo, S., Patanjali, S.R., Shukle, H., Chaplin, D.D. and Weisman, S.M. (1991) cDNA selection: efficient PCR approach for the selection of cDNAs encoded in large chromosomal DNA fragments. *Proc. Natl. Acad. Sci. (USA)*, **88**, 9623–9627.

Raudsepp, T., Frönicke, L., Scherthan, H., Gustavsson, I. and Chowdhary, B.P. (1996) Zoo-FISH delineates conserved chromosomal segments in horse and man. *Chromosome Research*, **4**, 218–225.

Rettenberger, G., Klett, C., Zechner, U., Kunz, J., Vogel, W. and Hameister, H. (1995) Visualization of the conservation of the synteny between pigs and humans by heterologous chromosomal painting. *Genomics*, **26**, 372–378.

Robbins, L.S., Nadeau, J.H., Johnson, K.R., Kelly, M.A., Roselli-Rehfuss, L., Baack, E. *et al.* (1993) Pigmentation phenotypes of variant extension locus alleles result from point mutations that alter MSH receptor function. *Cell*, **72**, 827–834.

Rohrer, G.A., Alexander, L.J., Hu, Z., Smith, T.P.L., Keele, J.W. and Beattie, C.W. (1996) A comprehensive map of the porcine genome. *Genome Research*, **6**, 371–391.

Rudolph, J.A., Spier, S.J., Byrns, G., Rojas, C.V., Bernoco, D. and Hoffman, E.P. (1992) Periodic paralysis in Quarter Horses: a sodium channel mutation disseminated by selective breeding. *Nature Genet.*, **2**, 144–147.

Sherrington, R., Rogaev, E.I., Liang, Y., Rogaeva, E.A., Levesque, G., Ikeda, M. *et al.* (1995) Cloning of a gene bearing missense mutations in early-onset familial Alzheimer's disease. *Nature*, **375**, 754–760.

Shuster, D.E., Kehrli, M.E. Jr., Ackermann, M.R. and Gilbert, R.O. (1992) Identification and prevalence of a genetic defect that causes leukocyte adhesion deficiency in Holstein cattle. *Proc. Natl. Acad. Sci. (USA)*, **89**, 9225–9229.

Solinas-Toldo, S., Lengauer, C. and Fries, R. (1995) Comparative genome map of man and cattle. *Genomics*, **27**, 489–496.

Zhang, Y., Proenca, R., Maffei, M., Barone, M., Leopold, L. and Friedman, J.M. (1994) Positional cloning of the mouse *obese* gene and its human homologue. *Nature*, **372**, 425–432.

6. MARKER ASSISTED SELECTION

P.M. VISSCHER [1,*], S. VAN DER BEEK [2,3], and C.S. HALEY [3]

[1] *University of Edinburgh, Institute of Ecology and Resource Management, West Mains Road, Edinburgh EH9 3JG, UK*
[2] *Wageningen Agricultural University, PO Box 338, 6700 AH Wageningen, Netherlands*
[3] *Roslin Institute, Roslin, Midlothian EH25 9PS, UK*

Traditional selection methods using phenotypic information have been successful in improving the profitability of livestock species. However, these methods have biological constraints in that some traits are sex or age limited or difficult and/or expensive to measure. Genetic markers can potentially ameliorate problems with traditional selection methods because they can be measured at any time, in both sexes. Linkage maps of the genomes of all major livestock species have been developed and are publicly available. These maps are the framework for artificial selection aided by markers. In crossbreeding introgression schemes, markers can be used to tag alleles to be introgressed and to speed up the genome recovery of the recurrent breed. Alternatively, marker alleles can be associated with phenotypic variation in recently created synthetic populations. In livestock populations, these methods are being applied at present, using marker alleles for colour, litter size, and disease resistance. Marker assisted selection in non-crossbred populations is more difficult, because associations between marker alleles and trait variation have to be traced within families. However, if markers are used to alter the design of breeding schemes, or to select where previously selection was at random, genetic progress can be increased substantially. Besides the 'straightforward' use of markers in selection programmes, markers can be used in quality control programmes, to control the rate of inbreeding, and to utilise non-additive genetic variation.

KEY WORDS: genetic marker; marker assisted selection; marker assisted introgression; linkage disequilibrium.

INTRODUCTION

Naturally occurring genetic variation underlies responses to the artificial selection imposed by mankind. This selection has resulted in the diversity of appearance and performance between different breeds of domestic animals, from dogs to cattle. In recent years such variation has been systematically and effectively exploited in national and commercial livestock breeding programmes to enhance quality and to reap substantial economic rewards in terms of improved efficiency.

Most traits of importance in animal (and plant) breeding are of a quantitative nature, i.e. observations do not fall into a few distinct classes, but can take any value within the range for that trait. For many traits, for example milk yield in dairy cattle and growth rate in pigs, the phenotypes typically follow an approximately normal distribution. The accepted explanation is that a phenotype is influenced by both the genotype and environment particular to an individual, and that across the population, genotypes and environmental effects can take

---
*Corresponding author: Tel.: +44-131-535-4052. Fax: +44-131-667-2601.
E-mail: peter.visscher@ed.ac.uk.

many different values, so that the resulting distribution is continuous (and often normal).

It is often assumed that many genes contribute to the variation in a quantitative trait. How many of such quantitative trait loci (QTLs) exist, and what are their effects? At present, we do not have a satisfactory answer to that question. Typically, a mammalian genome consists of 50,000 to 100,000 genes. One extreme hypothesis is that very few of the genes are QTLs, with each having a moderate or large effect, whereas at the other end of the spectrum we could hypothesise that most genes are QTLs with individually very small effects. As we will see later on, the number of QTLs which contribute to variation between and within breeds has large implications for QTL mapping experiments and marker assisted selection (MAS) programmes.

Traditionally, livestock improvement programmes have utilised selection based on phenotypic information on animals and their relatives. Such selection programmes have been successful, in that they have resulted in annual genetic gains of about 1–3% of the mean performance (e.g. Smith, 1984). For example, continued selection for growth rate in broilers has resulted in chickens that are three to four times heavier at the same age in a period of about 30 years (Havenstein *et al.*, 1995). In the last couple of decades, improved statistical methodology to separate genetic and environmental effects, for example Best Linear Unbiased Prediction (BLUP, e.g. Henderson, 1973) and Residual Maximum Likelihood (REML, Patterson and Thompson, 1971), and its adoption by the livestock industry, has led to increased rates of genetic gain in many livestock species.

There are nonetheless biological constraints on many of the traits of economic importance in livestock species which limit how much genetic gain can be achieved using phenotypic information alone. For example, traits such as milk yield in dairy cattle and litter size in pigs are so-called sex-limited, because they can only be measured on one sex. Other traits such as carcass quality and longevity may be termed age-limited, since they can only be measured when the animals are relatively old (or dead). For these traits it is either impossible to select candidates on which measurements were taken (as in the case of carcass traits), or the generation intervals would become very long if old animals were chosen to become parents for the next generation (as in the case of longevity). There is a third category of traits which are difficult to improve using traditional selection methods, and these are traits such as disease resistance, which are difficult or expensive to measure on a routine basis.

A further limitation of using phenotypic information only is that relatives of the same degree which neither have records themselves nor progeny with records obtain the same estimated breeding value. An example is that of full-sib dairy bulls entering a progeny test, which have the same estimated breeding value until the records of their daughters become available. In such cases we can not explain any of the genetic variation within families until progeny information becomes available.

Genetic markers can potentially ameliorate all of these problems, since they can be measured at any time, in both sexes, and can separate which chromosome segments full or half-sibs inherited from their parents. The essence of using genetic markers in breeding programmes is that they mark chromosomal regions (and sometimes individual genes), and so can follow the inheritance of these regions from parents to offspring. Thus if we know which chromosomal segments contain alleles of value, markers may be used to help identify animals that have inherited these alleles and hence the best of the genetic variation, whether or not we have phenotypic records or progeny information on the animals.

Recently, linkage maps of the genomes of most livestock species have been developed. For the pig, approximately 1000 markers are now publicly available (Archibald *et al.*, 1995; Ellegren *et al.*, 1994; Rohrer *et al.*, 1994). A similar number of markers is available for the bovine genome (e.g. Barendse *et al.*, 1994), and the chicken genome is approaching 500 markers (Burt *et al.*, 1995). The current status of the ovine genome map is that roughly 250 markers have been mapped (Crawford *et al.*, 1995).

We will discuss the use of these markers in selection programmes in this chapter. For presentation purposes, we have distinguished between the use of markers in populations recently derived from a crossbreeding event and in outbred populations with no recent crossbred origin, but it can be argued that such a separation is arbitrary. We briefly discuss the use of markers for quality control and for exploiting heterosis.

MARKERS IN CROSSBREEDING SCHEMES

No single commercial line or breed is likely to contain all of the best alleles for all traits of economic importance. If alleles of superior value for one or a few traits can be identified in breeds which are inferior in overall economic performance, an efficient crossing programme using genetic markers to help select for the best alleles might increase overall economic performance substantially. Although the starting point of any such programme may be well defined, i.e. a cross between two breeds or lines, the end point (a commercial product) can be reached through many different routes. For example, if one line is inferior for all but one or a few alleles, we might use marker assisted introgression. This is the process of introgressing particular alleles for trait loci from one breed or line (the donor line) into another (the recipient), with the aid of genetic markers, by repeated backcrosses to the superior line. At some point crosses within the backcross line would be used to fix the introgressed allele, and then selection would continue within the line. On the other hand, if the two lines are of similar genetic merit we might consider selecting the best alleles from both lines directly from an F_2 intercross with the aid of genetic markers. In between these two extremes there is a continuum of possibilities with varying numbers of rounds of backcrossing prior to intercrossing the animals and selecting within the intercross. The two extreme options have received some attention, but little attention has been paid to which point in the continuum is optimum for particular circumstances.

Marker Assisted Introgression

Genetic markers could be used in two ways in an introgression programme: (i) to tag the gene which is to be introgressed and aid identification of individuals carrying that gene (ii) to select for (or against) a particular background genotype and hence speed the recovery of the recipient genome. In most recent studies (Hillel *et al.*, 1990, 1993; Hospital *et al.*, 1992; Groen and Timmermans, 1992; Groen and Smith, 1995) it was assumed that the genotype at the gene to be introgressed was known exactly, hence there was no need to use markers to aid its introgression and attention was focused on the background genotype. In fact the genotype of genes to be introgressed will not usually be known as these will often be QTLs, which can only be genotyped imprecisely, if at all, using phenotypic information, or major loci (e.g. coat colour), which more often than not have dominance/recessive relationships and hence heterozygotes can not be distinguished from one of the homozygotes.

Markers can be used to select for a certain genetic background because whole segments of chromosomes are inherited. Hence, in the progeny of a particular cross, the segment of chromosome around a marker allele which originates from one breed is also more likely to come from that breed. However, the association between a marker and genes linked to it will be eroded over time due to recombination.

Having located a desired gene and genetic markers associated with it in an inferior breed, the aim of the introgression phase is to fix the favourable alleles in the commercial population with as little as is possible of the remainder of the genome from the inferior breed. Fixation of favourable alleles refers to the QTL or major gene and not to the markers, because fixing marker alleles is not an aim in itself. The route usually proposed (e.g. Smith *et al.*, 1987; Hillel *et al.*, 1990; Hospital *et al.*, 1992; Groen and Timmermans, 1992) is a number of generations of backcrossing of a population which carries the allele to be introgressed (from the donor population, i.e. the inferior breed) to a recipient population (i.e. the commercial breed), followed by an *inter se* cross to make the desired allele homozygous. In Figure 6.1, the proportion of individuals having one copy of the desired allele during the backcrossing phase is shown when no markers, a single marker at 5 cM distance from the gene, or two markers flanking the gene location are used to aid introgression. When no markers are used, the frequency of the desired allele halves each generation due to the random assortment of chromosomes. With a single marker, the frequency slowly reduces because of recombination between the gene of interest and the marker. With two flanking markers, the frequency stays very close to the desired 50%.

The efficiency of a marker assisted introgression programme depends on the frequency of the introgressed allele in the final population and the genetic progress for traits of economic benefit. As most studies have assumed that the allele to be introgressed can be identified without error by a single marker, the frequency of the allele during the backcross phase remains at 50%. In practice, a single marker or a marker bracket (a pair of markers flanking the region of the

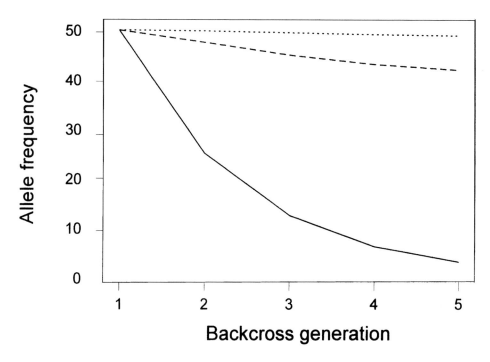

Figure 6.1 Marker assisted introgression using different numbers of markers. The position of the gene to be introgressed relative to the marker is assumed to be known exactly. The markers are fully informative (i.e. fixed for alternative alleles in the donor and recipient breeds). Solid line, no markers. Dashed line, using a single marker 5 cM from the introgressed gene. Dotted line, using two markers 5 and 15 cM on either side of the introgressed gene.

gene of interest) associated with the QTL or major gene is likely to be used, so that the frequency of the allele may be substantially less than 50% after a few generations of backcrossing (Visscher *et al.*, 1996). For example, assuming that the standard deviation of predicting the location of a QTL was 6 cM, which is reasonable for many QTL mapping experiments, and using only a single marker to aid the introgression, the proportion of animals that carried one copy of the QTL was reduced from 50 to about 20% in the 5th backcross generation (Visscher *et al.*, 1996).

In addition to following the fate of the introgressed allele, we need to consider what is happening to the background genotype. The donor line (or breed) is likely to be inferior for a number of traits of economic importance. For example, although the Meishan pig breed is superior to commercial European pig breeds for litter size and related traits, it is inferior with respect to lean growth and fatness traits. One criterion for comparison is the performance of the animals carrying the introgressed allele and the mean of the recipient line at the start of the programme. However, during the backcrossing and intercrossing phase the recipient (commercial) line will normally undergo selection, so that a better comparison is to compare the population carrying the allele with the commercial population at the same point in time. This is analogous to the problem studied by Haley (1991) and extensively by Gama *et al.* (1992), who calculated the genetic lag for economic performance for various backcross and intercross programmes when introgressing a transgene in a nucleus pig population. In that study it was assumed that the transgene genotype was known and genetic markers were not used to distinguish between the background genome of the founder transgenic animal and the rest of the population. These authors concluded that a gene would need an economic effect equivalent to 1–2 generations of selection to make its introgression worthwhile.

A number of studies have looked at marker assisted introgression using theoretical derivations or stochastic simulation. Hillel *et al.* (1990, 1993) proposed that DNA fingerprints could be used for introgression of alleles in backcross populations by selecting for or against a certain genomic background. Their theory is based on a number of 'chromosome segments', which effectively are unlinked loci. Groen and Timmermans (1992) presented a simulation study on the use of genetic markers to increase the efficiency of introgression through selection for the background genotype. When comparing phenotypic selection and selection using markers in a backcross programme, they conclude that not much benefit is to be expected from using markers. However, as pointed out by the authors, this conclusion depends on the parameters used (in particular on how effective phenotypic selection is). Using the parameters of Groen and Timmermans (1992), selection using markers has a small advantage over phenotypic selection for at least the first 3 backcross generations. The thorough study of Hospital, Chevalet, and Mulsant (1992) deals in detail with introgression in backcross breeding programmes. One of the main conclusions of this work was that retrieving the recipient's genome was approximately two generations faster if markers were used. Groen and Smith (1995) followed on from the study of Groen and Timmermans (1992), and studied the efficiency of phenotypic selection and selection on markers in backcross and intercross programmes. Selection was in two stages: firstly, animals were selected carrying the allele to be introgressed, and among those animals, those with the best phenotype or those with the largest number of markers from the recipient line were selected. For a number of scenarios studied, these authors concluded that selection using markers is always inferior to selection for phenotypes. This was most likely the case because the two populations did not differ widely in allele frequency of the QTLs.

MAS in a Synthetic Population

The efficiency of MAS in commercial populations depends heavily on whether it can be assumed that the association between certain markers and quantitative traits is the same in different families (Beckmann and Soller, 1983; Smith and Simpson, 1986). If this is the case we speak of linkage disequilibrium throughout

the population, and animals can be selected on the basis of their marker genotypes across families. Smith and Smith (1993) argued that effort should be
devoted to finding markers which are so close to the QTL that recombination
between them and the QTL can be ignored, so that selection can be across families. One way to achieve this in an outbred population where disequilibrium is not
widespread is to use a very high density of markers. An obvious way to generate
widespread disequilibrium, and hence require less markers, is to cross two
different lines. Thus we might cross two commercial lines and begin selecting a
new commercial line from the intercross.

Marker assisted selection from a line cross has been studied by Lande and
Thompson (1990), using theoretical derivations, and Zhang and Smith (1992,
1993) and Gimelfarb and Lande (1994), using simulation results. All studies
assumed linkage disequilibrium throughout the population and considered the
simplest situation; a cross between inbred lines. Marker assisted selection from
the intercross (an F_2 in these studies) then proceeds in two phases, (i) a number
of markers associated with the trait(s) of interest are chosen based on estimates
from a marker-quantitative trait association study (e.g. by analysis of associations
in the F_2), and (ii) animals are selected based on their marker genotype and their
phenotypes (and/or the phenotypes of their relatives). For the first phase, an
important question is how to select the markers which explain some of the genetic
variance in the population. A simple multiple regression approach will result in
an overestimate of the total variance explained by the markers (Wishart, 1931).
Therefore, Lande and Thompson (1990) proposed a two-stage procedure. In the
first stage, a set of promising markers are selected from all available markers. In
the second stage, estimates of the regression coefficients for the selected markers
are obtained from a new (independent) sample of animals. In this case, the
marker effects are unbiased (Lande and Thompson, 1990). However, as pointed
out by Visscher (1995), the total amount of variance explained by the selected
group of markers may still be biased upwards. Zhang and Smith (1992, 1993)
showed that with modelling marker effects as random effects, the problem of
overestimation might be reduced. However, the amount by which estimates of
marker effects are shrunk back to the overall mean depends on prior information
regarding the true amount of variation which is associated with the markers.
Usually, that information is not available.

Lande and Thompson (1990) give examples of the theoretical relative efficiency of marker assisted selection (including both marker information and
phenotypic observations) compared to traditional index selection, and show that
MAS performs much better for traits with low heritability (h^2) and large common
family effects (c^2 = proportion of total phenotypic variance due to common family
effects). For example, for a trait with $h^2 = 0.10$ and $c^2 = 0.25$, MAS is theoretically
approximately 50% more efficient than a selection index based on individual and
full-sib performance if the markers explain 20% of the genetic variance. If the
markers explain 40% of the genetic variance, MAS is about 3.5 times more
efficient than index selection for $h^2 = 0.05$ and $c^2 = 0.25$. A number of simulation
studies suggest that the theoretical predictions of Lande and Thompson (1990)

are too optimistic, especially if the time horizon is more than one generation. Gimelfarb and Lande (1994) contrasted MAS with just phenotypic selection by simulation and found that MAS was more efficient for at least 5 generations of selection for a single trait. If the regression coefficients for selected markers were re-estimated each generation, MAS was more efficient for the first 10 generations of selection. Surprisingly, practically all the weight in the index combining marker information and phenotypes was put on the marker information (Gimelfarb and Lande, 1994). Even with re-estimation of the marker effects, this is unexpected, since after a few generations of selection most genetic variance will be within rather than between marker genotypes.

Zhang and Smith (1992, 1993) compared the efficiency of MAS (using only marker information), with selection on BLUP breeding values and selection on an optimum combination of marker and phenotypic information. In Figure 6.2, results from Zhang and Smith (1992) are shown by comparing the response to MAS from selection on markers alone, selection on phenotypes using BLUP breeding values, or an optimum combination of the two sources of information.

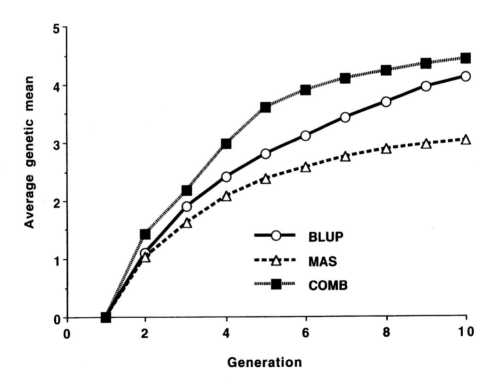

Figure 6.2 Marker assisted selection from a synthetic population. Based on data presented by Zhang and Smith (1992). Selection from an F_2 population for a trait with a heritability of 0.25. Selection was on markers (Δ), BLUP breeding values (○), or a combination of marker and phenotypic information (■).

It clearly shows an increased efficiency of 10–20% of combined selection over BLUP selection, at least until generation 10. Zhang and Smith (1993) also showed the loss in efficiency of estimating the marker effects with imprecision. For example, reducing the population size in which marker–QTL associations were estimated from 1000 to 100 reduced response to selection by about 50%. Similarly, Gimelfarb and Lande (1994) concluded that population size was the main parameter in determining the relative efficiency of MAS. In contrast, Lande and Thompson (1990) concluded that estimating the marker effects with error did not significantly reduce response to selection. However, these authors assumed that the appropriate markers (i.e. the ones most closely associated with QTLs) were included in the selection index, and that it was only the genetic variance associated with the markers that was subject to error, an unrealistic assumption, as in reality selected markers may not be those closest to QTLs.

All the above studies used a cross between inbred lines as their starting point. In livestock species, that is not possible as inbred lines are not available. Thus the question is whether the results hold for a cross between divergent outbred lines. When using outbred lines, the markers will generally not be completely informative, i.e. the two founder population may have some marker alleles in common. Thus it is not possible to determine from which breed marker alleles in an individual originated without following them through the pedigree back to their origin, and even this is often impossible for lowly informative markers. Using less informative markers implies that QTL mapping experiments and marker assisted selection programmes will be less efficient than in inbred lines using the same number of markers. However, in practice one would use more markers to ameliorate the problem of informativeness, and since so many markers are available from the linkage maps, lack of informative markers in a cross between divergent lines should not be a great problem. However, relative to working with inbred lines, the selection programmes would be more expensive. Another implication of using outbred lines is that detectable QTL may be segregating within each of the lines or breeds. Also, as for inbred lines, the 'inferior' breeds may harbour QTL alleles which improve the trait. From plant experiments there is evidence that for up to 20% of QTLs detected in crosses between wild and cultivated species the positive allele was from the line with the lower performance. There seems to be a direct relation (which can be predicted) between the difference between wild and cultivated species, and the probability that the wild species contains alleles with positive effects (De Vicente and Tanksley, 1993).

Scope in Livestock Populations

At present, there are already a number of genes which are candidates for introgression programmes, and synthetic populations also exist which are suitable for MAS programmes.

In beef cattle, genetic markers very close to the polled locus have recently been identified (Schutz et al., 1996; Brenneman et al., 1996). Polling is an important trait in cattle husbandry for welfare and economic reasons (the total economic cost for dehorning cattle in the UK is in the order of millions of pounds (Haley *et al.*, 1996). In many cattle breeds the recessive horned allele is at a high frequency, so introgression programmes could create a population homozygous polled. However, some populations, like the Holstein–Friesian dairy breed, are very much superior for the main trait of economic merit, i.e. milk yield, and have much larger rates of genetic gain than any potential donor breeds, so that it is difficult to see how an economically viable introgression programme could be initiated in that breed unless polling becomes a necessity on welfare grounds.

In pigs, at least one company is already introgressing chromosome regions associated with litter size from the Chinese Meishan into white breeds using genetic markers, and are using the same markers to select within commercial dam lines (Southwood *et al.*, 1996). In France, markers around a dominant major gene decreasing the yield of cured ham have been identified in Hampshire derived populations (Milan *et al.*, 1995). Resistance to the K88 strain of *E. Coli* is known to be determined by a recessive gene (Gibbons *et al.*, 1977), and pigs lacking the receptor for K88 are resistant to neonatal diarrhoea caused by this strain of *E. Coli*. Markers linked to K88 resistance are currently marketed for use in pig breeding programmes. Many UK abattoirs penalise slaughter pigs with coloured spots, so there is an economic incentive at present to breed for pure white pigs. The colour white is dominant in pigs and the gene responsible has been mapped to chromosome 8 and linked markers are known (Johansson *et al.*, 1992) and more recently the gene and causal mutation have been identified (Moller, 1995). The advantage of using a DNA based test in this case is that heterozygotes for the white allele (who themselves are phenotypically white) can be identified. Using classical selection without any markers will still result in the occasional coloured pig, since heterozygotes will remain in the population for a long time, and so the occasional homozygote for the colour allele will be produced.

Synthetic populations are predominantly found in pig, beef cattle, and sheep breeding programmes. Such populations are ideal for the application of MAS if the hybridisation was relatively recent, because then the degree of linkage disequilibrium is largest and an association between marker genotype and phenotype can be done across the whole population. However, at each generation of breeding since the hybridisation, the association between markers and QTL is reduced due to recombination. Substantial associations after T generations of mating are expected if the recombination rate (r) is, roughly, $r < 1/T$ (Lande and Thompson, 1990). Many synthetic populations in livestock breeding programmes are about 5 to 10 generations away from the original hybridisation process, so that QTL with large effects will be detected through their association with markers if the recombination rate between the QTL and the nearest marker is less than 10–20 cM. This is achievable with the density of the current linkage maps. Further technological developments could allow easy production of high density maps of markers and hence allow effective MAS for many more generations after a hybridisation event.

MARKER ASSISTED SELECTION IN AN OUTBRED POPULATION

A reasonable starting assumption is that, within an outbred population, markers and QTLs are in linkage equilibrium. This means that even for a marker that is closely linked to a QTL, across the population there is no overall association between the marker and the trait affected by the QTL. Thus, the source of association that is utilised when applying MAS in a crossbreeding scheme, is absent in an outbred population. If we focus, however, not on the population level but zoom in to the family level, then linkage disequilibrium reappears. Within the progeny of an animal heterozygous for both marker and QTL (say, the animal has genotype MQ/mq), the expectation of individuals inheriting allele M differs from that of individuals inheriting allele m. Therefore, although across population linkage disequilibrium is absent in an outbred population, marker assisted selection can be applied by aiming at within family associations.

Dentine (1992) pointed out that we can see a breeding value of an animal as the sum of the family average plus its individual deviation from the family average. Usually, sufficient information is available to estimate the family average, but the within family deviation can either not be estimated (e.g. in nucleus breeding for sex-limited or carcass limited traits where no record on the animal is available), is estimated based on own performance only, or is only estimable after waiting a long period (progeny testing). From this it follows that the efficiency of MAS in an outbred population should not be greatly hampered from the fact that between family differences are not picked up by the marker as these are already relatively well estimated. The efficiency of MAS only depends on the ability to explain within family variance. The variance explained by the marker depends on two factors: (1) the size of the QTL linked to the marker, and (2) the information available to estimate the effects of the marker alleles segregating within a family. We saw previously that the number of observations available to estimate the effect of a marker is a major determinant of the efficiency of MAS, and that even above 100 observations per marker class, increasing the number of observations has a large effect. We can therefore safely predict that within families, where the number of offspring is limited, amount of information will be a critical parameter.

Increases in selection response from MAS within outbred populations obtained from simulation studies described in literature vary from 0 to more than 60%. Ruane and Colleau (1995) found a zero response when selecting for a trait that was independent of sex and carcass and when performance was tested before selection. Meuwissen and Goddard (1996) found a response of 64% when MAS was for a trait measured on carcasses, when selection was performed before measuring the trait. In the latter case, an important assumption was that at the moment MAS is implemented, marker genotype information is available for five ancestral generations. For a trait expressed in all animals but recorded after selection, additional response was 37% when five ancestral generations were recorded, but only 6% when only the grandparental generations were marker typed. The results of Ruane and Colleau (1995) and Meuwissen and Goddard (1996) were for nucleus breeding. Kashi, Hallerman, and Soller (1990) studied a progeny testing scheme where markers were used to select the young sires that enter the progeny test, i.e. markers were used in an extra selection step to preselect young bulls. This resulted in an extra response of up to 30%. Van der Beek and Van Arendonk (1996) studied an outbred poultry breeding nucleus with selection for a sex-limited trait where only a limited number of male full-sibs were allowed to be selected. In their study additional response to MAS was 6–12%, where most of the additional response was due to replacing a random selection of male full-sibs by a marker assisted pre-selection step within each full-sib family.

All studies report a decline in additional response over generations. Additional response is due to an accelerated increase of the frequencies of favourable QTL alleles. As soon as the favourable allele reaches a frequency above 0.5, an accelerated increase of QTL allele frequency results in an accelerated reduction of variance explained by the QTL, and therefore in reduced impact of MAS. Meanwhile, due to improved selection for the marked QTL, more selection intensity is focused on the QTL, and consequently less on the other genes. Therefore, in the long term, MAS might even result in reduced cumulative genetic gain since MAS only results in accelerated fixation of the QTL, which is only an improvement in time, but not in absolute level (as phenotypic selection would also ultimately fix the QTL), and decreases polygenic response. This phenomenon was most clearly demonstrated by Gibson (1994). From this observation no general conclusion on the effect of MAS on long term response should be drawn. Firstly, reduced long term response does not occur when MAS is applied at a stage or within a group of animals where normally no or random selection is applied. For example pre-selection of young bulls entering a progeny test does not influence selection pressure and hence response for genes not associated with a marker. Secondly, adapted selection strategies can be introduced. Instead of selecting animals with the maximum estimated breeding value, an index can be created in which the weight of selection on QTLs is reduced.

In the previous sections we saw that the benefits from MAS are highest when selection takes place at stages or in groups of animals where previously no selection was possible. The introduction of a new technology such as MAS requires a re-optimisation of the breeding programme and should provoke breeders to alter their breeding strategies. One of the first alterations suggested was pre-selection of young bulls entering the progeny test. A second alteration is to select before recording instead of after recording, which shows much promise. Massey and George (1992) took this idea to the extreme by suggesting 'Velogenetics'. In this scheme embryo's obtained from donor cows are genotyped for markers, and only embryos with favourable marker alleles are implanted into recipient cows. Van der Beek (1996) suggested multipurpose use of markers for a poultry breeding system. Currently, breeding hens are mated to one male only, because otherwise the sire of hatched chickens would be unknown. If markers would be applied for parentage control, however, this problem would disappear. So, hens can be mated to several sires when markers are used for parentage control. The same markers can also be used for marker assisted selection. The resulting breeding system has both the advantages of factorial mating and of marker assisted selection. Similar schemes can be developed for other species.

Marker assisted selection in outbred populations can generate a substantial increase in genetic response. This increase, however, can only be obtained under specific conditions and at the cost of many marker typings. In simulation studies the highest responses were realised when many offspring from one parent could be obtained, or if information of many generations preceding the generation of selection was available. Most promising are those systems where generation interval can be reduced significantly, as in Velogenetics, or when several uses of markers can be combined.

MARKERS AND QUALITY CONTROL

In addition to the use of markers through their linkage with genes affecting traits of economic importance, genetic markers can be used in many other ways. One possible use is to uniquely identify individuals (in parentage testing or, in humans, in forensic science), or, since genotypes can be obtained from any product containing DNA, to identify the source of animal products. For example, since species and breeds differ in their marker allele frequency, it should be possible to test the origin of an animal product using a specified set of genetic markers. So, it should be possible to test whether a piece of meat is from cattle, ostriches, or emus, and if from cattle, from which breed (was your steak really from an Aberdeen Angus?). Incidentally, discriminating between animal products from different species would probably be done using mitochondrial DNA markers.

In dairy cattle production, genetic markers could be used for random tests of parentage using non-invasive sampling techniques, e.g. using milk samples. The latter source of DNA also gives an interesting quality control measure for the milk recording organisations, since they could check the accuracy of their recording process by verifying the genotype of an individual cow from different milk samples.

MARKERS AND NON-ADDITIVE MODES OF INHERITANCE

As discussed already noted, for Mendelian traits displaying dominance, it would be impossible to distinguish between the heterozygote and one of the homozygotes without the use of genetic markers or progeny testing. In general, genetic markers could also greatly assist selection in the case of non-additive QTL. For example, markers might be used to improve heterosis in crossbred animals. If there are genes of large effects which are clearly over-dominant, i.e. the heterozygote is superior to either homozygote, then markers could be used to genotype animals for the gene and separate (sire and dam) parent lines could be created which are fixed for alternative alleles at the locus. It is not clear whether over-dominance for single loci (or for chromosomal segments comprising a number of linked loci) is a common phenomenon in livestock species and hence whether such an approach is worthwhile. Future QTL studies will clarify this point, but at least in some plant species, overdominance for chromosomal segments appears widespread (Stuber *et al*., 1992) and the manipulation of heterotic chromosome segments using markers seems to hold promise. However, in general it is very difficult to distinguish between true overdominance due to a single QTL and apparent overdominance due to several linked QTLs which display dominance but not overdominance (Eshed and Zamir, 1994, 1995).

If genetic markers can be used to aid selection decisions regarding the crossing of lines or breeds, it should also be possible to use them to control inbreeding within outbred populations. For example, markers can be used to determine a more exact inbreeding coefficient than calculations solely based on pedigree information. In any mating between related animals the average inbreeding coefficient of the progeny can be predicted, however, because whole segments of chromosomes are inherited, some progeny will be 'more inbred' than others. For example in a 'typical mammal', among full-sibs produced by a sire-daughter mating, the average inbreeding coefficient will be 25% and the expected standard deviation of the inbreeding coefficient approximately 7% (from Hill, 1993), so that some animals will have an actual level of homozygosity by descent of 10%, while others will be 40% inbred. In a recent study, Christensen *et al*. (1994) looked at 21 informative genetic markers (i.e. markers which can be traced backed from progeny to parents unequivocally) in progeny of a sire-daughter mating in pigs and among 37 animals found realised inbreeding as assessed using the markers varied from 6 to 42%, with a mean of 25% (i.e. as expected). Furthermore, growth performance appeared negatively related to the realised inbreeding. The study by Christensen *et al*. (1994) suggests that markers should allow the actual inbreeding coefficient of animals to be assessed and hence, if desired, animals could be selected from within families on the basis of their realised inbreeding coefficient. However, the extent to which such selection is of value in reducing the long term accumulation of inbreeding without jeopardising progress under selection is not clear. There is a potential conflict between using markers for selecting the best animals within a family (which are likely to be related) and selecting the least related to minimise inbreeding and this subject needs further study. However, many recent studies on increasing long-term response to selection using index and BLUP selection have shown that there is scope for decreasing levels of inbreeding substantially without sacrificing response to selection (Brisbane and Gibson, 1995; Wray and Goddard, 1994; Villanueva *et al*., 1995).

Very recently, a major gene called Calipyge was discovered in sheep which displays an inheritance mode called polar overdominance (Cockett *et al*., 1994). Sheep which receive a single copy of this gene from their sire display the Calipyge phenotype (i.e. large buttocks), whereas individuals receiving a copy from their dam do not show the phenotype. Furthermore, if an individual receives two copies of the gene, it again does not show the phenotype. This mode of inheritance would be nearly impossible to discover without the use of genetic markers, and it would also be impossible to exploit the phenotype properly in a selection programme without the use of markers. This is because mating individuals with superior growth characteristics and hind quarters, i.e. individuals carrying one copy of the Calipyge gene (inherited from their sire) using conventional pheno-typic selection would result in only one quarter of their progeny showing the desired phenotype.

CONCLUSIONS

The present use of genetic markers to aid selection decisions are dominated by markers linked to major genes and markers linked to qualitative traits (e.g. colour, disease resistance). However, the ESR marker (Rothschild *et al.*, 1994) in pig breeding provides a first example where a QTL is being exploited in popula-tion recently derived from a crossing event.

The use of markers linked to QTL in outbred populations is much more difficult. Firstly, because designs to map QTL in outbred populations are less powerful than mapping experiment from crossing divergent lines (e.g. Knott *et al.*, 1996), and secondly because conventional selection methods are competi-tive in the rate of fixation for positive QTL alleles. The potential strength of using genetic markers within outbred populations is to select where previously selection was random, for example by discrimination between estimated breeding value of full-sib dairy bulls before they enter a progeny test, and by radically changing the design of the breeding programme.

For the medium and long term we foresee that the cost of genotyping will become similar or even less than the cost of phenotyping and number or density of markers will not be a limiting factor. In that scenario, the bottleneck will be the number of animals with phenotypes, since they will provide information on the association between markers and quantitative traits and developing methods that are available to deal effectively with the vast wealth of information generated by such new technologies.

ACKNOWLEDGEMENTS

This work was partially funded by the Marker Assisted Selection Consortium of the British Pig Industry. SvdB was supported by the EU and Euribrid B.V. CSH acknowledges support from the BBSRC, MAFF, and the EU.

REFERENCES

Archibald, A.L., Brown, J.F., Couperwhite, S., McQueen, H.A., Nicholson, D., Haley, C.S. *et al.* (1995) The PiGMaP Consortium linkage map of the pig (*Sus scrofa*). *Mammalian Genome*, **6**, 157–175.
Barendse, W., Armitage, S.M., Kossarek, L.M., Shalom, A., Kirkpatrick, B.W., Ryan, A.M. *et al.* (1994) A genetic linkage map of the bovine genome. *Nature Genetics*, **6**, 227–235.

Beckmann, J.S. and Soller, M. (1983) Restriction fragment length polymorphisms in genetic improvement: methodologies, mapping and costs. *Theoretical and Applied Genetics*, **67**, 35–43.

Brisbane, J.R. and Gibson, J.P. (1995) Balancing selection response and rate of inbreeding by including genetic relationships in selection decisions. *Theoretical and Applied Genetics*, **91**, 421–431.

Brenneman, R.A., Davis, S.K., Sanders, J.O., Burns, B.M., Wheeler, T.C., Turner, J.W. *et al.* (1996) The polled locus maps to BTA1 in a Bos indicus × Bos taurus cross. *Journal of Heredity*, **87**, 157–161.

Burt, D.W., Bumstead, N., Bitgood, J.J., Ponce de Leon, F.A. and Crittenden, L.B. (1995) Chicken genome mapping: a new era in avian genetics. *Trends in Genetics*, **11**, 190–194.

Christensen, K., Fredholm, M., Winterø, A.K. and Andersen, S. (1994) Effect of identical homozygosity on growth in pigs. *Proceedings of the 5th World Congress on Genetics Applied to Livestock Production*, **19**, 155–158.

Cockett, N.E., Jackson, S.P., Shay, T.L., Nielsen, D., Moore, S., Steele, M.R. *et al.* (1994) Chromosomal localization of the callipyge gene in sheep (Ovis aries) using bovine DNA markers. *Proceedings of the National Academy of Sciences of the United States of America*, **91**, 3019–3023.

Crawford, A.M., Dodds, K.G., Ede, A.J., Pierson, C.A., Montgomery, G.W. and Garmonsway, H.G. (1995) An autosomal genetic linkage map of the sheep genome. *Genetics*, **140**, 703–724.

De Vicente, M.C. and Tanksley, S.D. (1993) QTL analysis of transgressive segregation in an interspecific tomato cross. *Genetics*, **134**, 585–596.

Dentine, M.R. (1992) Marker-assisted selection in cattle. *Animal Biotechnology*, **3**, 81–93.

Ellegren, H., Chowdhary, B.P., Johansson, M., Marklund, L., Fredholm, M., Gustavsson, I. *et al.* (1994) A primary linkage map of the porcine genome reveals a low rate of genetic recombination. *Genetics*, **137**, 1089–1100.

Eshed Y. and Zamir D. (1994) Introgressions from Lycopersicon pennelii can improve the soluble-solids yield of tomato hybrids. *Theoretical and Applied Genetics*, **88**, 891–897.

Eshed Y. and Zamir D. (1995) An introgression line population of Lycopersicon pennellii in the cultivated tomato enables the identification and fine mapping of yield associated QTL. *Genetics*, **141**, 1147–1162.

Gama, L.T., Smith, C. and Gibson, J.P. (1992) Transgene effects, introgression strategies and testing schemes in pigs. *Animal Production*, **54**, 427–440.

Gibbons, R.A., Selwood, R., Burrows, M. and Hunter, P.A. (1977) Inheritance of resistance to neonatal *E. Coli* diarrhoea in the pig: examination of the genetic system. *Theoretical and Applied Genetics*, **51**, 65–70.

Gibson, J.P. (1994) Short-term gain at the expense of long-term response with selection of identified loci. *Proceedings of the 5th World Congress on Genetics Applied to Livestock Production*, **21**, 201–204.

Gimelfarb, A. and Lande, R. (1994) Simulation of marker assisted selection in hybrid populations. *Genetical Research*, **63**, 39–47.

Groen, A.F. and Timmermans, M.M.J. (1992) The use of genetic markers to increase the efficiency of introgression — a simulation study. *Proceedings of the XIX World's Poultry Congress*, **1**, 523–527.

Groen, A.F. and Smith, C. (1995) A stochastic simulation study on the efficiency of marker-assisted introgression in livestock. *Journal of Animal Breeding and Genetics*, **112**, 161–170.

Haley, C.S. (1991) Considerations in the development of future pig breeding programs. *Australasian Journal of Animal Science*, **4**, 305–328.

Haley, C.S., Williams, J., Woolliams, J.A. and Visscher, P.M. (1996) Gene mapping and its place in livestock improvement. British Cattle Breeders Club, *Digest no. 51*.

Havenstein, G.B., Ferket, P.R., Scheideler, S.E. and Rives, D.V. (1994) Carcass composition and yield of 1991 vs 1957 broilers when fed typical 1957 and 1991 broiler diets. *Poultry Science*, **73**, 1795–1804.

Henderson, C.R. (1973) Sire evaluation and genetic trends. *Proceedings of the animal breeding and genetics symposium in honour of Dr. J.L. Lush*, 10–40.

Hill, W.G. (1993) Variation in genetic composition in backcrossing programs. *The Journal of Heredity*, **84**, 212–213.

Hillel, J., Schaap, T., Haberfield, A., Jeffreys, A.J., Plotzky, Y., Cahaner, A. *et al.* (1990) DNA fingerprints applied to gene introgression in breeding programs. *Genetics*, **124**, 783–789.

Hillel, J., Verrinder Gibbins, M., Etches, R.J. and Shaver, D. McQ. (1993) Strategies for the rapid introgression of a specific gene modification into a commercial poultry flock from a single carrier. *Poultry Science*, **72**, 1197–1211.

Hospital, F., Chevalet, C. and Mulsant, P. (1992) Using markers in gene introgression breeding programs. *Genetics*, **132**, 1199–1210.

Johansson, M., Ellegren, H., Marklund, L., Gustavsson, U., Ringmar-Cederberg, E., Andersson, K. *et al.* (1992) The gene for dominant white color in the pig is closely linked to ALB and PDGFRA on chromosome 8. *Genomics*, **14**, 965–969.

Moller, M. (1995) Comparative genome analysis in the pig. Ph.D. Thesis. Swedish University of Agricultural Sciences, Uppsala, Sweden.

Kashi Y., Hallerman E. and Soller, M. (1990) Marker assisted selection of candidate bulls for progeny testing programmes. *Animal Production*, **51**, 63–74.

Knott, S.A., Elsen, J.M. and Haley, C.S. (1996) Methods for multiple marker mapping of quantitative trait loci in half-sib populations. *Theoretical and Applied Genetics*, **93**, 71–80.

Lande, R. and Thompson, R. (1990) Efficiency of marker assisted selection in the improvement of quantitative traits. *Genetics*, **124**, 743–756.

Massey, J.M. and Georges, M. (1992) Genmark's approach to marker-assisted selection. *Animal Biotechnology*, **3**, 95–109.

Meuwissen, T.H.E. and Goddard, M.E. (1996) The use of marker haplotypes in animal breeding. schemes. *Genetics Selection Evolution*, **28**, 161–176.

Milan, D., Le Roy, P., Woloszyn, N., Caritez, J.C., Elsen, J.M., Sellier, P. *et al.* (1995) The RN locus for meat quality maps to pig chromosome 15. *Genetics Selection Evolution*, **27**, 195–199.

Patterson, H.D. and Thompson, R. (1971) Recovery of interblock information when block sizes are unequal. *Biometrika*, **58**, 545–554.

Rohrer, G.A., Alexander, L.J., Keele, J.W., Smith, T.P. and Beattie, C.W. (1994) A microsatellite linkage map of the porcine genome. *Genetics*, **136**, 231–245.

Rothschild, M.F., Jacobson, C., Vaske, D.A., Tuggle, C.K., Short, T.H., Sasaki, S. *et al.* (1994) A major gene for litter size in pigs. *Proceedings of the 5th World Congress on Genetics Applied to Livestock Production*, **21**, 225–228.

Ruane, J. and Colleau, J.J. (1995) Marker assisted selection for genetic improvement of animal populations when a single QTL is marked. *Genetical Research*, **66**, 71–83.

Schmutz, S.M., Marquess, F.L.S., Berryere, T.G. and Moker, J.S. (1995) DNA marker-assisted selection of the polled condition in Charolais cattle. *Mammalian Genome*, **6**, 710–713.

Smith, C. (1984) Rates of genetic change in farm livestock. *Research and Development in Agriculture*, **1**, 79–85.

Smith, C. and Simpson, S.P. (1986) The use of polymorphisms in livestock improvement. *Journal of Animal Breeding and Genetics*, **103**, 205–217.

Smith, C. and Smith, D.B. (1993) The need for close linkages in marker-assisted selection for economic merit in livestock. *Animal Breeding Abstracts*, **61**, 197–204.

Smith, C., Meuwissen, T.H.E. and Gibson, J.P. (1987) On the use of transgenes in livestock improvement. *Animal Breeding Abstracts*, **55**, 1–10.

Southwood, O.J., Hoste, S., Short, T.H., Mileham, A.J. and Cuthbert-Heavens, D. (1996) Evaluation of genetic markers for litter size in Meishan synthetic and Large White pigs. *Proceedings of the British Society of Animal Science winter meeting*, **18**.

Stuber, C.W., Lincoln, S.E., Wolff, D.W., Helentjaris, T. and Lander, E.S. (1992) Identification of genetic factors contributing to heterosis in a hybrid from two elite maize inbred lines using molecular markers. *Genetics*, **132**, 823–839.

Van der Beek, S. and Van Arendonk, J.A.M. (1996) Marker-assisted selection in an outbred poultry breeding nucleus. *Animal Science*, **62**, 171–180.

Van der Beek, S. (1996) The use of genetic markers in poultry breeding. Ph.D. Thesis, Wageningen Agricultural University, Wageningen, The Netherlands.

Villanueva, B., Woolliams, J.A. and Simm, G. (1994) Strategies for controlling rates of inbreeding in MOET nucleus schemes for beef cattle. *Genetics Selection Evolution*, **26**, 517–535.

Visscher, P.M. (1995) Bias in genetic R^2 from halfsib designs. *Genetics Selection Evolution*, **27**, 335–345.

Visscher, P.M., Haley, C.S. and Thompson, R. (1996) Marker-assisted introgression in backcross breeding programs. *Genetics*, **144**, 1923–1932.

Wishart, J. (1931) The mean and second moment coefficient of the multiple correlation coefficient in samples from a normal population. *Biometrika*, **22**, 353–361.

Wray, N.R. and Goddard, M.E. (1994) Increasing long-term response to selection. *Genetics Selection Evolution*, **26**, 431–451.

Zhang, W. and Smith, C. (1992) The use of marker assisted selection with linkage disequilibrium. *Theoretical and Applied Genetics*, **83**, 813–820.

Zhang, W. and Smith, C. (1993) The use of marker assisted selection with linkage disequilibrium: the effects of several additional factors. *Theoretical and Applied Genetics*, **86**, 492–496.

7. COMPARATIVE GENOME MAPPING — THE LIVESTOCK PERSPECTIVE

ALAN L. ARCHIBALD*

Roslin Institute (Edinburgh), Roslin, Midlothian, EH25 9PS, Scotland, UK

The genomes of farmed animals, such as pigs, cattle and chickens are being mapped in order to identify genes controlling traits of economic importance. There is evidence of extensive conservation of genome organisation amongst higher vertebrates including these farm animals and more extensively characterised species, such as humans and mice. The primary goal of comparative mapping is to define relationships between species in terms of chromosomal evolution by mapping break-points and gene evolution by evaluating the structural and functional similarities between homologous genes. Amongst the benefits of comparative genome mapping are that a gene mapped in one species is effectively mapped in all other species for which the conserved genome structures have been identified. The observed conservation of genome organisation will allow the wealth of information being generated by the Human Genome Project to be exploited in the search for trait genes in farmed animals. Thus, comparative genome mapping in livestock will not only contribute to the understanding of genome evolution but is critical to current strategies for trait gene identification.

KEY WORDS: gene mapping; comparative gene mapping; genome; livestock; pigs; cattle; poultry.

INTRODUCTION

Comparative genome mapping and analysis are key facets of the Human Genome Project. Genome research on model organisms such as yeast, *C. elegans* and mouse is not only useful for the development of new techniques but also generates results that inform our interpretation of the relationship between genes and function. For example, the complete DNA sequence of the yeast *Saccharomyces cerevisiae* has been determined. This simple organism is estimated to have only 6000 genes, i.e. about one tenth of the genetic repertoire of humans and other mammals (Goffeau *et al.*, 1996). Yet many basic molecular functions, in terms of intermediate metabolism, protein synthesis and DNA replication are common to yeast and higher organisms. Thus, it is anticipated that the understanding of the genetic control of essential life parameters acquired from studying simpler organisms, which can be manipulated experimentally, will be applicable to humans and other higher vertebrates.

Comparisons of sequences both at the nucleotide and protein levels are useful in elucidating the relationships between gene or protein structure and function. Such sequence comparisons are not only valuable in determining how genes or proteins fulfill their specific functions but also contribute to the definition of sequences motifs. Such sequence motifs whether written in the four letter alphabet of DNA or in the twenty letter alphabet of proteins represent key

*Tel.: +44 (131) 527 4200. Fax: +44 (131) 440 0434. E-mail: Alan.Archibald@bbsrc.ac.uk.

elements or words in the language of life. The resulting lexicon can be used in attempts to decipher unknown DNA sequences, such as those generated by the yeast sequencing project. However, comparative genome analysis is held together with more than just the knowledge that this particular consensus sequence has a high affinity for a particular transcription factor or encodes a binding domain for a particular substrate. The similarities between chicken and sheep hemoglobin are not coincidences but are present because they are encoded by genes that are linked through evolution.

The DNA sequence of an organism is often referred to as the ultimate genome map. However, comparative genome analysis is also possible with maps of lower resolution. Genes that are found close to each other in one species are also often found close to each other in other species. This conservation of the spatial relationships between genes is also the result of shared evolutionary history.

Thus, comparative genome analysis and mapping only really makes sense in an evolutionary context. If there were no evolutionary relationships between organisms there would be no point in comparative genome analysis or mapping. The primary goal of comparative mapping is to define those relationships in terms of chromosomal evolution (map break-points) and gene evolution (structure and function) and thus comparative mapping can be justified in terms of understanding basic biological questions. Amongst the benefits of comparative genome mapping are that a gene mapped in one species is effectively mapped in all other species for which the conserved genome structures have been identified. For example, trait genes mapped in experimental animals including farm animals will provide candidate phenotypes for the thousands of expressed sequence tags (EST) of unknown function being mapped in humans and mice. Similarly the catalogue of mapped human and murine ESTs will provide candidate genes to explain traits being mapped in livestock.

In this chapter I will restrict myself to a consideration of comparative genome mapping of farm animals. For the sake of brevity I have not included farmed or harvested species of fish. The emphasis on examples from studies of the pig genome reflects my research interests and is meant to be illustrative rather than proscriptive.

GENES AND EVOLUTION — HOMOLOGY

Genes evolve divergently through mutation and gene duplication. Genes that share a common evolutionary past can be considered to be homologous. New genetic material can arise by gene duplication, either by regional duplication or by tetraploidization. Both these mechanisms of gene duplication give rise to 'paralogous' genes through subsequent divergent evolution (see Lundin, 1993, for discussion of paralogous and orthologous genes). Thus, paralogous genes exist within a species, have a common ancestral gene and explain the existence of gene families. Orthologous genes are found in different species and have diverged from a common ancestral gene as part of the process of speciation and separate evolution. The two concepts may be described as "species phylogeny" of "orthologous" genes between species and "gene phylogeny" of "paralogous" genes within a species (Bishop, 1994). The presence of extensive gene families makes it difficult to establish the orthologous relationships between genes in different species. The difficulties are compounded by the presence of pseudogenes which are supposed to be nonfunctional relics of members of gene families and by the loss of genes during evolution. The essence of comparative genome analysis is to establish the evolutionary history and links between genes in different species. The trees developed to explain these histories need to be developed without access to the intermediate ancestral species.

Criteria for Assessing Homology Relationships

As the ancestral species that provide the evolutionary links between current species are missing homology between genes in different species can only be inferred. The strength of the inference or claim of homology is dependent upon the quality of supporting evidence. Scientists engaged in comparative genome mapping have developed a series of criteria for evaluating homology relationships (Lalley *et al.*, 1989; O'Brien, 1991; O'Brien and Graves, 1991; Andersson *et al.*, 1996). The criteria are subject to constant review to take account of changes in technology and in our understanding of gene and genome evolution. The latest criteria are published in the report from the 1st International Workshop on Comparative Genome Organization (Andersson *et al.*, 1996). The revised criteria are (the most stringent are marked *):

Gene or other DNA sequence
- similar nucleotide sequence*
- cross-hybridization to the same molecular probe*
- conserved map position*
- similar transcription profile

Protein
- similar amino acid sequence*
- similar subunit structure and formation of functional heteropolymer
- immunological cross-reaction
- similar expression profile
- similar subcellular location
- similar substrate specificity
- similar response to specific inhibitors

Phenotype
- similar mutant phenotype
- complementation of function*

Nucleotide or amino acid sequence similarity as determined directly by sequence comparison or indirectly by cross-hybridization with molecular probes are the core criteria in assessing homology. Amongst the advantages of these criteria are the scope for quantitative rather than solely qualitative comparisons. The degree of sequence similarity can be expressed in terms of percentage identity in a defined region. For protein sequences pairs of amino acids in the aligned sequences, which are similar (e.g. phenylalanine and tryptophan are both aromatic and hydrophobic) rather than identical can also contribute to the overall comparison.

Complementation of function has been added to the latest list of criteria as transgenic technology now allow complementation tests to break the species barriers.

The most recent report from the committee on comparative gene mapping "recommends that comparative gene mapping papers should always state the criteria used to assess homology" (Graves *et al.*, 1996). I would extend the scope of this recommendation to papers that describe the mapping of *genes* in any species. In such gene mapping papers the use of a particular locus or gene symbol or name carries the implication that the gene described is homologous to a gene with the same symbol or name mapped earlier in another species. These implied claims of homology through the use of common nomenclature are then picked up and promulgated by the authors of comparative gene mapping review papers, database editors and even in the reports of the committee on comparative gene mapping.

Map Position as Evidence of Homology

The reasoning behind adding conserved map position to the list of criteria for assessing homology between genes in the context of comparative gene mapping can appear circular. Gene A_x and gene B_x are found tightly linked in species X. The map location of the homologue of gene A_x (A_y) is known in species Y. A gene, B_y, with some similarity to gene B_x is mapped close to gene A in species Y. Therefore, it is concluded that B_y is homologous to B_x and is cited as evidence of conservation of the A–B region. I have been outspoken in arguing that conserved map location was an inappropriate criteria for assessing homology between genes when the inferred homologies are then used to define conserved chromosomal regions. However, I now agree with Andersson *et al.* (1996) that "(the) overwhelming evidence for linkage conservation among mammal and vertebrate species" justifies the inclusion of "conserved map position" as "an important criterion of homology" that may be "particularly valuable in distinguishing between members of a gene family".

COMPARATIVE GENOME MAPPING

Terminology

As in many emerging fields of research and indeed with language itself there is scope for confusion in the careless use of words to describe new concepts. For the sake of clarity it is worth restating the meaning of some key terms. First, *synteny* means on the same chromosome. Thus, whilst two loci may be syntenic within a species, gene A in species X cannot be syntenic with gene B in species Y. However, syntenic relationships can be conserved across species. Thus, *conserved synteny* is a syntenic relationship between two or more homologous genes that is conserved in two or more species. As genes are syntenic merely if they are on the same chromosome a conserved synteny does not imply that all, or indeed any, of the genes that lie between the homologous loci will be conserved in both species. In a *conserved segment* two or more homologous genes in two or more species are found together in a contiguous block in which it is assumed that the genes are conserved in both species. The term *conserved order* covers cases where three or more homologous loci are found in the same order on one chromosome in each of the species under consideration. Finally, O'Brien *et al.* (1993) proposed the term smallest conserved evolutionary unit segment (SCEUS) as the shortest set of homologous genes on a conserved segment in two or more species regardless of gene order. Ordered SCEUS are a subclass of SCEUS in which the gene order is also conserved across all the species of interest. These terms are illustrated in Figure 7.1.

ZOO-FISH — The Big Picture

An overview of the conservation of synteny between two species can be revealed by heterologous chromosome painting. This elegant technique was initially demonstrated by painting chromosomes from primates with human chromosome-specific probes (Weinberg *et al.*, 1990; Jauch *et al.*, 1992). Probes generated from chromosome-specific libraries were used in chromosomal *in situ* suppression (CISS) hybridization to examine chromosomal rearrangements that have occurred in the recent evolution of primate species. Screthan *et al.*, (1994) extended this approach to the analysis of quite distantly related mammals, including human, mice, Muntjacs and whales.

The first reported use of heterologous chromosome painting or ZOO-FISH in a farmed animal species concerned the pig (Rettenberger *et al.*, 1995). These ZOO-FISH experiments in which pig chromosomes were painted with human chromosome-specific probes revealed 47 blocks of conserved synteny between humans and pigs (see Figure 7.2). Although these results are largely confirmed by data from Fronïcke *et al.* (1996), there are some differences between the two reports. For example, Fronïcke *et al.* (1996) report that the pig X chromosome is successfully painted with a human X chromosome-specific probes as would be expected from knowledge of the conservation of the X chromosome amongst Eutherian mammals. Fronïcke *et al.* (1996) also argue that Rettenberger *et al.* (1995) have misidentified the arms of pig chromosome 10 and that HSA10 paints SSC10p rather than SSC10q. The results of Fronïcke *et al.* (1996) with the HSA10 paint are confirmed by Goureau *et al.* (1996). Similarly, Fronïcke *et al.* (1996) report that amongst other regions the HSA1 probes paints SSC10q rather than SSC10p as recorded by Rettenberger *et al.* (1995). In contrast, the HSA1 probe

Species X

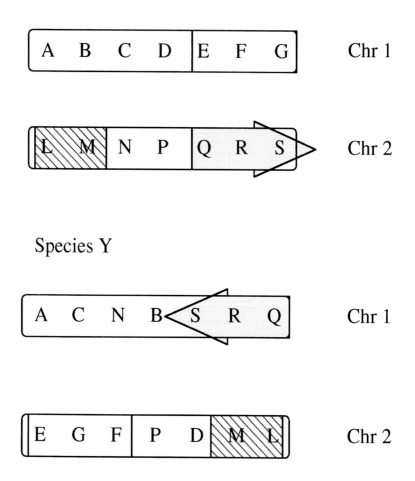

Species Y

Figure 7.1 Illustration of terms — synteny, conserved synteny, conserved segment and conserved order. The arrangements of homologous genes in two species are shown. In species X — A, B, C, D, E, F and G are syntenic or constitute a synteny group as they are located on a single chromosome. As A, B and C are syntenic in both species X and Y they represent a conserved synteny group, conserved syntenic relationship or simply a conserved synteny. Other examples of conserved synteny in this diagram include — [D, E, F, G]; [L, M, P] and [N, Q, R, S]. E, G and F constitute a conserved segment as this group in species Y is not interrupted by genes which are not also syntenic in species X. Q, R and S constitute a conserved orders — a special category of conserved segments in which the gene order is conserved in the species under consideration. As three or more loci are required to define order M and L can only be classified as a conserved segment. When gene order and syntenic relationships are compared across more than two species the segments conserved across all species are termed SCEUs or smallest conserved evolutionary unit segments.

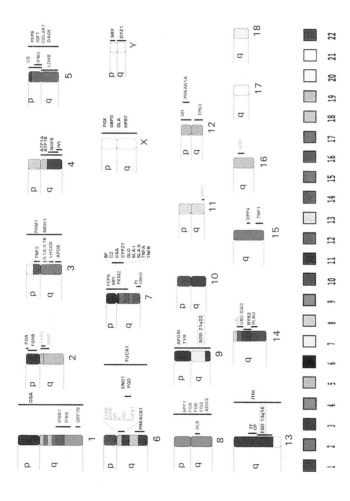

Figure 7.2 Visualization of conserved synteny between the human and porcine genomes (after Rettenberger *et al.*, 1995). This figure summarises the results of 22 separate heterologous chromosome painting experiments, in which human chromosome-specific probes were used for fluorescent *in situ* hybridization to pig chromosomes. For example, the human chromosome 4 specific probes only hybridised to pig chromosome 8; the human chromosome 7 probes hybridised to pig chromosome 18 and a region on the long arm of pig chromosome 9 (SSC9q11–q21). Gene map assignments at the time of the original publication are shown to the right of each pig chromosome. [From Rettenberger *et al.*, 1995. Reproduced with the kind permission of the authors and of Academic Press, *Genomics* **26**, 372–378].

used by Goureau *et al.* (1996) failed to yield a signal on SSC10 or on SSC14. Most of the remaining differences between these reports concern the delineation of the boundaries between blocks of conserved synteny.

There is agreement that four human autosome-specific probes each lit up all of a single pig chromosome — HSA4–SSC8; HSA13–SSC11; HSA17–SSC12 and HSA20–SSC17. Thus, we can conclude that these pairs of human and porcine chromosomes represent blocks of conserved synteny. The remaining human chromosome-specific probes lit up either more than two regions of the porcine genome or only part of a pig chromosome. From these latter data it is not possible to identify unambiguously the specific genomic segments that are conserved between humans and pigs. These conserved regions can be defined by repeating the heterologous chromosome painting in the opposite direction, i.e. painting human chromosomes with porcine chromosome-specific probes. Goureau *et al.* (1996) have partially completed this bi-directional analysis — human on pig and pig on human.

The conservation of synteny between humans and cattle and between humans and horses has also been addressed by chromosome painting (Solinas-Toldo *et al.*, 1995; Hayes *et al.*, 1995; Chowdhary *et al.*, 1996; Raudsepp *et al.*, 1996). Chowdhary *et al.* (1996) identified 46 homologous chromosomal segments conserved between humans and cattle. Studies are currently in progress to compare the bovine and porcine genomes by heterologous chromosome painting (Gerard Frélat, personal communication). Chromosome painting has also been used to determine the correspondence between the chromosomes of the domestic pig (*Sus scrofa*) and the chromosomes of babirusa (*Babyrousa bayrussa*) which is a distantly related member of the *Suidae* family (Bosma *et al.*, 1996). Briefly, by comparison of conventionally banded karyotypes it is possible to match 13 of the 18 autosomal pairs of babirusa chromosomes with specific domestic pig chromosomes or chromosome arms. The babirusa homologues of pig chromosomes 1, 3 and 6 cannot be determined in this manner. Probes specific for pig chromosomes 1, 3 and 6 painted babirusa chromosomes 15, 12+17, and 6+14 respectively and allowed the completion of the comparison of the pig and babirusa karyotypes (Bosma *et al.*, 1996).

The summary of conservation of synteny as revealed by heterologous chromosome painting is generally supported by map locations of homologous loci in the species of interest. Given the prior knowledge of conserved syntenies from comparative gene mapping data one might speculate that the interpretation of the inprecise chromosome painting images was shaped by this knowledge. The validity of the ZOO-FISH data is therefore most effectively tested where there was a lack of prior gene mapping data. For example, Rettenberger *et al.* (1995) and Fronïcke *et al.* (1996) identified a segment conserved on HSA18 and SSC6q in the absence of map locations for porcine homologues of HSA18 loci. The recent mapping to SSC6q of the porcine homologue of TTR, which maps to HSA18, confirms the predictions of the ZOO-FISH data (Archibald *et al.*, 1996a).

Conservation of Synteny Can Also Be Revealed by Gene Mapping Studies

The remarkable conservation of synteny between farmed mammals and human revealed by ZOO-FISH experiments was already evident from earlier gene mapping studies. In particular, the work of Womack and others at Texas A&M University indicated that there was greater conservation of synteny between the human and bovine genomes than between the human and murine genomes (Womack and Moll, 1986; Fries *et al.*, 1989; Womack, 1994; Womack and Kata, 1995). A panel of cattle-hamster somatic hybrid cells was established by fusing bovine white blood cells with HPRT deficient Chinese hamster cells and selecting for the presence of an active HPRT gene. The resulting hybrid cells lose bovine chromosomes at random. Initially the panel was examined for the presence of enzymes encoded by cattle genes retained in some, but not all hybrids. Twenty-eight enzyme-encoding loci were assigned to 21 syntenic groups (Womack and Moll, 1986). The authors aligned these and other published bovine synteny groups with the then current human and murine gene maps. There were fewer discordancies in syntenic relationships between humans and cattle than between humans and mice. Womack and Moll (1986) concluded that the organisation of the human and bovine genomes are more conserved than those of the human and murine genomes. The somatic hybrid cell panel has subsequently been used extensively for synteny mapping in cattle employing molecular techniques. Through the use of this panel Womack's group has made a major contribution to gene mapping in cattle and confirmed the early conclusion of extensive conservation of synteny between humans and cattle. Recently, Womack and Kata (1995) have stated that the difference in the degree of conservation between (a) humans and mice and (b) humans and cattle was not as great as originally predicted by Womack and Moll (1986).

Similar synteny mapping studies in sheep have demonstrated that there is also considerable conservation of synteny between humans and sheep. Conventional somatic hybrid cells have not been used to the same extent for gene mapping in pigs and not at all in chickens.

Quantifying Conservation of Synteny

From an analysis of less than 83 homologous loci mapped in both humans and mice Nadeau and Taylor (1984) estimated that the average length of conserved autosomal segments as 8.1 ± 1.6 centimorgans. Using information from fifteen times as many mapped homologous loci Copeland *et al.* (1993) concluded that segments conserved between humans and mice have an average length of 8.8 cM, thus confirming the validity of Nadeau and Taylor's model. One hundred and five conserved autosomal segments and eight conserved segments on the X chromosome have been identified by examining mapping data for over 1747 homologous loci in humans and mice (Andersson *et al.*, 1996). In contrast, the heterologous chromosome painting experiments summarised above indicate that there are about fifty (i.e. fewer and larger) genomic segments conserved between humans and representative Artiodactyls such as cattle and pigs.

Bengtsson *et al.* (1993) have developed methods for quantifying the degree of reorganisation between species. More recently, Law and Burt (1996) have written a computer program for calculating these measures of genome reorganisation from mapping data.

Conservation of Synteny Does Not Mean Conservation of Gene Order

Uni-directional heterologous chromosome painting and synteny mapping in somatic hybrid cell allows the definition of conserved syntenies between species. Conserved segments within conserved syntenies can be delineated by the application of bi-directional heterologous chromosome painting (Goureau *et al.*, 1996). These methods, however, do not indicate whether the gene order within the conserved regions is also conserved. Comparative gene order is critical both to understanding chromosome evolution and in exploiting comparative gene mapping to identify trait genes as described below. There is a tendency to assume conservation of gene order on the basis of conserved synteny. Nadeau (1989) explicitly distinguishes between conservation of syntenic relationships and conservation of gene order. He uses *linkage conservation* in place of *conserved order* as defined above.

Heterologous chromosome painting results using human probes to paint porcine chromosomes and *vice versa* demonstrate that human chromosome 8 and porcine chromosome 4 represent not only a conserved synteny but also a conserved segment (Rettenberger *et al.*, 1995; Fronïcke *et al.*, 1996; Goureau *et al.*, 1996). Gene mapping data, with one exception support this conclusion. The exception concerns chromogranin A (CHGA), which maps to HSA 14, but which has also been mapped to SSC8. A restriction fragment length polymorphism (RFLP) revealed with a porcine chromogranin A probe (Couperwhite *et al.*, 1993) was mapped by linkage analysis to SSC8 (Archibald *et al.*, 1995). More recently, CHGA has been mapped by fluorescence *in situ* hybridization to SSC7q24–q26 as would be predicted from comparative mapping data (Kojima *et al.*, 1996). These recent data suggest that the earlier linkage, RFLP data should be checked, as should the identity of the probe used for the RFLP experiments.

Although human chromosome 8 and porcine chromosome 4 appear to represent a conserved segment, the order of genes within this segment is not conserved (Ellegren *et al.*, 1993, see Figure 7.3). Similar, differences in gene order within human–pig conserved segments are described by Johansson *et al.* (1995).

Developing Ordered Gene Maps for Comparative Mapping

As noted above, conservation of synteny does not equate with conservation of gene order. In order to implement the comparative positional candidate gene approach described below for isolating trait genes in livestock it will be necessary to develop ordered gene maps for farm animals.

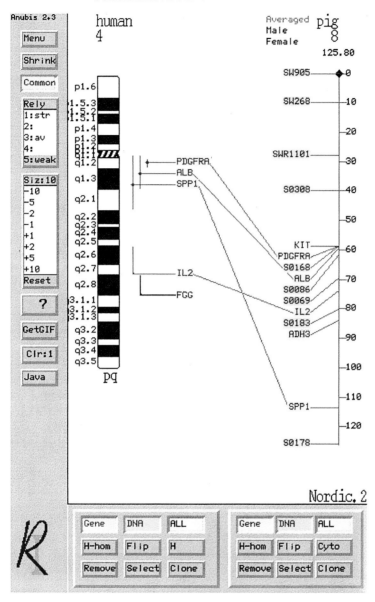

Figure 7.3 Comparison of human chromosome 4 and pig chromosome 8. A linkage map of pig chromosome 8 (Marklund *et al.*, 1996) is shown aligned to a very simplified cytogenetic map of human chromosome 4. The map alignment was effected with the Anubis map viewer (Mungall, 1996; http://www.ri.bbsrc.ac.uk/cgi-bin/anubis). Within the conserved synteny between human chromosome 4 and pig chromosome 8, the inversion of the IL2-SPP1 interval is evident (see Johansson *et al.*, 1992). This image was downloaded from the prototype of The Comparative Animal Genome database mounted on the Roslin Institute's World Wide Web genome server.

There are two approaches for developing genome-wide ordered gene maps — linkage or radiation hybrid mapping. Linkage mapping has proved an effective means of constructing high resolution gene maps in mice by exploiting the polymorphism between the *Mus musculus* and *Mus spretus* species (Copeland *et al.*, 1993). Over 2000 genes have now been mapped in the Frederick cross. Crosses between genetically divergent stocks exemplified by the Wild Boar × Swedish Yorkshire (Marklund *et al.*, 1996) or the Chinese Meishan × European breeds (Archibald *et al.*, 1995) used for pig linkage mapping have proved useful for mapping genes. For example, about 200 genes have been mapped by the PiGMaP Linkage Consortium. However, the genetic differences between these pig breeds is not as great as the differences between the *Mus musculus* and *Mus spretus* species. Thus, even in these breeds it has been difficult to develop polymorphic markers for genes and the limited degree of polymorphism means that many of the markers associated with genes are not mapped robustly. These difficulties highlight the paradox of mapping genes by linkage analysis. Genes represent the conserved portions of the genome yet variation or polymorphism is an absolute requirement for linkage mapping.

Mapping by irradiation and fusion gene transfer (IFGT), also known as radiation hybrid mapping, is not limited by the need for polymorphic markers and thus could make a valuable contribution to gene mapping and comparative gene mapping in livestock (Walter and Goodfellow, 1993; Walter *et al.*, 1994). Briefly, donor cells (e.g. pig fibroblasts) are irradiated and fused to hamster A23 (*TK⁻*) recipient cells (Walter *et al.*, 1994). A radiation dose of about 3–5 Krads is used to generate fragments of the appropriate size range for a map of 1 Mbp resolution. Selection in HAT medium will yield radiation hybrid clones which have retained random fragments of the donor (e.g. pig) genome in addition to the donor genome's *TK* locus. A panel of radiation hybrids are established which are scored for the presence or absence of DNA sequences from the donor genome, usually by PCR. As the hybrids are only assayed for the presence or absence of the donor DNA sequences there is no requirement for polymorphism. Thus, genes can be mapped readily assuming that the donor genes can be distinguished from those of the rodent recipient cells. By focusing on the 3′UT regions of genes this problem can be minimised. Whole genome radiation hybrids have made a major contribution to the recently published human gene map which encompasses 16,000 genes (Schuler *et al.*, 1996). In collaboration with Professor Peter Goodfellow's laboratory, my group are developing a radiation hybrid map of the porcine genome. Womack and colleagues are also developing radiation hybrids for mapping in cattle (Schlöpfer *et al.*, 1996).

CATS — A Framework for Comparative Genome Mapping?

The alignment of genome maps from different animal species is not only limited by the relative paucity of mapped genes in species other than humans and mice, but also by the proportion of mapped genes that are mapped in more than one species. As a first attempt to address the need for a common set of reference loci for comparative gene mapping O'Brien *et al.* (1993) identified a set of so-called anchored reference loci. The 321 anchored reference loci were selected on the basis that they were cloned human and mouse genes which were well distributed throughout the human and mouse genome. Where known, the map locations of the homologous loci in cattle and domestic cats were cited. Although the proportion of these loci which were mapped in other species increased, the hopes of O'Brien and his collaborators that all 321 anchored reference loci would be rapidly mapped in a wide range of animals were not fulfilled.

In order to facilitate the establishment of a common framework for comparative gene mapping in animals Lyons *et al.* (1997) have attempted to develop evolutionary conserved (PCR) primer pairs for amplification of anchor loci from any mammalian DNA source. The so-called *comparative anchor tagged sequences (or CATS)* were developed from alignments of DNA sequences of homologous genes from several species. The PCR primer pairs designed from these sequence alignments were optimised for the amplification of domestic cat DNA. The optimised PCR conditions were also tested on DNA from twenty other mammalian species. Of 410 CATS primers, 318 were optimised for the cat. Eighty-five percent of the resulting cat PCR products exhibited sequence similarity to the expected locus. Lyons *et al.* (1997) claim that 32–52% of the 318 CATS primers optimised on cat DNA yield a single PCR product under the same conditions when used for PCR on other mammalian DNA. The CATS primers were widely distributed prior to publication to scientists engaged in gene mapping in other species (Raney *et al.*, 1996; Zhang *et al.*, 1996). Results to date have been mixed with some laboratories reporting fewer than expected single PCR products and the sequences of some PCR products exhibiting no relationship to the expected sequence. Moreover, if mapping in radiation hybrids is to be the method of choice for gene mapping, there is a potential difficulty in using the CATS markers which have been designed for amplification from all mammalian DNA. The difficulties arise because there may be problems distinguishing between the PCR products generated from the recipient (rodent) genome and from the donor genome.

STATUS OF COMPARATIVE GENE MAPS
WITH RESPECT TO LIVESTOCK

There are a plethora of comparative gene mapping publications. In essence many authors attempt to add substance to papers describing the mapping of gene(s) by discussing the impact of the new mapping data on comparative gene mapping. It is not necessary to refer specifically to comparative gene mapping papers in order to evaulate the current status of comparative gene maps. The number of genes mapped in the species of interest is indicative of the quality of the respective comparative gene maps. The resulting predictions concerning the comparative maps should be qualified by an evaluation of the number of (homologous) genes mapped in common in the species of interest. As genes are being added to the maps of farmed animals on a daily basis it is no longer prudent to quote figures for the number of genes mapped in these species. Rather, the reader should refer to the genome databases discussed below. These sources indicate that ~400 genes have been mapped in cattle, ~ 300 in pigs, ~ 240 in sheep and ~ 140 in chickens. The information in the livestock genome databases is currently (March, 1997) not completely up to date. Following a period of database development efforts are being made to enter a backlog of data.

The Bovine Genome Is a Model for Sheep and Goats and Perhaps Deer Also

The karyotypes of cattle, sheep and goats are similar (Hayes *et al.*, 1991). Indeed, the similarity in banding pattern between bovine and ovine chromosomes has been cited as evidence of conservation of genome organisation between these species (Hediger *et al.*, 1991). The predicted homologies between cattle and sheep chromosomes are further supported by gene mapping data (Echard *et al.*, 1994; Broad *et al.*, 1996). The conservation of sequences between cattle and sheep and also between cattle and goats includes anonymous DNA sequences such as microsatellite markers (Moore *et al.*, 1991; Kemp *et al.*, 1995). Microsatellites that are polymorphic in one of these species tend to be monomorphic in the others. The study of these markers between species may be useful in understanding the evolution of these polymorphic loci. However, I am not convinced about the merits of using a panel of the same microsatellite markers for genetic diversity studies within each species.

The value of the extensive conservation between the bovine and ovine genomes was demonstrated recently by the use of bovine microsatellite markers to map the callipyge muscle hypertrophy gene in sheep (Cockett *et al.*, 1994).

The bovine genome map may also serve as a model for the genome maps of other advanced pecorans, including buffalo and deer. Comparative cytogenetic studies of chromosomes from a range of bovid species (Gallagher and Womack, 1992; Iannuzzi and DiMeo, 1995) and advanced pecorans (Gallagher *et al.*, 1994) have revealed extensive conservation of banding patterns and karyotypes. Artiodactyls encompass the suborders Suiformes (including pigs), Tylopoda (including camels and llamas) and Ruminantia. Within the Ruminantia suborder the Pecora include antelopes, buffalo, cattle, deer, giraffes and sheep. In a comparative gene mapping study in sheep and deer a linkage group assigned to sheep chromosome 24 and the order of genes within it was found to be conserved, in deer (Broom *et al.*, 1996). Thus, whilst a high resolution gene map of the bovine genome is required for comparative positional candidate gene cloning as discussed below, low resolution gene maps may be sufficient for other commercially exploited ruminants such as buffalo, deer, sheep and goats. The detailed bovine genome map would be used as an interface for transfers of map information between the gene-rich maps of humans and mice and the relatively gene-poor maps of these other ruminants.

The Avian Genome — A Special Case

Birds and mammals shared a common ancestor about 350 million years ago. The organization of avian genomes as exemplified by the chicken karyotype is quite different from that of mammals. The chicken karyotype ($2n=78$) is characterised by 10 macrochromosomes and 29 microchromosomes. The nucleotide composition of the macro- and microchromosomes appear to differ with the latter being G/C rich. Recent studies suggest that the microchromosomes may also be relatively gene rich, in as much as chicken CpG islands appear to be preferentially located on the microchromosomes (McQueen *et al.*, 1996). One might reasonably predict that there would be little evidence of conservation of synteny between the chicken and mammalian genomes.

Conservation of synteny between chicken chromosomes (both macro- and micro-) and human chromosomes has been reported (e.g. Klein *et al.*, 1996; Pitel *et al.*, 1996; Jones, *et al.*, 1997, see also Burt *et al.*, 1995). Burt *et al.* (1996) have identified 19 chicken syntenic groups, each involving between two and six loci, which are conserved in mammals. Further improvements in the resolution and gene content of the chicken genome maps are required in order to determine whether some of these conserved syntenies include large conserved segments or even conserved gene.orders. For example, Burt and his colleagues consider that the avian microchromosomes could represent highly conserved genomic segments (Jones *et al.*, 1997). As the chicken genome is about half the size of mammalian genomes but is thought to contain a similar number of genes, the gene density is expected to be greater. Thus, this more compact genome may be particularly useful for comparative genome mapping studies aimed at unravelling the mysteries of vertebrate genome evolution.

BIOINFORMATICS

Genome research now generates too much data for individual scientists to assimilate and exploit without the use of computing systems. Computers are required for the storage, retrieval and analysis of the burgeoning genome data.

Databases

Databases have been developed to meet the needs of livestock genome mappers. Clearly, it was necessary for individual laboratories to create database systems to handle their experimental data. Here, however, I will restrict myself to the genome databases developed to hold and summarise published genome mapping information. This function is met for the human genome project by the Genome Database (GDB) and for the mouse mapping community by the Mouse Genome Database (MGD). The first livestock genome database was PiGBASE which was developed as a clone of the Jackson Laboratory's mouse genome database — GBASE, the predecessor of MGD. The GBASE model was subsequently implemented for sheep and chicken. Several genome databases have been established for cattle, including BOVMAP and BovGBASE. The PiGBASE, BOVMAP, ChickBASE and Sheepmap (SheepGBASE) are recognised by the International Society of Animal Genetics (ISAG) as the genome databases for pigs, cattle, chicken and sheep respectiively in a manner analogous to the recognition accorded to GDB and MGD. The GBASE model used for some livestock genome databases has recently been replaced with a generic single species genome database, Arkdb, developed at the Roslin Institute (Archibald *et al.*, 1996b).

The livestock genome databases are accessible on the World Wide Web with multiple nodes to circumvent the problems from slow international networks links. The URLs for the livestock genome databases and other key genome resources are listed in Table 7.1.

Although all these genome databases attempt to address issues of comparative genome mapping and analysis their primary foci are on their species of interest. The comparative mapping data in each of the databases is limited, often to a note of the putative homologous locus in humans. Thus, there is a need for comparative genome databases that address the multiple dimensions possible in comparative analyses — human–cattle, cattle–sheep, cattle–pig, pig–sheep and so on. A number of databases have been developed to address this need.

The most extensive of the current comparative genome databases concerned with animals is the homology component of the MGD [URL = http://mgd.hgmp. mrc.ac.uk/homology.html]. Although the MGD includes information on homologous genes in 61 species, including cattle, pig, sheep, goat and horse, it is limited to consideration of mammalian homology and thus does not encompass poultry. MGD, however, does include homology data for some of the less well characterised mammals that are exploited economically such as the silver fox, kangaroos, rabbits and mink. Whilst the earlier homology query system was limited in using the mouse genome as the universal benchmark to which all other genomes could be compared one at a time, the current system allows comparisons of any pair of the 61 species in the database. The information retrieved from such comparisons include the locus symbols and chromosome locations of each pair of homologous in the two species of interest, plus relevant citations. The cited literature includes the references to the mapping of each locus in each species of interest. Where there is a genome database for the species of interest there are hot links to the relevant locus entries in those databases. Unfortunately, the MGD mammalian homology system does not record or cite the evidence to support the claim of homology between the pairs of loci.

The Comparative Animal Genome database (TCAGdb) recently developed at the Roslin Institute will not only record the homology statements and their sources, but also the supporting evidence. As with the MGD model, detailed information on individual loci will not be held in TCAGdb. Rather links will be provided to the relevant genome database. Where such a genome database does not exist an Arkdb single species database will be created and populated with the minimal requirements for the functioning of TCAGdb. Such minimalist single species genome databases will be offered to genome mappers in these species of interest. Amongst the tools being developed in the context of TCAGdb is the Anubis map manager currently used by the Arkdb livestock genome mapping and BOVMAP databases (Mungall, 1996). The Anubis map viewer is currently used

Table 7.1 Genome databases and other genome related bioinformatics resources.

Database name	Description	URL(s)
PiGBASE	Pig genome database, Arkdb series, contains interactive map displays and experimental details and references	UK (primary) node: http://www.ri.bbsrc.ac.uk/pigmap/pigbase/pigbase.html USA node: http://tetra.gig.usda.gov:8400/pigbase/manager.html
SheepBASE	Sheep genome database, Arkdb series, contains interactive map displays and experimental details and references	New Zealand (primary) node: http://dirk.invermay.cri.nz/ UK node: http://www.ri.bbsrc.ac.uk/sheepmap/ USA node: http://tetra.gig.usda.gov:8400/sheepgbase/manager.html
ChickBASE	Chicken genome database, Arkdb series, contains interactive map displays and experimental details and references	UK (primary) node: http://www.ri.bbsrc.ac.uk/chickmap/chickgbase/manager.html USA node: http://tetra.gig.usda.gov:8400/chicgbase/manager.html
BovGBASE	Cattle genome database, Arkdb series, contains interactive map displays and experimental details and references	USA (primary) node: http://tetra.gig.usda.gov:8400/bovgbase/manager.html UK node: http://www.ri.bbsrc.ac.uk/genome_mapping.html
BOVMAP	Cattle genome database, experimental details, references, homology query, intercative map displays	France: http://locus.jouy.inra.fr/cgi-bin/bovmap/intro.pl
Mouse Genome DataBase (MGD)	Comprehensive mouse genome database, references, maps, mammalian homology query system with links to single species genome databases	USA (primary) node: http://www.informatics.jax.org/ UK node: http://mgd.hgmp.mrc.ac.uk/ France node: http://www.pasteur.fr/Bio/MGD Japan node: http://mgd.niai.affrc.go.jp
Genome Data Base (GDB)	Comprehensive human genome databases	USA (primary) node: http://gdbwww.gdb.org/ UK node: http://www.hgmp.mrc.ac.uk/gdb/gdbtop.html Australia node: http://morgan.angis.su.oz.au/gdb/

Table 7.1 (*Continued*)

Database name	Description	URL(s)
		Japan node: http://www.gdb.gdbnet.ad.jp/ There are also further mirror sites in France, Germany, Israel, The Netherlands and Sweden
The Comparative Animal Genome database (TCAGdb)	Comparative animal genome database, interactive map displays, evidence for homology claims, references for homology claims, references, links to single species databases	http://www.ri.bbsrc.ac.uk/tcagdb.html
Human/Mouse Homology Relationships	Summary of human/mouse homology relationships, with comparative maps	http://www3.ncbi.nlm.nih.gov/Homology/
Livestock Genome Mapping	Cluster of livestock and comparative genome databases mounted at the Roslin Institute, Scotland, UK	http://www.ri.bbsrc.ac.uk/genome_mapping.html
Livestock Animal Genome Database	Cluster of livestock genome databases mounted at the National Agricultural Laboratory, USA	http://tetra.gig.usda.gov:8400/
MRC HGMP RC	UK MRC Human Genome Mapping Project Resource Centre — has extensive collection of genome databases and other resources with good links to other genome sites worldwide	http://www.hgmp.mrc.ac.uk/

for studying chromosome maps within a single species. Multiple map views are available for comparison of maps of the same chromosome. These views are being extended to accommodate homology information from TCAGdb. Prototype SCEUS displays, which show conserved evolutionary segments between multiple species, and Oxford-grid style displays have been developed. Anubis version 2.2 is in use with the livestock genome databases (URL=http://www.ri.bbsrc.ac.uk/genome_mapping.html). An alpha version of Anubis version 3.0 is also available (URL=http://www.ri.bbsrc.ac.uk/anubis3).

THE VALUE OF COMPARATIVE GENOME MAPPING IN FARMED ANIMALS

Comparative genome analysis will have a key role in the isolation and characterization of trait genes in the farmed animal species. Recent years have seen initiatives to map the large complex genomes of many animals, including cattle, deer, pigs, sheep and poultry in addition to the widely studied human and murine genomes. The rationale for genome mapping in farm animals is that it offers a way of understanding the genetic control, of complex traits such as growth and reproduction. Genetic (linkage) mapping or genome scanning allows regions of the genome influencing the trait of interest to be identified (e.g. Andersson *et al.*, 1994). However, in order to understand how the trait gene acts or exploit the gene through gene transfer it will be necessary to isolate the trait locus.

There are two strategies for moving from linked markers to the gene itself i.e. 'positional' cloning or a 'positional candidate gene' approach (Collins, 1995). The latter approach has been more productive in the cloning of human disease genes and is likely to be similarly effective in livestock. The identification of the ryanodine receptor gene (*RYR1*) as the gene responsible for malignant hyperthermia in pigs (see below, and Fujii *et al.*, 1991) confirms that this strategy is equally valid in the livestock species. A well populated *gene* map of the species of interest is an essential prerequisite for the 'positional candidate gene' approach. Although over 1200 loci have been mapped in the pig, only ~300 are associated with functional genes. The genome maps of other livestock species are similarly deficient in genes. In contrast, over 16,000 expressed sequences and genes have been mapped in humans (Schuler *et al.*, 1996) and over 5000 genes in mice (Andersson *et al.*, 1996).

Comparative Positional Candidate Gene Cloning

Comparative gene mapping provides a means to circumvent the limitations of the gene content of current livestock genome maps. Comparative mapping provides a framework for transferring information from 'map-rich' species (e.g. humans and mice) to relatively 'map-poor' species such as farm animals.

I consider that a comparative positional candidate gene approach will be an effective strategy for identifying trait genes in livestock. Briefly, in QTL-mapping experiments animals recorded for the trait of interest will be genotyped with a panel of polymorphic anonymous DNA markers (microsatellites or simple tandem repeat loci). This initial genome scan will reveal QTL or regions of the genome influencing the trait of interest. These regions will be defined by the flanking microsatellite markers and will generally span at least 20 cM which could correspond to 20 megabases or more. By inspection of either the international reference linkage maps (e.g. the PiGMaP Linkage consortium or the International Bovine Reference Panel maps) or radiation hybrid maps the nearest flanking genes to the QTL can be identified. By consideration of the homologous loci in other species, especially humans and mice, it may be possible to identify the homologous chromosomal regions in these other species. Thus, the extensive catalogue of genes and expressed sequence tags mapped in the other species can be added to the list of genes that can be considered as candidates for the trait genes of interest.

Case Study 1 — The 'Halothane' Story

Malignant hyperthermia (MH) in Man and pigs provides a useful example of the candidate gene approach and demonstrates the value of comparative gene mapping. Halothane-induced malignant hyperthermia (MH) is a feature of the so-called porcine stress syndrome that also encompasses sudden stress deaths and a predisposition to yield pale soft exudative (PSE) meat (for reviews see MacLennan and Phillips, 1992; Archibald, 1991). In pigs susceptibility to halothane-induced malignant hyperthermia has been shown to be controlled by a recessive gene at a single autosomal locus (*HAL*) with both alleles exhibiting variable penetrance. Linkage analyses assigned the *HAL* locus to a linkage group that included S, GPI, *EAH*, *A1BG*, and *PGD* (see Archibald and Imlah, 1985; Archibald, 1991). The HAL locus was subsequently mapped to chromosome 6 through *in situ* hybridization assignments for the two linked markers (*GPI* and *PGD*) (Davies *et al.*, 1988; Yerle *et al.*, 1990).

Of the linked markers the human homologues of *GPI*, *A1BG* and *PGD* could be readily identified. In humans *GPI* and *A1BG* map to chromosome 19 and *PGD* to chromosome 1. Thus, the eventual mapping of MH in humans to chromosome 19q was predictable if one regarded human and porcine MH as arising from mutations in homologous genes (McCarthy *et al.*, 1990). The risks inherent in this assumption are evident from the subsequent identification of some inherited malignant hyperthermia in humans are not linked to chromosome 19 (Deufel *et al.*, 1992; Levitt *et al.*, 1992).

When the gene encoding the skeletal muscle sacroplasmic reticulum Ca^{2+} release channel protein, also known as the ryanodine receptor (*RYR1*) was mapped to human chromosome 19q, it was considered as a candidate for two human disorders that can be viewed as myopathies — myotonic dystrophy and malignant hyperthermia. Linkage studies excluded the former and supported the latter (Mackensie *et al.*, 1990; MacLennan *et al.*, 1990). Subsequent studies identified a C to T transition at nucleotide 1843 in the *RYR1* gene which causes an arginine to cysteine substitution. This point mutation was correlated with susceptibility to MH in five pig breeds and cosegregated with the *HAL n* allele in informative backcrosses (Fujii *et al.*, 1990; Otsu *et al.*, 1991). The mapping of the porcine *RYR1* locus to chromosome 6 (Harbitz *et al.*, 1990) and evidence that the calcium release channels isolated from MH susceptible pigs are slower to close (Mickelson *et al.*, 1988) support the conclusion that the C1843T mutation is responsible for susceptibility to halothane-induced malignant hyperthermia in pigs.

Strikingly a corresponding C1840T mutation in the human *RYR1* gene is associated with some inherited forms of malignant hyperthermia, whilst in another pedigree MH is associated with a different *RYR1* mutation (Galliard *et al.*, 1991, 1992).

Case Study 2 — Dominant White Colour in Pigs

Most commercial pigs in Europe are white. White coat colour in pigs has been shown to be genetically determined by a single dominant allele (see Ollivier and Sellier, 1982). Andersson and his colleagues have used European Wild Boar × Large White mapping pedigrees to map and identify the gene responsible for white coat colour (Johansson *et al.*, l992). Their mapping efforts were guided by a consideration of mapped coat colour genes in the mouse. The dominant white spotting (*W*), patch (*Ph*) and rump-white (*Rw*) genes all map to murine chromosome 5. Johansson *et al.* (1992) developed polymorphic markers for the porcine *PDGFRA* and *ALB* loci whose murine homologues are closely linked to *W*, *Ph* and *Rw* and tested them as markers for coat colour in pigs. The porcine dominant white colour locus was shown to be linked to *PDGFRA* and *ALB* and mapped to SSC8 through an *in situ* hybridization assignment of the *ALB* locus. Evidence from other species suggested that *PDFRA* and *KIT* were both candidate genes for dominant white in pigs. However, recombination between *PDGFRA* and dominant white eliminated *PDGFRA*. As no variation at the *KIT* locus could be detected in the initial study, its candidature could not be tested.

In follow up studies an single stranded conformational polymorphism (SSCP) within the *KIT* locus was used to demonstrate tight linkage between *KIT* and dominant white (Johansson Moller *et al.*, 1996). The SSCP analysis revealed that the *KIT* locus was duplicated in pigs carrying the dominant white allele. As yet, the extent of the duplication has not been determined nor the causal link between the duplication and the dominant white coat colour phenotype. The genetic control of coat colour in pigs is of more than academic interest. At least in Europe coloured pigs incur a financial penalty at slaughter.

Case Study 3 — The 'Booroola' Gene — Still Looking

The 'Booroola' gene (*FecB*) is a major gene influencing fecundity in sheep which was first identified in Australian Merinos. One copy of the *FecB* allele increases litter size, on average, by one extra lamb. By segregation analysis *FecB* has been mapped to a linkage group on ovine chromosome 6 (Montgomery *et al.*, 1993, 1994). There is extensive conservation between ovine chromosome 6 and human chromosome 4. Thus, ovine homologous of genes mapped to human chromosome 4 and HSA4q in particular can be considered candidates for the *FecB* fecundity gene. As different Booroola genotypes exhibit differences in plasma gonadotrophin-releasing hormone (GnRH) levels and differing pituitary responses to exogenous GnRH, the gene encoding the gonadotrophin-releasing hormone receptor (GNRHR) and which maps to HSA4q13.1–q21.1 was a candidate for *FecB*. However, although an RFLP marker for ovine *GNRHR* maps to OAR6 it is at least 20 cM away from *FecB* (Montgomery *et al.*, 1995). Presumably, the human gene map (Schuler *et al.*, 1996) of this region is currently being scoured for alternative candidate genes. The search will be hampered by the fact that as with pig chromosome 8, the order of the genes on HSA4 is not conserved in the corresponding region on sheep chromosome 6. *FecB* maps to an interval between *EGF* and *SPP1* on sheep chromosome 6 (Montgomery *et al.*, 1993, 1994). Unfortunately, some genes that map to the interval between *EGF* and *SPP1* on HSA4q, specifically *KIT* and *PDGFRA*, map outside the *EGF* and *SPP1* interval sheep (Montgomery *et al.*, 1995). Thus, the need for high resolution gene maps in order to define the regions of conserved order is evident.

Amongst the other major genes in livestock for which comparative positional candidate gene searches are being pursued are the *RN* meat quality gene in pigs (Milan *et al.*, 1996), the callipyge muscular hypertrophy gene in sheep (Cockett *et al.*, 1994) and the poll gene in cattle (Georges *et al.*, 1993). As the latter gene influences horn development there may be some difficulties identifying likely human homologues.

FUNCTIONAL, COMPARATIVE GENOMICS

Finally, comparative genomics provides a means of characterising (trait) genes once they have been identified. One of the most effective means of validating the link between genotype and phenotype is by manipulating the former and recording the consequences. Whilst such genetic manipulation is routine in lower organisms including bacteria and yeast, it is both more demanding and more expensive in higher animals, especially in the farm animal species. Genetic manipulation by homologous recombination in embryo-derived stem cells in mice provides a practicable means of tackling this problem for livestock trait genes. Transgenic mice in which candidate (livestock) trait genes have been manipulated may be particularly effective models for pigs as both species are monogastrics and have litters of multiple offspring. For example, a transgenic mouse carrying the C1843T mutation in its ryanodine receptor gene could be used to determine whether this so-called 'HAL' mutation causes both susceptibility to malignant hyperthermia and reductions in fat or only the former phenotype.

CONCLUSIONS

The livestock genome projects are both contributors to and exploiters of comparative genome mapping. Gene mapping in relatively closely related species such as cattle and sheep will inform our understanding of genome evolution over shorter timescales than the much studied human–mouse interval. Similarly, the chicken which shared a common ancestor with the mammals over 350 million years ago will make a valuable contribution to unravelling the evolution of vertebrate genomes. As argued above, comparative positional candidate approaches are likely to provide the most effective means to isolate economically important trait genes. A comparative genomics perspective will not only allow provide candidate trait genes for livestock from the wealth of mapped human and murine genes but will also provide candidate phenotypes for mapped expressed human sequences of unknown function.

ACKNOWLEDGMENTS

I am grateful to my colleagues Dave Burt and Andy Law for stimulating discussions on issues of comparative genome analysis especially during the designing of the Arkdb and TCAGdb databases to which David Nicholson, Chris Mungall and Jian Hu contributed from the computing side. I thank Alan Hillyard, formerly of The Jackson Laboratory and now of Base4 Bioinformatics for stimulating these discussions and guiding us along the way. I thank Ian Franklin for his clear and simple explanation of the importance and sense in comparative mapping i.e. "comparative genome mapping only makes sense in an evolutionary context" as expounded at the 1st HUGO Comparative Genome Workshop (Andersson *et al.*, 1996). I am grateful to the Biotechnology and Biological Sciences Research Council who fund my comparative genome mapping research and support the livestock genome databases at Roslin.

REFERENCES

Andersson, L., Haley, C.S., Ellegren, H., Knott, S.A., Johansson, M., Andersson, K., Andersson-Eklund, L., Edfors-Lilja, I., Fredholm, M., Hansson, I., Håkansson, J. and Lundström, K. (1994) Genetic mapping of quantitative trait loci for growth and fatness in pigs. *Science*, **263**, 1771–1774.

Andersson, L., Archibald, A., Ashburner, M., Audun, S., Barendse, W., Bitgood, J., Bottema, C., Broad, T., Brown, S., Burt, D., Charlier, C., Copeland, N., Davis, S., Davisson, M., Edwards, J., Eggen, A., Elgar, G., Eppig, J.T., Franklin, I., Grewe, P., Gill III, T., Graves, J.A.M., Hawken, R., Hetzel, J., Hillyard, A., Jacob, H., Jaswinska, L., Jenkins, N., Kunz, H., Levan, G., Lie, O., Lyons, L., Maccarone, P., Mellersh, C., Montgomery, G., Moore, S., Moran, C., Morizot, D., Neff, M., Nicholas, F., O'Brien, S., Parsons, Y., Peters, J., Postlewait, J., Raymond, M., Rothschild, M., Schook, L., Sugimoto, Y., Szpirer, C., Tate, M., Taylor, J., VandeBerg, J., Wakefield, M., Wienberg, J. and Womack, J. (1996) Comparative genome organisation of vertebrates. *Mammalian Genome*, **7**, 717–734.

Archibald, A.L. (1991) Halothane-induced malignant hyperthermia in pigs. In: *Breeding for disease resistance in farm animals*, edited by J.B. Owen and R.F.E. Axford, pp. 449–466. Wallingford: CAB International.

Archibald, A.L. and Imlah, P. (1985) The halothane sensitivity locus and its linkage relationships. *Animal Blood Groups and Biochemical Genetics*, **16**, 253–263.

Archibald, A.L., Haley, C.S., Brown, J.F., Couperwhite, S., McQueen, H.A., Nicholson, D., Coppieters, W., Van de Weghe, A., Stratil, A., Winterø, A.K., Fredholm, M., Larsen, N.J., Nielsen, V.H., Milan, D., Woloszyn Robic, A., Dalens, M., Riquet, J., Gellin, J., Caritez, J.-C., Burgaud, G., Ollivier, L., Bidanel, J.-P., Vaiman, M., Renard, C., Geldermann, H., Davoli, R., Ruyter, D., Verstege, E.J.M., Groenen, M.A.M., Davies, W., Høyheim, B., Keiserud, A., Andersson, L., Ellegren, H., Johansson, M., Marklund, L., Miller, J.R., Anderson Dear, D.V., Signer, E., Jeffreys, A.J., Moran, C., Le Tissier, P., Muladno Rothschild, M.F., Tuggle, C.K., Vaske, D., Helm, J., Liu, H.-C., Rahman, A., Yu, T.-P., Larson, R.G. and Schmitz, C.B. (1995) The PiGMaP consortium linkage map of the pig (*Sus scrofa*). *Mammalian Genome*, **6**, 157–175.

Archibald, A.L., Couperwhite, S. and Jiang, Z.H. (1996a) The porcine *TTR* locus maps to chromosome 6q. *Animal Genetics*, **27**, 351–353.

Archibald, A.L., Hu, J., Mungall, C., Hillyard, A.L., Burt, D.W., Law, A.S. and Nicholcon, D. (1996b) A generic single species genome database. XXVth International Conference on Animal Genetics, 21–25 July 1996, Tours, France, *Animal Genetics*, **27**, Suppl. 2, 55.

Bengtsson, B.O., Klinga Levan, K. and Levan, G. (1993) Measuring genome reorganisation from synteny data. *Cytogenetics and Cell Genetics*, **64**, 198–200.

Bishop, M. (1994) Comparative mapping and sequencing. In: *Guide to Human Genome Computing*, edited by M.J. Bishop, pp. 159–189. London: Academic Press.

Bosma, A.A., de Haan, N.A., Mellink, C.H.M., Yerle, M. and Zijlstra, C. (1996) Chromosome homology between the domestic pig and the babirusa (family Suidae) elucidated with the use of porcine painting probes. *Cytogenetics and Cell Genetics*, **75**, 32–35.

Broad, T.E., Lambeth, M., Burkin, D.J., Jones, C., Pearce, P.D., Maher, D.W. and Ansari, H.A. (1996) Physical mapping confirms that sheep chromosome 10 has extensive conserved synteny with cattle chromosome 12 and human chromosome 13. *Animal Genetics*, **27**, 249–253.

Broom, J.E., Tate, M.L. and Doods, K.G. (1996) Linkage mapping in sheep and deer identifies a conserved pecora ruminant linkage group orthologous to two regions of HSA 16 and a portion of HSA7q. *Genomics*, **33**, 358–364.

Burt, D.W., Bumstead, N., Bitgood, J.J., Ponce de Leon, A. and Crittenden, L.B. (1995) Chicken genome mapping: a new era in avian genetics. *Trends in Genetics*, **11**, 190–194.

Burt, D.W., Jones, C.T., Morrice, D.R. and Paton, I.R. (1996) Mapping the chicken genome — an aid to comparative studies. *Animal Genetics*, **27**, Suppl. 2, 66.

Chowdhary, B.P., Fronïcke, L., Gustavsson, I. and Scherthan, H. (1996) Comparative analysis of the cattle and human genomes: detection of ZOO-FISH and gene mapping-based chromosomal homologies. *Mammalian Genome*, **7**, 297–302.

Cockett, N.E., Jackson, S.P., Shay, T.L., Nielsen, D., Moore, S.S., Steele, M.R., Barendse, W., Green, R.D. and Georges, M. (1994) Chromosomal localization of the callipyge gene in sheep (*Ovis aries*) using bovine DNA markers. *Proceedings of the National Academy of Sciences, USA*, **91**, 3019–3022.

Collins, F.S. (1995) Positional cloning moves from perditional to traditional. *Nature Genetics*, **9**, 347–350.

Copeland, N.G., Jenkins, N.A., Gilbert, G.J., Eppig, J.T., Maltais, L.J., Miller, J.C., Dietrich, W.F., Weaver, A., Lincoln, S.E., Steen, R.G., Stein, L.D., Nadeau, J.H. and Lander, E.S. (1993) A genetic linkage map of the mouse; current applications and future prospects. *Science*, **262**, 57–66.

Couperwhite, S. and Archibald, A.L. (1993) An *Eco*RV RFLP at the porcine chromogranin A locus (*CHGA*). *Animal Genetics*, **24**, 331.

Davies, W., Harbitz, I., Fries, R., Stranzinger, G. and Hauge, J.G. (1988) Porcine malignant hyperthermia carrier detection and chromosomal assignment using a linked probe. *Animal Genetics*, **19**, 203–212.

Deufel, T., Golla, A., Iles, D., Meindl, A., Meitinger, T., Schindelhauer, D., de vries, A., Pongratz, D., MacLennan, D.H., Johnson, K.J. and Lehmann-Horn, F. (1992) Evidence for genetic hetero-geneity of malignant hyperthermia susceptibility. *American Journal of Human Genetics*, **50**, 1151–1161.

Echard, G., Broad, T.E., Hill, D. and Pearce, P. (1994) Present status of the ovine gene map (*Ovis aries*) — Comparison with bovine map (*Bos taurus*). *Mammalian Genome*, **5**, 324–332.

Ellegren, H., Fredholm, M., Edfors-Lilja, I., Winterø, A.K. and Andersson, L. (1993) Conserved synteny between pig chromosome 8 and human chromosome 4 but rearranged and distorted linkage maps. *Genomics*, **17**, 599–603.

Fries, R., Beckmann, J.S., Georges, M., Soller, M. and Womack, J. (1989) The bovine gene map. *Animal Genetics*, **20**, 3–29.

Fonïcke, L., Chowdhary, B.P., Scherthan, H. and Gustavsson, I. (1996) A comparative map of the porcine and human genomes demonsrtates ZOO-FISH and gene mapping-based chromosomal homologies. *Mammalian Genome*, **7**, 285–290.

Fujii, J., Otsu, K., Zorzato, F., De Leon, S., Khanna, V.K., Weiler, J.E., O'Brien, P.J. and MacLennan, D.H. (1991) Identification of a mutation in porcine ryanodine receptor associated with malignant hyperthermia. *Science*, **253**, 448–451.

Gallagher Jr. D.S. and Womack, J.E. (1992) Chromosome conservation in the *Bovidae*. *Journal of Heredity*, **83**, 287–298.

Gallagher Jr. D.S., Derr, J.N. and Womack, J.E. (1994) Chromosome conservation among the advanced pecorans and determination of the primitive bovid karyotype. *Journal of Heredity*, **85**, 204–210.

Galliard, E.F., Otsu, K., Fujii, J., Khanna, V.K., De Leon, S., Derdemezi, J., Britt, B.A., Duff, C.L., Worton, R.G. and MacLennan D.H. (1991) A substitution of cysteine for arginine 614 in the ryanodine receptor is potentially causative of human malignant hyperthermia. *Genomics*, **11**, 751–755.

Galliard, E.F., Otsu, K., Fujii, J., Duff, C., De Leon, S., Khanna, V.K., Britt, B.A., Worton, R.G. and MacLennan, D.H. (1992) Polymorphisms and deduced amino acid substitutions in the coding sequence of the ryanodine receptor (RYR1) gene in individuals with malignant hyperthermia. *Genomics*, **13**, 1247–1254.

Georges, M., Drinkwater, R., King, T., Mishra, A., Moore, S.S., Nielsen, D., Sargeant, L.S., Sorensen, A., Steele, MR., Zhao, X., Womack, J.E. and Hetzel, J. (1993) Microsatellite mapping of a gene affecting horn development in *Bos taurus*. *Nature Genetics*, **4**, 206–210.

Goffeau, A., Barrell, B.G., Bussey, H., Davis, R.W., Dujon, B., Feldmann, H., Galibert, F., Hoheisel, J.D., Jacq, C., Johnston, M., Louis, E.J., Mewes, H.W., Murakami, Y., Philippsen, P., Tettelin, H. and Oliver, S.G. (1996) Life with 6000 genes. *Science*, **274**, 546–567.

Goureau, A., Yerle, M., Schmitz, A., Riquet, J., Milan, D., Pinton, P., Frelat, G. and Gellin, J. (1996) Human and porcine correspondence of chromosome segments using bidirectional chromosome painting. *Genomics*, **36**, 252–262.

Graves, J.A.M., Wakefield, M.J., Peter, J., Searle, A.J., Archibald, A., O'Brien, S.J. and Womack, J.E. (1996) Report of the committee on comparative gene mapping. In: *Human Gene Mapping 1995 — A coppendium*, compiled by A.J. Cuticchia, M.A. Chipperfield and P.A. Foster with the assistance of the staff at the Genome Data Base, pp. 1351–1408. Baltimore and London: The John Hopkins University Press.

Harbitz, I., Chowdhary, B., Thomsen, P.D., Davies, W., Kaufmann, U., Kran, S., Gustavsson, I., Christensen, K. and Hauge, J.G. (1990) Assignment of the porcine calcium release channel gene, a candidate for the malignant hyperthermia locus to the 6p11–>q21 segment of chromosome 6. *Genomics*, **8**, 243–248.

Hayes, H. (1995) Chromosome painting with human chromosome-specific DNA libraries reveals the extent and distribution of conserved segments in bovine chromosomes. *Cytogenetics and Cell Genetics*, **71**, 168–174.

Hayes, H., Petit, E. and Dutrillaux, B. (1991) Comparison of RBG-banded karyotypes of cattle, sheep and goats. *Cytogenetics and Cell Genetics*, **57**, 51–55.

Hediger, R., Ansari, H.A. and Stranzinger, G.F. (1991) Chromosome banding and gene localizations support extensive conservation of chromosome structure between cattle and sheep. *Cytogenetics and Cell Genetics*, **57**, 127–134.

Iannuzzi, L. and DiMeo, G.P. (1995) Chromosomal evolution in bovids: a comparison of cattle, sheep and goat G- and R-banded chromosomes and cytogenetic divergences among cattle, goat and river buffalo sex chromosomes. *Chromosome Research*, **3**, 291–299.

Jauch, A., Weinberg, J., Stanyon, R., Arnold, N., Tofanelli, S., Ishida, T. and Cremer, T. (1992) Reconstruction of genomic rearrangements in great apes and gibbons by chromosomal painting. *Proceeding of the National Academy of Sciences, USA*, **89**, 8611–8615.

Johansson, M., Ellegren, H. and Andersson, L. (1995) Comparative mapping reveals extensive linkage conservation but with gene order rearrangements between the pig and human genomes. *Genomics*, **25**, 682–690.

Johansson, M., Ellegren, H., Marklund, L., Gustavsson, U., Ringmar-Cederberg, E., Andersson, K., Edfors-Lilja and Andersson, L. (1992) The gene for dominant white color in the pig is closely linked to *ALB* and *PDGFRA* on chromosome 8. *Genomics*, **14**, 965–969.

Johansson Moller, M., Chaudharyt, R., Hellmén, E., Høyheim, B., Chowdhary, B. and Andersson, L. (1996) Pigs with the dominant white coat color phenotype carry a duplication of the *KIT* gene encoding the mast/stem cell growth factor receptor. *Mammalian Genome*, **7**, 822–830.

Jones, C.T., Morrice, D.R., Paton, I.R. and Burt, D.W. (1997) Gene homologs on human chromosome 15q21–q26 and a chicken microchromosome identify a new conserved segment. *Mammalian Genome*, **8**, 436–440.

Kemp, S.J., Hishida, O., Wambugu, J., Rink, A., Longeri, M.L., Ma, R.Z., Da, Y., Lewin, H.A., Barendse, W. and Teale, A.J. (1995) A panel of polymorphic bovine, ovine and caprine microsatellite markers. *Animal Genetics*, **26**, 299–306.

Klein, S., Morrice, D.R., Sang, H., Crittenden, L.B. and Burt, D.W. (1996) Genetic and physical mapping of the chicken IGFl gene to chromosome 1 and conservation of synteny with other vertebrate genomes. *Journal of Heredity*, **87**, 10–14.

Kojima, M., Ohata, K., Harumi, T., Murakami, Y. and Yasue, H. (1996) Isolation and chromosomal assignment of four genes in the pig by fluorescence *in situ* hybridization. *Animal Genetics*, **27**, Suppl. 2, 80.

Lalley, P.A., Davisson, M.T., Graves, J.A.M., O'Brien, S.J., Womack, J.E., Roderick, T.H., Creau-Goldberg, N., Hillyard, A.L., Doolittle, D.P. and Rogers, J.A. (1989) Report of the committee on comparative mapping. *Cytogenetics and Cell Genetics*, **51**, 503–532.

Law, A.S. and Burt, D.W. (1996) qValue — A program to calculate comparative measures of genomic reorganisation from cytogenetic and/or linkage information. *CABIOS*, **12**, 181–183.

Levitt, R.C., Olckers, A., Meyers, S., Fletcher, J.E., Rosenberg, H., Isaacs, H. and Meyers, D.A. (1992) Evidence for the localization of a malignant hyperthermia susceptibility locus (*MHS2*) to human chromosome 17. *Genomics*, **14**, 562–566.

Lundin, L.G. (1993) Evolution of the vertebrate genome as reflected in paralogous chromosomal regions in man and the house mouse. Analytical review. *Genomics*, **16**, 1–19.

Lyons, L.A., Raymond, M.M. and O'Brien, S.J. (1994) Comparative genomics: the next generation. *Animal Biotechnology*, **5**, 103–111.

McCarthy, T.V., Healy, J.M.S., Heffron, J.J.A., Lehane, M., Deufel, T., Lehmann-Horn, F., Farrall, M. and Johansson, K. (1990) Localization of the malignant hyperthermia susceptibility locus to human chromosome 19ql2–13.2. *Nature*, **343**, 562–564.

Mackensie, A.E., Korneluk, R.G., Zorzato, F., Fujii, J., Phillips, M., Iles, D., Wieringa, B., Leblond, S., Bailly, J., Willard, H.F., Duff, C., Worton, R.G. and MacLennan, D.H. (1990) The human ryanodine receptor gene: its mapping to l9ql3.1, placement in a chromosome 19 linkage group, and exclusion as the gene causing myotonic dystrophy. *Americam Journal of Human Genetics*, **46**, 1082–1089.

MacLennan, D.H. and Phillips, M.S. (1992) Malignant hyperthermia. *Science*, **256**, 789–794.

MacLennan, D.H., Duff, C., Zorzato, F., Fujii, J., Phillips, M., Korneluk, R.G., Frodis, W., Britt, B.A. and Worton, R.G. (1990) Ryanodine receptor gene is a candidate for prediposition to malignant hyperthermia. *Nature*, **343**, 559–561.

McQueen, H.A., Fantes, J., Cross, S.H., Clark, V.H., Archibald, A.L. and Bird, A.P. (1996) CpG islands of chicken are concentrated on microchromosomes. *Nature Genetics*, **12**, 321–324.

Marklund, L., Johansson Møller, M., Høyheim, B., Davies, W., Fredholm, M., Juneja, R.K., Mariani, P., Coppieters, W., Ellegren, H. and Andersson, L. (1996) A comprehensive linkage map of the pig based on a wild pig–Large White intercross. *Animal Genetics*, **27**, 255–269.

Mickelson, J.R., Gallant, E.M., Litterer, L.A., Johansson, K.M., Rempel, W.E. and Louis, C.F. (1988) Abnormal sarcoplasmic reticulum ryanodine receptor in malignant hyperthermia. *Journal of Biological Chemistry*, **263**, 9310–9315.

Montgomery, G.W., Crawford, A.M., Penty, J.M., Dodds, K.G., Ede, A.J., Henry, H.M., Pierson, C.A., Lord, E.A., Galloway, S.M., Schmack, A.E., Sise, J.A., Swarbrick, P.A., Hanrahan, V., Buchanan, F.C. and Hill, D.F. (1993) The ovine Booroola fecundity gene (*FecB*) is linked to markers from a region of human chromosome 4q. *Nature Genetics*, **4**, 410–414.

Montgomery, G.W., Lord, E.A., Penty, J.M., Dodds, K.G., Broad, T.E., Cambridge, L., Sunden, S.L.F., Stone, R.T. and Crawford, A.M. (1994) The ovine Booroola fecundity (*FecB*) gene maps to sheep chromosome 6. *Genomics*, **22**, 148–153.

Montgomery, G.W., Penty, J.M., Lord, E.A., Brooks, J. and McNeilly, A.S. (1995) The gonadotrophin-releasing hormone receptor maps to sheep chromosome 6 outside of the region of the *FecB* locus. *Mammalian Genome*, **6**, 436–438.

Moore, S.S., Sargeant, L.L., King, T.J., Mattick, J.S., Georges, M. and Hetzel, D.J.S. (1991) The conservation of dinucleotide microsatellites among mammalian genomes allows the use of heterologous PCR primer pairs in closely related species. *Genomics*, **10**, 654–660.

Mungall, C. (1996) Visualisation tools for genome mapping — the Anubis map manager. XXVth International Conference on Animal Genetics, 21–25 July 1996, Tours, France, *Animal Genetics*, **27**, Suppl. 2, 56.

Nadeau, J.H. (1989) Maps of linkage and synteny homologies between mouse and man. *Trends in Genetiics*, **5**, 82–86.

Nadeau, J.H. and Taylor, B.A. (1984) Lengths of chromosomal segments conserved since divergence of man and mouse. *Proceedings of the National Academy of Sciences, USA*, **81**, 814–818.

O'Brien, S.J. (1991) Mammalian genome mapping: lessons and prospects. *Current Opinions in Genetics and Development*, **1**, 105–111.

O'Brien, S.J. and Graves, J.A.M. (1991) Report of the Committee on Comparative Gene Mapping. *Cytogenetics and Cell Genetics*, **58**, 1124–1151.

Ollivier, L. and Sellier, P. (1982) Pig genetics: a review. *Ann. Génét. Sél. Anim.*, **14**, 481–544.

O'Brien, S.J., Seuánez, H.N. and Womack, J.E. (1988) Mammalian genome organization: An evolutionary overview. *Annual Review of Genetics*, **22**, 323–351.

O'Brien, S.J., Womack, J.E., Lyons, L.A., Moore, K.J., Jenkins, N.A. and Copeland, N.G. (1993) Anchored reference loci for comparative genome mapping in mammals. *Nature Genetics*, **3**, 103–112.

Otsu, K., Khanna, V.K., Archibald, A.L. and MacLennan, D.H. (1991) Co-segregation in Fl generation backcrosses of porcine malignant hyperthermia and a probable causal mutation in the skeletal muscle ryanodine receptor gene. *Genomics*, **11**, 744–750.

Pitel, F., Fillon, V., Le Fur, N., Bumstead, N. and Vignal, A. (1996) Localization of the avian fatty acid synthase gene to a conserved region between a chicken microchromosome and human chromosome 17q. *Animal Genetics*, **27**, Suppl. 2, 67.

Raney, N., Graves, K.T., Flannery, A.R., Ennis, R., Bailey, E., Lyons, L.A., Laughlin, T.F. and O'Brien, S.J. (1996) Efficacy of comparative anchor-tagged sites (CATS) primers for synteny mapping the horse. *Animal Genetics*, **27**, Suppl. 2, 74.

Raudsepp, T., Fronicke, L., Scherthan, H., Gustavsson, I. and Chowdhary, B.P. (1996) ZOO-FISH delineates conserved chromosomal segments in horse and man. *Chromosomal Research*, **4**, 218–225.

Rettenberger, G., Klett, C., Zechner, U., Kunz, J., Vogel, W. and Hameister, H. (1995) Visualization of the conservation of synteny between humans and pigs by heterologous chromosomal painting. *Genomics*, **26**, 372–378.

Schlöpfer, J., Yang, Y., Rexroad, C.E. and Womack, J.E. (1996) Construction of a bovine whole-genome radiation hybrid panel. *Animal Genetics*, **27**, Suppl. 1, 63.

Schrethan, H., Cremer, T., Arnason, U., Weier, H.-U., Lima-de-Faria, A. and Fronïcke, L. (1994) Comparative chromosome painting discloses homologous segments in distantly related mammals. *Nature Genetics*, **6**, 342–347.

Schuler, G.D., Boguski, M.S., Stewart, E.A., Stein, L.D., Gyapay, G., Rice, K., White, R.E., Rodriguez-Tome, P., Aggarwal, A., Bajorek, E., Bentolila, S., Birren, B.B., Butler, A., Castle, A.B., Chiannilkulchai, N., Chu, A., Clee, C., Cowles, S., Day, P.J., Dibling, T., Drouot, N., Dunham, I., Duprat, S., East, C.,... Hudson, T.J. (1996) A gene map of the human genome. *Science*, **274**, 540–546.

Solinas-Toldo, S., Lengauer, C. and Fries, R. (1995) Comparative genome map of human and cattle. *Genomics*, **27**, 489–496.

Walter, M.A. and Goodfellow, P.N. (1993) Radiation hybrids: irradiation and fusion gene transfer. *Trends in Genetics*, **9**, 352–356.

Walter, M.A., Spillet, D.J., Thomas, P., Weissenbach, J. and Goodfellow, P.N. (1994) A method for constructing radiation hybrid maps of whole genomes. *Nature Genetics*, **7**, 22–28.

Weinberg, J., Stanyon, R., Jauch, A. and Cremer, T. (1990) Molecular cytotaxonomy of primates by chromosomal *in situ* suppression hybridization. *Genomics*, **8**, 347–350.

Womack, J.E. (1994) Chromosomal evolution from the perspective of the bovine gene map. *Animal Biotechnology*, **5**, 123–128.

Womack, J.E. and Moll, Y.D. (1986) Gene map of the cow: conservation of linkage with mouse and man. *The Journal of Heredity*, **77**, 2–7.

Womack, J.E. and Kata, S.R. (1995) Bovine genome mapping: evolutionary inference and the power of comparative genomics. *Current Opinion in Genetics and Development*, **5**, 725–733.

Yerle, M., Archibald, A.L., Dalens, M. and Gellin, J. (1990) Localization of PGD and TGFβ-1 to pig chromosome 6q. *Animal Genetics*, **21**, 411–417.

Zhang, W., Chen, Y. and Moran, C. (1996) Use of comparative ancor-tagged sequence (CATS) markers in the pig genome. *Animal Genetics*, **27**, Suppl. 2, 84.

Part 3
ENGINEERING THE GENOME

8. TECHNIQUES FOR THE PRODUCTION OF TRANSGENIC LIVESTOCK

W.H. EYESTONE

PPL Therapeutics, Inc., Virginia Tech Corporate Research Center, Blacksburg, Virginia 24060, USA

Recent advances in molecular biology and reproductive technology have generated the possibility to create transgenic livestock. Applications of transgenesis in farm animals include enhancing food and fiber production, disease resistance, producing recombinant proteins in the mammary gland and creating a source of organs for xenotransplantation into human beings. Transgenic founder animals are generated by injecting gene constructs into the pronuclei of fertilized eggs, which subsequently integrate permanently into the genome. Transgene expression is regulated by the use of gene constructs consisting of a tissue-specific promoter fused to the structural gene of interest. Dissemination of transgenes into a herd or flock is accomplished by established animal breeding techniques. Recent data on producing transgenic cattle are presented.

KEY WORDS: transgenic; microinjection; livestock; cattle; sheep; pigs.

INTRODUCTION

A transgenic animal may be defined as one whose genome has been permanently altered by the addition, deletion or modification of specific genes. This powerful technology can be used to accelerate the rate of genetic change relative to conventional selective breeding by modifying the expression of endogenous genes or to create entirely new genotypes by the introduction of novel genes. Transgenesis has been used to modify agricultural production traits and to direct the production of recombinant proteins in the milk of domestic animals. It is the aim of this paper to discuss methods of generating transgenic livestock, with particular emphasis on transgenic dairy cattle.

Historical Perspective

Mice were the first mammals to be rendered transgenic. In their pioneering work, Gordon *et al.* (1980) microinjected SV40 DNA directly into the pronuclei of fertilized mouse eggs, which were then transferred into recipient mice for the balance of gestation. Some of the resulting pups were shown by Southern blot analysis to harbor the SV40 DNA, providing evidence that the minute quantity of DNA injected into the pronuclei had indeed integrated into the genome. These exciting results were quickly repeated in several laboratories (Brinster *et al.*, 1981; Constantini and Lacy, 1981; Gordon and Ruddle, 1981). Others soon demonstrated that transgenes could be expressed in somatic tissue (Wagner *et al.*, 1981) and transmitted to offspring (Constantini and Lacy, 1981; Gordon and Ruddle,

1981; Palmiter *et al.*, 1982). The relative ease by which this approach yielded transgenic mice led to the adoption of pronuclear DNA injection as the method of choice for generating transgenic founder animals in several species, including livestock (Hammer *et al.*, 1985).

Transgene Integration and Inheritance

After pronuclear injection, transgenes usually integrate at a single chromosomal locus for which there is no corresponding allele; thus, transgenic animals generated by pronuclear DNA injection may considered "hemizygous" for a given integration locus. Most transgenic animals bear multiple copies of a transgene at the integration locus (Bishop and Smith, 1989; Bishop, 1997). Hemizygous transgenes are usually transmitted in simple Mendelian fashion to 50% of their offspring. Exceptions to this occur in cases of multiple-integration loci and mosaicism. The latter situation arises when integration occurs after zygotic DNA replication; thus, the transgene is present in only a portion of the cells that comprise the resulting founder animal (it has been estimated that at least 30% of founder generation transgenics are mosaic; Wall and Seidel, 1992). Multiple-site integrations and mosaicism are usually detected when transgenic founders fail to transmit the transgene in a Mendelian manner; alternatively, *in situ* hybridization using probes specific to the transgene can be used to detect mosaicism in specific cell populations. First generation transgenic offspring of single-integration site, mosaic founders are authentically hemizygous and will transmit the transgene to the expected 50% of offspring. If desired, transgenes may be introgressed to generate homozygous animals who will transmit to 100% of their offspring, though these offspring will again be hemizygous.

Phenotype Modification in Transgenic Animals

The primary objective for altering genotype via transgenesis is to achieve a con-comitant phenotypic modification. One of the first experiments to reveal the power of transgenesis for modifying phenotype aimed to enhance growth by overexpressing growth hormone from a transgene. A "fusion" construct consist-ing of the structural gene for rat growth hormone (rGH) driven by a mouse metallothionine-I (MT-I) promoter sequence (Palmiter *et al.*, 1982) was used to enhance growth hormone levels. Transgenic mice (as well as non-transgenic littermate controls) were fed a diet supplemented with zinc to activate the MT-I promoter (normally activated by heavy metal ions in hepatic tissue) in the fusion gene in order drive rGH expression. Some transgenics grew nearly twice as fast as their non-transgenic littermates. Further analysis revealed that rGH mRNA was present in hepatic tissue, and rGH was detected in blood serum. Thus, two key principles in transgenic animal technology were established: (1) the ability to drive gene expression in a target tissue by fusing its structural sequence to the promoter of a gene normally expressed in the target tissue and (2) the ability to modify phenotype as a direct consequence of transgene expression.

The authors of that report (Palmiter *et al.*, 1982) described their results as "dramatic"; indeed they were, so much so that they were inspired to venture that "[transgenesis] has implications...as a way to accelerate animal growth...and as a method of farming valuable gene products". They further suggested that transgenes could be expressed in livestock to enhance growth and lactation, or as a means of producing large quantities of protein or "genetic farming". In these statements, they spelled out what has since become a substantial portion of the transgenic livestock agenda to this day.

TECHNIQUES FOR PRODUCING TRANSGENIC LIVESTOCK

Transgenic Founder Generation by Pronuclear Injection

Hammer *et al.* (1985) generated the first transgenic livestock by pronuclear DNA injection. However, the difficulties encountered by these and other workers who attempted to produce transgenic livestock gave substance to the prediction of Palmiter *et al.* (1982) that "applying these techniques to large animals will be more difficult" (compared to mice). Some of these problems were: (1) difficulty in visualizing pronuclei, especially in pig and cow zygotes (due to zygote lipid content that rendered them opaque), (2) markedly reduced embryo development and pregnancy rates after pronuclear DNA injection and (3) reduced transgene integration efficiency, especially in sheep, goats and cattle (Table 8.1).

The current method of choice for generating transgenic livestock employs direct injection of DNA into one pronucleus of a fertilized zygote (Figure 8.1). The methods used to generate transgenic livestock are based on those developed for mice (Gordon *et al.*, 1981) and described in detail by Hogan *et al.* (1986), Gordon (1993) and Pinkert (1994) with some important modifications to accommodate species differences (Martin and Pinkert, 1994). Zygotes for pronuclear DNA injection may be obtained from the oviducts of superovulated females; alternatively, they may be generated *by in vitro* oocyte maturation and fertilization, a common practice for making transgenic cattle (Figure 8.1). Pronuclei in sheep and goats can be visualized directly using phase contrast, Nomarski differential

Table 8.1 Efficiency of making transgenic livestock compared to mice. Figures given for mice are broad averages, while those for livestock are ranges derived from the listed references.

Species	Integration frequency		Reference
	% of eggs injected	% of offspring	
Mice	~3	~15	Wall, 1996
Sheep	0.1–2	1–14	Brem, 1992
Goats	0–1	0–10	Brem, 1992; Ebert and Schindler, 1993
Cattle	0.01–0.5	0–11	Brem, 1992; Eyestone, 1994; this chapter.
Pigs	0.04–4	2–35	Brem, 1992

interference contrast or Hoffmann interference contrast optics. Bovine and porcine zygotes must first be centrifuged for several minutes at $\sim 13,000 \times g$ to displace cytoplasmic lipid vesicles that otherwise obscure the pronuclei (Wall and Hawk, 1988). After centrifugation, lipid vesicles accumulate to one side of the zygote, and since they are less dense than pronuclei, come to occupy a portion of the zygote where they no longer obscure the pronuclei. Fortunately, this seemingly harsh treatment has little affect on embryo development (Wall et al., 1985; Wall and Hawk, 1988; Gagne et al., 1990; Peura et al., 1994a) though it may result in reduced cell numbers in morulae (Wall et al., 1985; Wall and Hawk, 1988). In general, several picoliters of a solution containing several hundred copies of construct DNA are injected directly into a pronucleus through an extremely fine glass needle. Most workers inject DNA in a buffered solution of 0.1 mM Tris-HCl with 0.1–0.25 mM EDTA at DNA concentration of 2–4 ug/ml. Higher DNA concentrations have been associated with lower embryo developement (Brinster et al., 1985; Bondioli et al., 1991). The pronucleus swells visibly during injection and will remain so after the needle is withdrawn (Figure 8.1). In principle, the microinjection process is quite simple; in practice, success depends on operator skill, quality of the injection needles, DNA quality, zygote quality and ability to visualize pronuclei. Complete technical protocols for the microinjection procedure (micromanipulation equipment, microtool manufacture and pronuclear microinjection) are available elsewhere (Hogan et al., 1986; Gordon, 1993) and will not be detailed here.

Offspring obtained from microinjected zygotes must be evaluated for the presence of the transgene. Confirmation of transgene integration is obtained with polymerase chain reaction (PCR) and Southern blotting using construct-specific probes and by analyzing tissues to which expression was targeted for the corresponding mRNA and protein. The latter aspect is particularly important since transgene expression is known to vary greatly between individuals and transgenic lines. The protein may be further analyzed for correct structure and bioactivity. Germline transgenesis is confirmed by breeding the animals and analyzing their offspring for transgenesis in the manner just described. Finally, analyses appropriate to the desired phenotypic modification (e.g. enhanced growth, modification of milk composition) must be performed.

Evaluation of Transgenic Lines

A primary aim of transgenesis is to establish a new genetic line in which the transgenic modification is stably transmitted and expressed both within and between generations. Selection of a particular line of transgenic livestock must be based on several criteria: (1) ability to transmit the transgene stably and predictably to subsequent generations, (2) maintenance of stable transgene expression level and desired phenotype both within and between generations, and (3) absence of undesirable genetic or phenotypic side effects resulting from the genetic modification. Since founder lines are likely to differ according to these criteria, several founders must be made and tested for each construct to ensure the generation of a useful line.

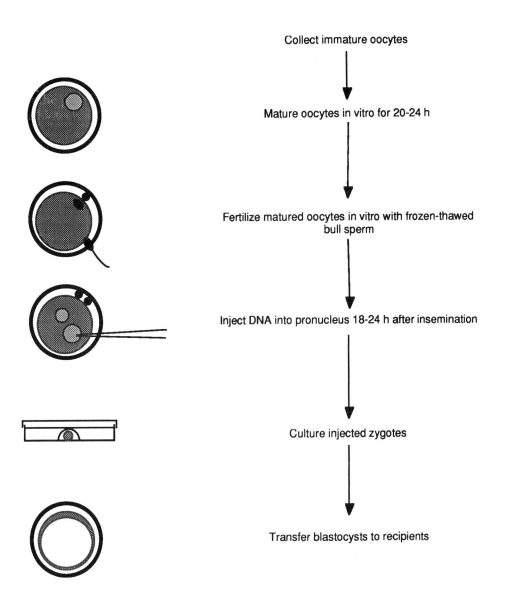

Figure 8.1 Method used to produce transgenic bovine embryos using *in vitro* embryo production. See text for details.

PRODUCTION OF RECOMBINANT PROTEINS IN
THE MILK OF TRANSGENIC LIVESTOCK

The notion of producing valuable proteins in the milk of transgenic animals was first presented in detail by Lathe *et al.* (1985). These authors argued that the mammary gland was nearly ideal for "genetic farming" in view of its ability to synthesize and secrete large quantities of protein in an exocrine fashion. Indeed, the mammary gland has several advantages over alternative systems that employ genetically modified bacteria, yeast or cultured mammalian cells to produce recombinant proteins. For example, proteins requiring complex post-translational modifications for biological activity (e.g. glycosylation, gamma-carboxylation or phosphorylation) may be difficult or impossible to produce in simple microbial systems and it is often difficult to obtain large quantities of recombinant protein from cultured mammalian cells. Moreover, the projected costs of producing recombinant proteins in the mammary gland are far lower than those associated with microbial or cell culture based systems (Datar *et al.*, 1993; Bremel *et al.*, 1996).

Producing recombinant proteins in milk requires a construct consisting of the promoter sequence of a major milk protein gene fused to the structural gene of interest. Such a construct will direct and restrict expression to the mammary gland during lactation. Heterologous gene expression in the mammary gland has been achieved with promoter sequences of several milk protein genes, including mouse whey-acidic protein (Andres *et al.*, 1987; Gordon *et al.*, 1987; Archibald *et al.*, 1990; Wall *et al.*, 1991; Ebert *et al.*, 1991; Velander *et al.*, 1992), bovine alpha-s_1 casein (Meade *et al.*, 1990; Platenburg *et al.*, 1994) and ovine beta-lactoglobulin (Archibald *et al.*, 1990; Wright *et al.*, 1991).

The choice of species in which to produce a particular protein depends on a number of factors, including the quantity of protein required and the time-scale on which the protein is to be made. Sheep or goats have been selected to produce relatively high value proteins required in small or moderate quantities, or when the desired timescale to production is relatively short (alpha-1-anti-trypsin: Carver *et al.*, 1993; tissue plasminogen activator: Ebert *et al.*, 1991; see Table 8.2 for detailed species comparison). Cattle have been considered for producing lower value proteins required in large quantities (e.g. human serum albumin: Wall, 1996) or for modifying milk composition for human consumption (human lactoferrin: Krimpenfort *et al.*, 1991; human alpha-lactalbumin, see later in this chapter). However, the time required to produce and obtain milk from transgenic cattle is nearly twice that for sheep and goats (Table 8.2).

Generation of Transgenic Cattle for Production of
Recombinant Proteins in Milk

Due its prodigious capacity for protein production, the cow may be considered the ultimate among livestock species for mammary production of recombinant proteins. High-merit dairy cows can produce in excess of 10,000 liters of milk per

Table 8.2 Interval from zygote microinjection to onset of lactation, total lactation milk volume and estimated recombinant protein production capacity in sheep, goats and cattle. The interval from microinjection to lactation includes gestation, interval from birth to breeding and interval from breeding to parturition. Lactation volumes are broad averages: actual apounts may vary greatly between breeds and individuals.

Species	Interval from microinjection to lactation (years)	Milk volume/ lactation (liters)	Recombinant protein capacity (g)/lactation[1]
Sheep	1.5	300	600
Goats	1.5	600	1,200
Cattle	2.8	10,000	20,000

[1] Assumes expression level of 2.0 grams/liter.

305-day lactation (Table 8.2). Even at rather modest expression levels of a around 2 grams/liter, a single cow could produce up to 20 kg of recombinant protein per year. Moreover, production costs are estimated to be around $10/gram, compared to ~$10,000/gram to ~ $20,000/gram for cell culture or microbial production systems, respectively (Datar *et al.*, 1993; Bremel, 1996).

Despite this encouraging prospect, progress on the generation and utilization of transgenic cattle has been slow compared to that in other species. Although a small number of transgenic cattle have been reported (Roschlau *et al.*, 1988, 1989; Bondioli *et al.*, 1991; Krimpenfort *et al.*, 1991; Hill *et al.*, 1992; Bowen *et al.*, 1994; Hyttenin *et al.*, 1994), in only one case has transgene expression been documented (c-ski gene: Bowen *et al.*, 1994) and there are no published reports of transgene transmission through the germline. Relative lack of progress in these areas is due to unique difficulties encountered in generating transgenic cattle, including long generation interval, monotocous reproductive pattern, high animal acquisition and maintenance expense and low frequency of generating transgenic calves from microinjected zygotes. Indeed, the logistical and financial burden imposed by these issues has discouraged the widespread establishment of large-scale, sustained transgenic cattle programs.

Zygote Source

Early efforts aimed at producing transgenic cattle utilized zygotes recovered from superovulated donors produced *in vivo*. Zygotes were flushed from the oviducts *in situ* (McEvoy and Sreenan, 1990) or *ex situ* after salpingectomy (Roschlau *et al.*, 1988, 1989; Massey, 1990; Bondioli *et al.*, 1991; Hill *et al.*, 1992). About four injectable zygotes were recovered per donor. Since only 0.09% of the injected zygotes yielded transgenic calves, around 300 donors were required to obtain the ca. 1100 zygotes needed to ensure the birth of a single transgenic calf (reviewed by Eyestone, 1994). The acquisition and maintenance of a zygote donor herd to support a large-scale transgenic program requires a tremendous logistical effort and financial commitment. The high costs of running a zygote donor represent a major obstacle to basing a transgenic cattle production program on this approach.

Most recent attempts to produce transgenic cattle have utilized zygotes produced by *in vitro* maturation and fertilization of oocytes (Figure 8.1) obtained cheaply and in large numbers from freshly-killed cows at slaughterhouses (Krimpenfort *et al.*, 1991; Hill *et al.*, 1992; Bowen *et al.*, 1994; Hyttenin *et al.*, 1994; Jura *et al.*, 1995; Behboodi *et al.*, 1993, 1995). In this approach, immature oocytes are aspirated from ovaries obtained at slaughter, then matured and fertilized *in vitro;* zygotes are microinjected 16–24 h after insemination. The relative ease and economy of this approach has led to the virtual abandonment of the superovulated donor as a zygote source for large-scale transgenic cattle programs.

Information on genetic background and specific health status of slaughterhouse donors is nearly impossible to obtain, though it is often possible to utilize oocytes from slaughterhouses that process primarily either beef or dairy animals. However, if maternal genetics or health status is critical, immature oocytes can be recovered non-surgically from known donors by transvaginal echoscopy, then matured and fertilized *in vitro* to provide zygotes for pronuclear DNA injection (de Loos *et al.*, 1996). Indeed, the developmental potential of zygotes generated in this fashion may be higher than those derived from slaughterhouse material (de Loos *et al.*, 1996). While the transvaginal approach will likely provide fewer zygotes on a daily basis than a slaughterhouse-based program, it does allow for the repeated use of specific donors and thus combines some advantages of both *in vivo* and *in vitro* zygote production schemes.

Pronuclear DNA Injection

Injectable pronuclei of *in vitro*-derived zygotes generally appear between 16 and 26 h after insemination. Interestingly, pronuclei are present in zygotes between 8 and 26 h post-insemination as determined by aceto-orcien staining; their optimum visibility for pronuclear DNA injection occurs during a relatively brief "injection window" between about 18 and 24 h post-insemination (Peura *et al.*, 1994a). Thus, most injections of *in vitro*-derived bovine zygotes are probably performed during the mid to late S-phase of the cell cycle (Eyestone and First, 1988; Barnes and Eyestone, 1990). One model for the mechanism of transgene integration states that integration occurs during the S-phase (Bishop and Smith, 1989; Wall, 1996). Indeed, murine zygotes are generally injected during G1, leading some workers to speculate that higher integration frequencies are obtained in mice because zygotes are injected earlier in the cell cycle giving transgenes more opportunity to integrate (Wall *et al.*, 1996). However, results of experiments designed to address this issue in cattle have been equivocal (Krisher *et al.*, 1994a; Gagne *et al.*, 1995). Resolution of this problem in cattle must await development of methods (e.g. *in situ* hybridization) to reliably assess transgene integration in early stage embryos.

As in other species, embryo development in cattle is reduced by introduction of DNA into pronuclei. Although some zygotes may lyse immediately after injection (up to 40% in some cases: Thomas *et al.*, 1993), lysis does not fully account for all injection-related losses. The various zygote preparation and handling procedures associated with pronuclear DNA injection (centrifugation to stratify cytoplasm for pronuclear visualization, exposure to temperature changes, light and handling media) had little or no effect on subsequent development (Wall and Hawk, 1988; Gagne *et al.*, 1990; Peura *et al.*, 1994a). Mere introduction of the injection needle into the cytoplasm and pronucleus did not affect subsequent development (Peura *et al.*, 1994b). However, injection of water or DNA buffer alone into the pronucleus reduced subsequent embryo development; inclusion of DNA with the buffer reduced development even more (Peura *et al.*, 1994b). That DNA injected into the pronuclei reduces embryo viability is unfortunate, but it is something that must be put up with until an alternative means of generating transgenic animals is developed.

Embryo Culture

Microinjected bovine zygotes are generally cultured for 6–7 days before transfer to final recipients. This practice permits embryos to be transferred by simple, non-surgical means to the uterus and helps to deal with some of the major logistical issues of generating transgenic cattle. First, it avoids the laborious surgery involved in transferring individual (or even multiple) zygotes into the bovine oviduct. Second, it avoids the high risk of pregnancy loss and freemartinism associated with multiple-fetus pregnancies that often result from transferring multiple zygotes or embryos to recipient cattle. Finally, it provides an important developmental screen, since only normally developed embryos are selected for transfer to final recipients. Since only about 5–15% of injected zygotes develop to a transferable stage during this period, recipient requirements are reduced drastically (up to 95%) compared to direct transfer of one or even several zygotes to the oviducts of final recipients.

Microinjected zygotes have been successfully cultured *in vivo* and *in vitro*. *In vivo* systems include the bovine reproductive tract (Roschlau *et al.*, 1988, 1989; Reichenbach *et al.*, 1991) and the oviducts of rabbits (Hawk *et al.*, 1989; Gagne *et al.*, 1990; Reichenbach *et al.*, 1991; Thomas *et al.*, 1993; Bowen *et al.*, 1994), sheep (Biery *et al.*, 1988; Hill *et al.*, 1992; Bondioli *et al.*, 1991; Behboodi *et al.*, 1993, 1995), swine (Reichenbach *et al.*, 1991) and excised mouse oviducts maintained in organ culture (Peura *et al.*, 1994a). Several *in vitro* culture systems have also been utilized, including co-culture with oviductal tissue (Reichenbach *et al.*, 1991; Behboodi *et al.*, 1993, 1995; de Loos *et al.*, 1996) and buffalo rat liver cells (Krisher *et al.*, 1994a), oviduct tissue-conditioned medium (Krimpenfort *et al.*, 1991; Thomas *et al.*, 1993), diluted bovine oviductal fluid (Bondioli *et al.*, 1991) and semi-defined culture media (Peura *et al.*, 1994a,b). According to some studies, pronuclear-injected, *in vivo*-cultured zygotes develop better than their *in vitro*-cultured counterparts, and are regarded by some to be of higher

Table 8.3   Generation of transgenic cattle during a 3-month production campaign at PPL Therapeutics, Inc.

No. injected/ total (%)	No. developed (% of injected)	No. transferred (% of injected)	No. pregnant (% of transferred)	No. calves (% of transferred)	No. transgenic (% of calves)
5,717/ 10,339 (55)	404 (7)	278 (5)	81 (29)	47 (17)	5 (11)

morphological quality (Behboodi *et al.*, 1993, 1995). However, *in vitro* systems are far simpler to use and less expensive, and recovery rate after culture is always stable at 100%, compared to a highly variable 0–100% after *in vivo* culture.

Embryo Transfer and Fetal Development

Embryos developing to the compact morula and blastocyst stages are generally transferred by standard non-surgical methods to the uteri of recipient animals. Initial pregnancy rate is lower than that achieved with non-manipulated embryos (about 25% vs. 50%, respectively; reviewed by Eyestone, 1994; Table 8.3). Moreover, calving rate is far lower than for ordinary embryos (15–20%; reviewed by Eyestone, 1994; Table 8.3). Clearly, pronuclear DNA microinjection has latent affects on both embryonic and fetal development. The reason for this reduced embryonic and fetal survival are unknown, but it may result from chromosomal damage or insertional mutations induced during the microinjection process.

Production of Transgenic Cattle at PPL Therapeutics

Our laboratory has recently been engaged in large-scale efforts to produce transgenic cattle that express human milk proteins in their milk. Founder animal production campaigns have been conducted for two human alpha-lactalbumin constructs with the aim of producing at least 5 transgenic founders for each construct. The procedures employed, as well as some representative results, will be outlined in this section.

In vitro techniques were used to generate zygotes for microinjection and for their culture to the morula or blastocyst stage (Figure 8.1). Immature oocytes were aspirated from ovaries obtained from several slaughterhouses, matured according to Sirard *et al.* (1988) either in a laboratory incubator or in a portable, battery-powered incubator during overnight transit from two distant locations (Long *et al.*, 1994). After a 20–24 h maturation interval, oocytes were inseminated with frozen-thawed, swim-up separated bull sperm (Parrish *et al.*, 1986).

For pronuclear DNA injection, presumptive zygotes were stripped of cumulus cells approximately 16 h post-insemination (pi), centrifuged for ~6 min at 13,000g and examined for pronuclei on an inverted microscope under Nomarski interference contrast optics. Zygotes were then placed on a depression slide in ~200 ul of TL-hepes (Parrish *et al.*, 1988) covered with mineral oil to prevent evaporation. The medium was maintained at a temperature of 38.5°C during injection sessions.

Zygotes were injected between 16 and 24 h pi by introducing a finely-pulled glass injection needle into one of the two pronuclei (Figure 8.1).

Embryos were cultured *in vitro* for 6 days. Embryos that developed to the compact morula or blastocyst stage were transferred non-surgically to the uteri of recipients heifers in whom estrus had been synchronized to within ± 24 h of the day of *in vitro* fertilization. Pregnancy was diagnosed by trans-rectal ultrasonography at Day 30 of gestation and monitored monthly thereafter. To maximize perinatal survival, recipients were scheduled for elective Cesarean section 5–7 days prior to their anticipated due dates, though some calved naturally prior to this time. Transgene integration was assessed by PCR and Southern blotting of DNA extracted from a small piece of ear tissue and from white blood cells.

The results one three-month campaign are presented in Table 8.3. Using *in vitro* embryo production techniques, up to 800 zygotes could be injected per week. On average, 7% of the injected eggs developed to the morula or blastocyst stage by Day 7 pi. Up to 43 embryos were transferred during any given week. Initial pregnancy and calving frequencies (29% and 17%, respectively; Table 8.3) were similar to those reported by others (reviewed by Eyestone *et al.*, 1994). Five of 47 (11%) of the calves born were transgenic. The integration frequency obtained was higher than that previously reported (0–6%; reviewed by Eyestone, 1994); however, the efficiency of producing transgenic calves from microinjected zygotes (0.1%) was similar to that in other studies (reviewed by Eyestone, 1994).

FUTURE PROSPECTS

The production of transgenic livestock by the traditional methods described in this paper is a relatively inefficient process. Two technologies are currently being developed to alleviate some of this inefficiency. The first involves methods to screen embryos for transgenesis prior to transfer into recipients to reduce recipient logistics and cost. Embryos can be biopsied with minimal effect on subsequent development and the biopsy then analyzed for the transgene by PCR prior to transfer. This approach has been used to correctly predict the birth of transgenic calves (Bowen *et al.*, 1994; Hyttenin *et al.*, 1994). However, PCR analysis of microinjected embryos is plagued by high levels of false-positives, presumably due to the presence of non-integrated, injected DNA either in or on the embryos (Bowen *et al.*, 1994; Krisher *et al.*, 1994b), thus limiting its utility as an effective screening tool. An alternative screening approach would be to use fluorescent *in situ* hybridization (Lewis-Williams *et al.*, 1997) which, if performed on biopsied blastomeres in metaphase, should avoid the false-positive problems associated with PCR.

Perhaps the ultimate approach to making transgenic livestock involves the use of embryonic stem cells. Totipotent, or even pluripotent, cells could be genetically manipulated with great precision by homologous recombination, then incorporated into an embryo either by blastocyst injection (as is done for the mouse) or preferably, by nuclear transfer (Campbell *et al.*, 1996). By using homologous recombination, this approach would eliminate variation in transgene expression by allowing for site-specific and transgene integration; moreover, all embryos produced by this route would be transgenic, thus reducing recipient animal requirements. Although true embryonic stem cells have not been isolated from any livestock species to date, prospects for success remain optimistic since it has been possible to generate lambs after nuclear transfer from cultured inner cell mass cells (Campbell *et al.*, 1996).

The use of transgenic technology in livestock at this moment is an expensive and somewhat risky proposition. As a result, commercial investment in this area has been limited to those applications with a high potential for financial return, i.e. production of recombinant biomedical proteins in the mammary gland of dairy animals. It is likely that agricultural applications of transgenesis, which pose a somewhat reduced prospect for financial return, will not emerge until technical refinements (such as those mentioned above) reduce the costs of producing transgenic livestock.

REFERENCES

Andres, A., C. Schoenberger, B. Groner, L. Henninghausen, M. Lemeur and P. Gerlinger (1987) H-ras oncogene expression directed by a milk protein gene promoter: tissue specificity, hormonal regulation and tumor induction in transgenic mice. *Proc. Natl. Acad. Sci. USA* **84**, 1299–1303.

Archibald, A., M. McLenaghan, V. Hornsey, J. Simons and A. Clark (1990) High-level expression of biologically active human alpha-1 antitrypsin in the milk of transgenic mice. *Proc. Natl. Acad. Sci. USA* **87**, 5178–5182.

Barnes, F.L. and W.H. Eyestone (1990) Early cleavage and the maternal-zygotic transition. *Theriogenology* **33**, 141–152.

Behboodi, E., G. Anderson, S. Horvat, J. Medrano, J. Murray and J. Rowe (1993) Microinjection of bovine embryos with a foreign gene and its detection at the blastocyst stage. *J. Dairy Sci.* **76**, 3392–3399.

Behboodi, E., G. Anderson, R. BonDurrant, S. Cargill, B. Kreuscher, J. Medrano and J. Murray (1995) Birth of large calves that developed from *in vitro*-derived bovine embryos. *Theriogenology* **44**, 227–232.

Biery, K., K. Bondioli and J. DeMayo (1988) Gene transfer by pronuclear injection the bovine. *Theriogenology* **29**, 224 (abstract).

Bishop, J. and P. Smith (1989) Mechanism of chromosomal integration of microinjected DNA. *Mol. Biol. Med.* **6**, 283–289.

Bishop, J.O. (1997) Chromosomal insertion of DNA. *Reprod. Nutr. Dev.* **36**, 607–618.

Bondioli, K., K. Biery, K. Hill, K. Jones and J. DeMayo (1991) Production of transgenic cattle by pronuclear injection. In: *Transgenic Animals*, edited by N. First and F. Haseltine, pp. 265–273. Butterworth-Niemann, Boston.

Bowen, R., M. Reed, A. Schnieke, G. Seidel, Z. Brink, A. Stacey, W. Thomas and K. Kajikawa (1994) Transgenic cattle resulting from biopsied embryos: Expression of c-ski in a transgenic calf. *Biol. Reprod.* **50**, 664–668.

Brem, G. (1992) Gene transfer in farm animals. In: *Embryonic Development and Manipulation in Animal Development*, edited by A. Lauria and F. Gandolfi, pp.147–164. Portland Press, London.

Bremel, R. (1996) Potential role of transgenesis in dairy production and related areas. *Theriogenology* **45**, 51–56.

Brinster, R., H. Chen, M. Trumbauer, A. Senear, R. Warren and R. Palmiter (1981) Somatic expression of herpes simplex thymidine kinase in mice following injection of a fusion gene in eggs. *Cell* **27**, 223–231.

Brinster, R., H. Chen, M. Trimbauer and R. Palmiter (1985) Factors affecting the efficiency of introducing foreign DNA into mice by microinjecting eggs. *Proc. Natl. Acad. Sci. USA* **82**, 239–241.

Campbell, K.H.S., J. McWhir, W.A. Ritchie and I. Wilmut (1996) Sheep cloned by nuclear transfer from a cultured cell line. *Nature* **380**, 64–66.

Carver, A., M.A. Dalrymple, G. Wright, D. Cottom, D. Reeves, Y. Gibson, J. Keenan, J. Barrass, A. Scott, A. Colman and I. Garner (1993) Transgenic livestock as bioreactors: Stable expression of human alpha-1-antitrypsin by a flock of sheep. *BioTechnology* **11**, 1263–1270.

Constantini, F. and E. Lacy (1981) Introduction of rabbit B-globin gene into the mouse germ line. *Nature* (London) **294**, 92–94.

Datar, R., T. Cartwright and C. Rosen (1993) Process economics of animal cell and bacterial cell fermentations: A case study analysis of tissue plasminogen activator. *BioTechnology* **11**, 349–357.

de Loos, F., S. Hengst, F. Pieper and M. Saladdine (1996) Trans-vaginal oocyte recovery used for generation of bovine embryos for DNA microinjection. *Theriogenology* **45**, 349 (abstr.).

Ebert, K., J. Selgrath, P. DiTullio, J. Denman, T. Smith, M. Memon, J. Schindler, G. Monastersky and K. Gordon (1991) Transgenic production of a variant of human tissue plasminogen activator in goat milk: generation of transgenic goats and analysis of expression. *BioTechnology* **9**, 835–838.

Ebert, K.M. and J.E.S. Schindler (1993) Transgenic farm animals: A progress report. *Theriogenology* **39**, 121–136.

Eyestone, W.H. and N.L. First (1988) Cell cycle analysis of early bovine embryos. *Theriogenology* **29**, 243 (abstr.).

Eyestone, W.H. (1994) Challenges and progress in the production of transgenic cattle. *Reprod. Fertil. Dev.* **6**, 647–652.

Gagne, M., F. Pothier and M.-A. Sirard (1990) Developmental potential of early bovine zygotes submitted to centrifugation and microinjection following *in vitro* maturation of oocytes. *Theriogenology* **34**, 417–425.

Gagne, M., F. Pothier and M.-A. Sirard (1995) Effect of microinjection time during post-fertilization S-phase on embryonic development. *Mol. Reprod. Dev.* **41**, 184–194.

Gordon, J., G. Scagnos, D. Plotkin, J. Barbosa and F. Ruddle (1980) Genetic transformation of mouse embryos by microinjection of purified DNA. *Proc. Natl. Acad. Sci. USA* **77**, 7380–7384.

Gordon, J. and F. Ruddle (1981) Integration and stable germ line transmission of genes injected into mouse pronuclei. *Science* **214**, 1244–1246.

Gordon, J. (1993) "Production of transgenic mice" In: *Methods in Enzymology, vol. 225: Guide to Techniques in Mouse Development*, edited by P.M. Wasserman and M.L. DePamphilis, pp. 747–771.

Gordon, K., E. Lee, J. Vitale, A. Smith, H. Westphal and L. Henninghausen (1987) Production of human tissue plasminogen activator in transgenic mouse milk. *BioTechnology* **5**, 1183–1187.

Hammer, R., V. Pursel, C. Rexroad, R. Wall, D. Bolt, K. Ebert, R. Palmiter and R. Brinster (1985) Production of transgenic rabbits, sheep and pigs by microinjection. *Nature* **315**, 680–683.

Hawk, H.W., R.J. Wall and H.H. Conley (1989) Survival of DNA-injected cow embryos temporarily cultured in rabbit oviducts. *Theriogenology* **32**, 243–240.

Hill, K., J. Curry, F. DeMayo, K. Jones-Diller, J. Slapak and K. Bondioli (1992) Production of transgenic cattle by pronuclear injection. *Theriogenology* **37**, 222 (abstract).

Hogan, B., F. Constantini and E. Lacy (1986) *Manipulating the Mouse Embryo: A Laboratory Manual.* Cold Spring Harbor Laboratory, Cold Spring Harbor, New York.

Hyttenin, J.-M., T. Peura, M. Tolvanen, J. Aalto, L. Alhonen, R. Sinervirta, M. Halmekyto, S. Myohannen and J. Janne (1994) Generation of transgenic dairy cattle from transgene-analyzed and sexed embryos produced *in vitro*. *BioTechnology* **12**, 606–608.

Jura, J., J.J. Kopchick, W. Chen, T. Wagner, J. Modlinski, M. Reed, J. Knapp and Z. Smorag (1995) *In vitro* and *in vivo* development of bovine embryos from zygotes and 2-cell embryos microinjected with endogenous DNA. *Theriogenology* **41**, 1259–1266.

Krimpenfort, P., A. Rademakers, W. Eyestone, A. van der Schans, S. van den Brook, P. Kooiman, E. Kootwijk, G. Platenburg, F. Pieper, R. Strijker and H. de Boer (1991) Generation of transgenic dairy cattle by *in vitro* embryo production. *BioTechnology* **9**, 844–847.

Krisher, R.L., J.R. Gibbons, R.S. Conseco, J.L. Johnson, C.G. Russel, D.R. Notter, W.H. Velander and F.C. Gwazdauskas (1994a) Influence of the time of microinjection on development and DNA detection frequency in bovine embryos. *Transgenic Res.* **3**, 226–230.

Krisher, R., J. Gibbons, F. Gwazdauskas and W. Eyestone (1994b) DNA detection frequency in microinjected bovine embryos following extended culture *in vitro*. *Anim. Biotech.* **6**, 15–26.

Lathe, R., A. Clark, A. Archibald, J. Bishop, P. Simons and I. Wilmut (1985) Novel products from livestock. In: *Exploiting New Technologies in Animal Breeding*, edited by C. Smith, W. King and J. McKay. Oxford Science Publications, Oxford, U.K.

Lewis-Williams, J., Y. Sun, Y. Han, C. Ziomek, R.S. Denniston, Y. Echelard and R.A. Godke (1997) Birth of successfully identified transgenic goats using preimplantation stage embryos biopsied for FISH. *Theriogenology* **47**, 226 (abstr.).

Long, C.R., P. Diamani, C. Pinto-Correia, R.A. MacLean, R.T. Duby and J.M. Robl (1994) Morphology and subsequent development in culture of bovine oocytes matured *in vitro* under various conditions of fertilization. *J. Reprod. Fert.* **102**, 361–369.

Martin, M.J. and C.A. Pinkert (1994) "Production of transgenic swine" In: *Transgenic Animal Technology*, edited by C.A. Pinkert, pp. 315–338. Academic Press, San Diego.

Massey, J.M. (1990) Animal production in the year 2000 A.D. *J. Reprod. Fertil.* (Suppl. **41**), 199–208.

McEvoy, T. and J. Sreenan (1990) The efficiency of production, centrifugation, microinjection and transfer of one- and two-cell bovine ova in a gene transfer program. *Theriogenology* **33**, 819–828.

Meade, H., L. Gates, E. Lacy and N. Lonberg (1990) Bovine As1-casein gene sequences direct high level expression of active human urokinase in mouse milk. *BioTechnology* **8**, 443–450.

Palmiter, R., R. Brinster, R. Hammer, M. Trubaner, M. Rosenfeld, N. Birnberg and R. Evans (1982) Dramatic growth of mice that developed from eggs microinjected with metallothionine-growth hormone fusion genes. *Nature* **300**, 611–615.

Parrish, J.J., J.L. Susko-Parrish, M.L. Leibfried-Rutledge, E.S. Critser, W.H. Eyestone and N.L. First (1986) Bovine *in vitro* fertilization with frozen-thawed semen. *Theriogenology* **25**, 591–600.

Parrish, J.J., J. Susko-Parrish, M.A. Winer and N.L. First (1988) Capacitation of bovine sperm by heparin. *Biol. Reprod.* **38**, 1171–1180.

Peura, T., J.-M. Hyttenin, M. Tolvanen and J. Janne (1994a) Effects of microinjection-related treatments on the subsequent development of *in-vitro* produced bovine oocytes. *Theriogenology* **42**, 433–443.

Peura, T., M. Tolvanen, J.-M. Hyttenin and J. Janne (1994b) Effects of membrane-piercing and the type of pronuclear injection fluid on development of *in-vitro* produced bovine embryos. *Theriogenology* **41**, 273 (abstr.).

Pinkert, C. (1994) *Transgenic Animal Technology*, Academic Press, San Diego, CA.

Platenburg, G.J., E.P. Kootwijk, P.M. Koolman, S.L. Woloshuk, J.H. Nuijens, P.J. Krimpenfort, F.R. Pieper, N.A. de Boer and R. Strijker (1994) Expression of human lactoferrin in milk of transgenic mice. *Transgenic Res.* **3**, 99–104.

Reichenbach, H.-D., U. Berg and G. Brem (1991) *In vivo* and *in vitro* development of microinjected bovine zygotes and two-cell embryos obtained at slaughter after superovulation. *Proceedings of the 7th scientific meeting of the European Embryo Transfer Association*, Cambridge, U.K., pp. 196 (abstr.).

Roschlau, K., P. Rommel, D. Roschlau, H. Schiderski, R. Huhn, W. Kanitz and F. Rehbock (1988) Microinjection of viral vector into bovine zygotes. *Arch. Tierz. Berlin* **31**, 3–8.

Roschlau, K., P. Rommel, L. Andreewa, M. Zackel, D. Roschlau, M. Schwerin, R. Huhn and M. Gazarjan (1989) Gene transfer experiments in cattle. *J. Reprod. Fertil.* (Suppl. **38**), 153–160.

Sirard, M.-A., J.J. Parrish, C.B. Ware, M.L. Leibfried-Rutledge and N.L. First (1988) The culture of bovine oocytes to obtain developmentally competent embryos. *Biol. Reprod.* **39**, 546–552.

Thomas, W., A. Schnieke and G. Seidel (1993) Methods for producing transgenic bovine embryos from *in vitro* matured oocytes. *Theriogenology* **40**, 679–688.

Velander, W.H., L. Johnson, R.L. Page, C.G. Russel, A. Subramanian, T.D. Wilkins, F.C. Gwazdauskas, C. Pittius and W.N. Drohan (1992) High-level expression of a heterologous protein in the milk of transgenic swine using the cDNA encoding human protein C. *Proc. Natl. Acad. Sci. USA* **89**, 12003–12010.

Wagner, T.E., P.C. Hoppe, J.D. Jollick, D.R. Scholl, R.L. Hodinka and J.B. Gault (1981) Microinjection of a rabbit B-globulin gene into zygotes and its subsequent expression in adult mice and their offspring. *Proc. Nat. Acad. Sci.* **78**, 6376–6383.

Wall, R. (1996) Modification of milk composition in transgenic animals. In: *Beltsville Symposia in Agricultural Research XX: Biotechnology's role in the Genetic Improvement of Farm Animals*, edited by R.H. Miller, V.G. Pursel and H.D. Norman, pp. 165–188. American Society of Animal Science, Savoy, IL, USA.

Wall, R. and H. Hawk (1988) Development of centrifuged cow zygotes in cultured rabbit oviducts. *J. Reprod. Fertil.* **82**, 673–680.

Wall, R. and G. Seidel (1992) Transgenic farm animals: a critical analysis. *Theriogenology* **38**, 337–357.

Wall, R., V. Pursel, R. Hammer and R. Brinster (1985) Development of porcine ova that were centrifuged to permit visualization of pronuclei and nuclei. *Biol. Reprod.* **32**, 645–651.

Wall, R., V. Pursel, A. Shanay, R. McKnight, C. Pittius and L. Henninghausen (1991) High-level synthesis of a heterologous milk protein in the mammary glands of transgenic swine. *Proc. Natl. Acad. Sci.* **88**, 1696–1700.

Wright, G., A. Carver, D. Cottom, D. Reeves, A. Scott, P. Simons, I. Wilmut, I. Garner and A. Colman (1991) High-level expression of active human alpha-1-antitrypsin in the milk of transgenic sheep. *BioTechnology* **9**, 830–834.

9. MODIFICATION OF PRODUCTION TRAITS

VERNON G. PURSEL*

*U.S. Department of Agriculture, Agricultural Research Service,
Beltsville Agricultural Research Center, Gene Evaluation and Mapping Laboratory,
Beltsville, Maryland 20705, USA*

The ability to isolate, clone and transfer individual genes into farm animals provides the opportunity for scientists to modify the traits of farm animals in ways that were previously impossible. Productivity traits that may be amenable to genetic manipulation include rate of growth, efficiency of feed utilization, nutrient composition of meat and milk products, quality and quantity of wool, and resistance or susceptibility to diseases. Transfer of growth-related genes received the most attention in the beginning of the transgenic era, but progress has been slow and appears dependent on development of effective methods to tightly regulate expression of the transgenes. While alteration of milk composition has tremendous potential for producing entirely new milk products or improving the efficiency of manufacturing cheese, the high cost of producing transgenic cattle and the long generation interval have severely limited this effort. Considerable progress has recently been achieved on introduction of a cysteine biosynthetic pathway into the rumen, modification of wool keratin proteins, and stimulation of wool follicle growth in sheep. If initial success in stimulation of wool growth is substantiated as the transgenic sheep mature, wool may become the first animal product resulting from improvement of a production trait by transgenesis. Some progress has been made on transfer of genes for naturally occurring disease resistance, for preformed antibodies, and for viral envelope proteins. While several strategies to increase disease resistance have potential, additional research is required before these approaches can be applied in the field.

KEY WORDS: recombinant DNA; transgenesis; disease resistance; growth rate; carcass fat; wool growth; milk composition.

INTRODUCTION

As we approach the 21st century, those involved in food production may find it useful to think about the future. With the world's population increasing by nearly 100 million people each year, it boggles the mind to think about how all these people are going to be fed. Most certainly if this ever-increasing population is going to avoid massive waves of starvation or wars over agricultural resources we will need to harness all advantages that modern agricultural methods have to offer, and that certainly will include plant and animal biotechnology.

While some people will argue that there will be no place for animal agriculture as the world population continues to increase, recent trends indicate otherwise. In some western countries animal products contribute about two-thirds of the total protein in the food supply and provide almost three-fourths of the eight essential amino acids (National Research Council, 1988). While people in the developed countries in recent years have attempted to reduce their consumption

* Postal address: Building 200, Room 2, BARC-East, Beltsville, MD 20705, USA. Tel.: 301-504-8114. Fax: 301-504-8414. E-mail: vpursel@ggpl.arsusda.gov.

of animal protein, quite the reverse is seen in developing countries. It is well recognized that as per capita income increases so does the consumption of animal products; the same trend occurs as urbanization increases (De Boer *et al.*, 1994). Data from around the world show that on the whole the percentage of the population that can afford to consume animal products is increasing. Thus, unless this trend is reversed, we should expect to see the demand for animal products to increase tremendously during the coming decades. The use of genetic modification will be instrumental in providing a way for the animal industry to satisfy the increased demand for animal food and fiber products.

The following sections review the progress on genetic manipulation of productivity traits in farm animals as well as some of the areas that offer promise for manipulation in the future. These areas include stimulation growth rate, increased efficiency of animal production, development of new or improved meat, milk and fiber products, and enhanced resistance to diseases. At the outset it should be noted that the progress on manipulation of animal traits is far slower than originally envisioned by the early proponents of this technology. The main reasons for this slow progress are: firstly, most economically important traits are controlled by multiple genes, which are largely unknown at this time, and are, understandably, not amenable to manipulation. Secondly, the low efficiency of gene transfer in farm animals makes research on transgenesis quite costly, thus preliminary investigations are usually conducted in mice. Unfortunately, in many cases' results obtained in mice are not directly applicable to farm animals. Thirdly, the ability to regulate expression of transgenes is still far from adequate, even in the mouse, and frequently the regulation of expression obtained in transgenic mice is lacking when the same transgene is used in farm animals.

GROWTH RATE AND FEED EFFICIENCY

Much of the earlier transgenic farm animal research was conducted using a growth hormone (GH) or growth hormone releasing factor (GRF) genes because these peptide hormones regulate many of the physiological processes that influence growth rate and feed efficiency. This early work was fuelled by the results of Palmiter *et al.* (1982) that indicated transgenic mice expressing excess GH grew much faster and to a larger size than control mice. However, for farm animals increased size or growth rate is not nearly as important as improved efficiency of feed utilization or an increase in the proportion of lean body mass, which are economic traits that are altered when growth hormone is elevated.

GH and GRF Transgenics

A number of GH transgenic pigs and sheep were produced with human, bovine, rat, porcine or ovine GH under the control of several gene promoters as is shown in Table 9.1. Vise *et al.* (1988) reported that one pig expressing porcine GH (pGH) grew at an exceptionally rapid rate compared to littermates

Table 9.1 Growth-related genes transferred into genomes of farm animals.

Gene construct (promoter-coding sequence)	Abbreviation[a]	Animal	Reference
Albumin-growth hormone releasing factor	mALB-hGRF	Pig, Sheep	Pursel et al. (1989a); Rexroad et al. (1991)
Cytomegalovirus (LTR)-growth hormone	CMV-pGH	Pig	Ebert et al. (1990)
Mammary tumor virus (LTR)-growth hormone	MTV-bGH	Cattle	Roshlau et al. (1989)
Metallothionein-growth hormone	mMT-hGH	Pig, Rabbit, Sheep	Brem et al. (1985); Hammer et al. (1985)
	mMT-bGH	Pig, Sheep	Pursel et al. (1987); Rexroad et al. (1989)
	oMT-oGH	Sheep	Murray et al. (1989)
	hMT-pGH	Pig	Vize et al. (1988)
Metallothionein-growth hormone releasing factor	hMT-hGRF	Pig	Brem et al. (1988); Pursel et al. (1989b)
		Sheep	Rexroad et al. (1989)
Metallothionein-insulin-like growth factor-I	mMT-hIGF-I	Pig	Pursel et al. (1989b)
Moloney leukemia virus (LTR)-growth hormone	MLV-rGH	Pig	Ebert et al. (1988)
	MLV-pGH	Pig	Ebert et al. (1990)
Mouse sarcoma virus (LTR)-cellular SKI	MSV-cSKI	Pig, Cattle	Pursel et al. (1992); Bowen et al. (1994)
Phosphoenolpyruvate carboxykinase-growth hormone	rPEPCK-bGH	Pig	Wieghart et al. (1990)
Prolactin-growth hormone	bPRL-bGH	Pig	Polge et al. (1989)
αSkeletal actin-estrogen receptor	cASK-hER	Cattle	Massey (1990)
αSkeletal actin-insulin-like growth factor-I	cASK-hIGF-I	Cattle, Pig	Hill et al. (1992); Coleman et al. (1995b)
Transferrin-growth hormone	mTF-bGH	Pig, Sheep	Pursel et al. (1990a); Rexroad et al. (1991)

[a] Lowercase letters designate species from which DNA sequence was derived: v, bovine; c, chicken; h, human; m, murine; o, ovine; p, porcine; r, rat.

(1273 vs. 781 g/day), while Ebert *et al.* (1990) reported two transgenic pigs expressing pGH grew at the same rate as littermates. In a study involving the comparison of two lines of transgenic pigs expressing bovine GH (bGH) and sibling controls, Pursel *et al.* (1989b) found 11% and 14% faster growth rates and 18% increase in feed efficiency (Table 9.2). However, reduction in carcass fat as transgenic pigs approached market weight was the most consistent and dramatic effect of elevated GH as is shown in Figure 9.1.

Unfortunately, pigs that continuously expressed excess GH exhibited several notable health problems, which included lameness, susceptibility to stress, gastric ulcers, parakeratosis, lethargy, anestrus in gilts, and lack of a libido in boars (Pursel *et al.*, 1987; Ebert *et al.*, 1988; Pursel *et al.*, 1989b). In contrast, no increase

Table 9.2 Average daily gain and feed efficiency of MT-bGH transgenic and sibling control pigs (30–90 kg body weight)[a,b].

Line	Group	No.	Average daily gain g/day ± S.E.M	No.	Efficiency kg feed/kg gain ± S.E.M
37–06[c]	Control	23	813 ± 17	8	2.99 ± 0.12
37–06[c]	Transgenic	13	903 ± 23	5	2.45 ± 0.16
			(P = 0.002)		(P = 0.026)
31–04[d]	Control	7	869 ± 43		ND[e]
31–04[d]	Transgenic	7	988 ± 62		ND[e]
			(P = 0.15)		

[a] From Pursel *et al.*, 1990b; [b] Pigs were fed corn-soybean diet containing 18% crude protein plus 0.25% lysine; [c] G2 and G3 progeny of founder 37–06; [d] G2 progeny of founder 31–04; [e] Not determined because pigs were group fed.

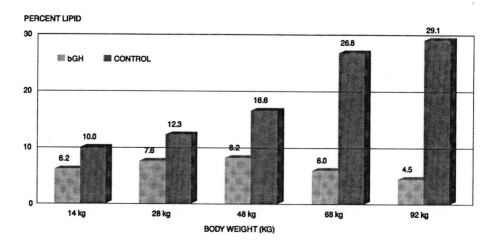

Figure 9.1 Least-squares mean total carcass lipid for four to six MT-bGH transgenic and sibling control pigs at each body weight (reprinted from Pursel and Solomon, 1993, p. 431 by courtesy of Marcel Dekker, Inc.).

in the incidence of these pathological conditions was observed in transgenic pigs carrying nonfunctional copies of GH transgenes or in transgenic pigs that expressed only low levels of bGH (Pursel *et al.*, 1987; Polge *et al.*, 1989).

In contrast to the GH transgenic pigs, transgenic lambs expressing elevated ovine GH (oGH) or bGH did not grow faster or utilize feed more efficiently than control lambs, but they were much leaner (Rexroad *et al.*, 1989; Murray *et al.*, 1989). In transgenic lambs, the lack of body fat may have been the result of hyperglycaemia and glycosuria (Rexroad *et al.*, 1989, 1991). Severely bowed front legs was a frequent anatomical abnormality observed in the transgenic lambs.

Transfer of a growth hormone releasing factor (GRF) transgene is an alternative approach to obtain elevated GH that has been investigated in swine and sheep. Transgenic lambs that expressed GRF had continuously elevated GH and were phenotypically indistinguishable from GH transgenic lambs. In contrast, GH concentrations were not elevated in pigs that expressed GRF because the GRF in blood plasma was the 3–44 metabolite rather than the 1–44 native peptide (Pursel *et al.*, 1989a).

It was recognized from the outset that regulation of transgene expression would be required to circumvent deleterious effects from continuous exposure of animals to elevated GH. While oGH transgenic mice expressed minimally without addition of zinc in the water, the same construct produced high concentrations of constitutive expression in sheep (Murray *et al.*, 1989) and swine (Pursel *et al.*, 1997). Similarly, expression of phosphoenolpyruvate carboxykinase-bGH (PEPCK-bGH) in mice could be regulated by altering the ratio of carbohydrate to protein in the diet of mice (McGrane *et al.*, 1988). However, dietary manipulation did not control the level of GH expression when PEPCK-bGH was transferred into swine (Weighart *et al.*, 1990). Recently, tetracycline- and ecdysone-regulated systems to switch transgene expression on and off in mice have been developed (Furth *et al.*, 1994; Gossen *et al.*, 1995; No *et al.*, 1996). These transgene switch systems show great promise but are not yet perfected. When improved gene switch constructs become available there is little doubt that additional research with GH or GRF transgenes will be conducted.

cSKI Transgenics

The *cSKI* transgene has also been investigated for potential stimulation of muscle development in swine and cattle. Initially, Sutrave *et al.* (1990) transferred the *cSKI* transgene into mice where expression was found to produce extensive hypertrophy of skeletal muscles and reduced body fat. A single transgenic calf was produced that exhibited considerable muscle hypertrophy at about two months of age, which was followed by progressive muscle degeneration over several weeks to the point where euthanasia was necessary (Bowen *et al.*, 1994). Expression of the *cSKI* transgene in swine resulted in a wide range of phenotypes among animals (Pursel *et al.*, 1992). Five transgenic pigs exhibited varying degrees of muscular hypertrophy, while five other *cSKI* transgenic pigs exhibited muscular atonia and weakness in both the front and rear legs. Skeletal muscles from these pigs had high levels of *cSKI* mRNA, while cardiac muscle contained low levels, and no transgene mRNA was detected in any other tissue. Histological examination of skeletal muscles from these myopathic pigs revealed that muscle fibres contained large vacuoles. When the *cSKI* transgene was transmitted to subsequent generations none of transgenic pigs developed muscle hypertrophy without also simultaneously exhibiting considerable myofibre degeneration (Pursel, V.G. unpublished observations). Consequently, no line of *cSKI* transgenic pigs has been developed with commercial potential. In the future possibly the *cSKI* gene may still have application, but evaluation of that potential is dependent upon development of an effective means of regulating expression to prevent myofibre degeneration. Alternatively, understanding the mechanism by which *cSKI* stimulates muscle mass might provide new approaches to enhance muscle development.

IGF-I Transgenics

Recently transgenic pigs have been produced with a fusion gene composed of avian skeletal α-actin promoter, first intron and 3′-noncoding flanking regions and insulin-like growth factor-I (IGF-I) coding region (Coleman *et al.*, 1995b; Pursel *et al.*, 1996). Coleman *et al.* (1995a) previously reported that this fusion gene directs high levels of expression specifically to striated muscle in transgenic mice and elicits myofibre hypertrophy. In the 12 transgenic pigs that have been investigated, muscle IGF-I concentrations varied from 20 to 1702 ng/g muscle compared to less than 10 ng/g muscle in non-transgenic control pigs. In marked contrast to previous experiences with GH transgenic pigs, definitive phenotypes for the IGF-I transgenic pigs were not detected, and no gross abnormalities, pathologies, or health-related problems were encountered. However, the investigators have not yet established whether a sufficient amount of the IGF-I is released from the muscle fibres in these transgenic pigs so that the autocrine or paracrine stimulation of myofibres can ensue. Comprehensive studies of growth characteristics, efficiency of feed utilization, hormonal profiles, myofibre composition, and carcass composition are in progress with progeny resulting from the transgenic founders.

MODIFICATION OF MILK COMPOSITION

Milk is widely considered one of nature's most perfect foods because of its high content of essential amino acids, essential fatty acids, vitamins and bioavailable calcium. This rich source of nutrients results in dairy products providing about 20% of the protein in the diet of several western countries (Gerrior and Zizza, 1994). Alteration of milk composition offers the dairy industry considerable potential for the future but has thus far received little research emphasis. A list of potential changes in milk components that have been suggested by various investigators is shown in Table 9.3.

About 80% of the protein in cow's milk is made up of the caseins (αS_1, αS_2, β and κ) while the whey fraction makes up the remainder. The caseins form the curds in cheese production and for that reason they are extremely important for dairy manufacturing. In contrast, the whey proteins (β-lactoglobulin, α-lactalbumin, serum albumin and γ-globulin) make up only 20% of the milk proteins and represent a less valuable biproduct in the manufacture of cheese. Selective elimination of β-lactoglobulin, which makes up about one-half of the whey, would be beneficial to cheese production since its presence in milk inhibits rennin's action on κ-casein (Yom and Bremel, 1993). Since β-lactoglobulin is responsible for some of the allergic reactions to cows' milk, its elimination from fluid milk would also be advantageous for some consumers. However, removal of β-lactoglobulin from cattle would require genetic engineering of embryonic stem cells, which presently are not developed for this species.

Table 9.3 Some proposed modifications of milk constituents[a].

Change	Consequence
Increase α- and β-caseins	Enhanced curd firmness for cheese-making, improved thermal stability, increased calcium content
Increase phosphorylation sites in caseins	Increased calcium content, improved emulsification
Introduce proteolytic sites in caseins	Increased rate of textural development (improved cheese ripening)
Increase κ-casein concentration	Enhanced stability of casein aggregates, decreased micelle size, decreased gelation and coagulation
Eliminate β-lactoglobulin	Decreased high temperature gelation, improved digestibility, decreased allergenic response, decreased primary source of cysteine in milk
Decrease α-lactalbumin	Decreased lactose, increase market potential of fluid milk, decreased ice crystal formation, compromise osmotic regulation of mammary gland
Add human lactoferrin	Enhanced iron absorption, protect against gut infections
Add human lysozyme	Increase antimicrobial activity, reduce rennet clotting time and increase cheese yield
Add proteolytic sites to κ-casein	Increased rate of cheese ripening
Decrease expression of acetyl CoA carboxylase	Decreased fat content, improved nutritional quality, reduce milk production costs
Express immunoglobulin genes	Protection against pathogens such as salmonella and listeria
Replace bovine milk proteins genes with human equivalents	Mimic human breast milk

[a] Adapted from Jinenez-Flores and Richardson (1985); Yom and Bremel (1993); Maga and Murray (1995).

Caseins

Since caseins are extremely important to the manufacture of cheese, modification of the relative amount or composition of the caseins may offer considerable economic value. One meritorious manipulation that has been suggested is to introduce extra copies of the αS_1-casein gene in cows to increase its proportion in milk. Jimenez-Flores and Richardson (1985) suggest that such a alteration would enlarge the micelles and enhance textural development and curd characteristics. Alternatively, introduction of a chymosin-sensitive region in the αS_1-casein gene by site-specific mutagenesis may accelerate the rate of textural development (Jimenez-Flores and Richardson, 1985).

Increasing the ratio of κ-casein to β-lactoglobulin might also be accomplished by inserting additional copies of the κ-casein gene. Such an alteration may be effective in reducing the size of casein micelles and improve the thermal stability of proteins in canned, sterilized milk products. In addition, Jimenez-Flores and Richardson (1985) suggest deletion of a phosphate group from β-casein would yield a softer cheese with higher moisture content, while addition of a phosphate group would yield a firmer cheese with less moisture and provide improved emulsifying properties. Each change would result in milk with characteristics that would be advantageous for specific market products.

Reduction in Butterfat

Nutrition- and diet-conscious consumers are increasingly shunning products that have high fat levels. As a result of this declining demand either surplus butterfat accumulates or the price declines sufficiently to stimulate consumption. Reduced butterfat production would provide a solution to this problem. Traditional genetic selection is not a suitable means of reducing fat content in milk because the genetic and phenotypic correlations for fat and protein yields are estimated at .86 and .93, respectively (Bremel, 1996). Bremel, Yom and Bleck (1989) suggest de novo fat synthesis from acetate might be reduced by blocking acetyl CoA carboxylase gene expression. The potential of this concept has been tested by transfecting preadipocytes with a ribozyme gene directed against acetyl CoA carboxylase mRNA (Ha and Kim, 1994). The rate of fatty acid synthesis in transfected cells was 30–70% that of the control adipocytes. If transfer of this ribozyme gene had a similar effect on butterfat production in the mammary gland there is the potential to have a dramatic influence on the fat content of milk. Since a gram of fat has 2.25 times the amount energy as a gram of carbohydrate or protein, reduction in fat output in milk would greatly reduce the energy required to produce milk. Yom and Bremel (1993) have suggested that reducing the fat content of milk from 3.8% to 2% would permit dairy farmers to increase the proportion of forage in the diet from about 60% to 83%. Consequently, the concentrate portion of the lactation ration would be reduced by 50%, and the farmers' feed bill for lactating cows would be reduced by 22%.

Lactose

Lactose is a major component of cows milk that makes it an unacceptable food source for a sizable portion of the adult human population deficient in β-galactosidase and unable to hydrolyse lactose (Mercier, 1986). In addition, the low solubility of lactose is responsible for grittiness defects in ice cream. These problems might be alleviated by the partial inhibition of the α-lactalbumin gene, which is an essential cofactor in the synthesis of lactose. Since lactose is responsible for the movement of water through the secretory cells, a reduction in α-lactalbumin and lactose would partially reduce total milk volume, with no reduction in overall production of milk protein. Such an inhibition of lactalbumin expression might be accomplished by transfer of an antisense sequence of the α-lactalbumin gene ligated to a mammary-specific promoter (Yom and Bremel, 1993).

Conversely, Bleck *et al.* (1996) have suggested that enhanced expression of α-lactalbumin in sow milk may increase milk production and boost pre-weaning growth rates in piglets. An increase in α-lactalbumin should elevate the lactose synthase activity in the mammary gland and stimulate lactose content in sow milk. An increase in lactose content early in lactation might provide a valuable energy source for the newborn piglet. In addition, the increased lactose content should increase the total quantity of milk produced. The investigators have produced transgenic swine with the bovine α-lactalbumin gene and experiments are in progress to test this hypothesis (Bleck *et al.*, 1996).

Human Milk Proteins

The introduction of several human milk protein genes into dairy cows or replacement of these bovine genes with human genes may one day play an important nutritional role in human infants that are now unable to receive milk from their mother. Milk from cows and humans differ considerably and consequently cows' milk is not an ideal source of food for human infants. Total protein content of human milk is low (0.9%) and whey proteins predominate, while cows' milk contains about 3.3% protein with 80% of it being casein (Bounous *et al.*, 1988). In addition, bovine β-lactalbumin is quite allergenic to many human infants, and the concentration of lactoferrin in human milk is three-times that of cows' milk.

Lactoferrin provides antimicrobial activity to the human infant and may be an important source of bioavailable iron and other minerals (Mercier, 1986). Therefore, enhancing the concentration of lactoferrin in cows' milk or expression of human lactoferrin in cows' milk may result in a milk product that is more suitable for human infants. Krimpenfort *et al.* (1991) reported the birth of a bull calf with a fusion gene composed of bovine αS_1-casein regulatory region and human lactoferrin coding sequences. Information has not been published regarding the expression of the transgene in milk.

Human milk contains about 3000 times as much lysozyme as is present in cows' milk. Although the biological function of lysozyme in human milk is not known, its antimicrobial activity is considered to be part of the natural defense against food microorganisms, and it may protect the mammary gland against bacterial infection (see review by Maga and Murray, 1995). In addition, research by Giangiacomo et al. (1992) showed that addition of lysozyme to cows' milk was beneficial for rennet clotting time, yield and syneresis in cheese processing. Therefore, enhanced expression of lysozyme in milk may be beneficial for infant formulations and cheese production.

WOOL PRODUCTION

Australia and New Zealand have large expanses of grazing lands that are used to convert forage to wool, which is a high quality textile fibre that is a valuable exportable commodity. The importance of wool to the economies of these countries has led investigators to attempt to improve the efficiency of wool production and enhance its characteristics as a textile fibre. Thus far three research approaches have been undertaken to improve wool production.

Synthesis of Cysteine

Production of high quality wool is dependent upon an abundant supply of amino acids and cysteine in particular. The keratins are the major structural proteins of the wool fibre and a large amount of cysteine is required to form the extensive disulphide bridges that link the keratins as the fibres grow. Cysteine is the rate limiting amino acid for the production of wool. Addition of cysteine to the diet does not increase wool production because the rumen degrades proteins and sulphur is lost as hydrogen sulphide. Bacterial genes are capable of synthesizing cysteine from the hydrogen sulphide and serine, both of which are available in the rumen. This limitation for wool production has led Australian investigators to attempt a genetic engineering approach to overcome this obstacle.

Serine transacetylase (cys E) and o-acetylserine sulfhydrylase (cys M or K) are required for the synthesis of cysteine from rumen substrates, hydrogen sulphide and serine. Bacterial genes for these enzymes have been isolated, sequenced and cloned for Escherichia coli (Ward et al., 1989) and Salmonella typhimurium (Rogers, 1990). These linked bacterial genes (cys E-cys M or K) were used to form transgenes with three gene promoters that give broad expression, sheep metallothionein-Ia (oMT), Rous sarcoma virus long terminal repeat (RSV LTR) and mouse phosphoglycerate kinase-1 (mPgk-1).

The cys E-cys M or K transgenes with oMT, RSVLTR and mPgk-1 promoters were first tested in vitro in tissue culture cells and then in transgenic mice. While these transgenes expressed well in cultured mammalian cells (Sivaprasad et al., 1995), only the transgenic mice with the oMT promoter or the mPgk promoter expressed sufficient enzyme levels in stomach and intestines to support significant cysteine synthesis in vitro (Bawden et al., 1995). Concurrently, these fusion genes were transferred into sheep zygotes and the resulting transgenic lambs were evaluated for expression of the enzyme genes (Bawden *et al.*, 1995; Powell *et al.*, 1994). These three promoters were ineffective in directing expression of the bacterial enzymes in the rumen of the transgenic sheep. However, low levels of expression were detected in skeletal muscle of three of 23 RSVLTR lambs and one of 10 mPgk-1 lambs (Bawden *et al.*, 1995).

Subsequently, Rogers and coworkers (Powell *et al.*, 1994) isolated a rumen-specific gene from a sheep rumen cDNA library. This gene encodes a small proline-rich protein (oSPR) that is highly expressed specifically in the ruminal epithelium. The *cys E-cys M or K* transgene with oSPR promoter was then transferred into sheep zygotes. Of seven transgenic sheep evaluated, only one expressed the transgene in the rumen at a low level at three months of age, and it lacked expression when reevaluated at six months of age.

Wool Keratin Proteins

The second approach to improved wool production that has been undertaken is to modify the protein composition of the wool fibres. The genes for many of the keratin proteins have been sequenced (reviewed by Powell and Rogers, 1990a; Powell *et al.*, 1994). Rogers and coworkers suggest that increasing the abundance of the keratin filament proteins might alter the wool-dyeing properties and the wool crimp characteristics (Powell *et al.*, 1994). Alternatively, increasing the quantity of cysteine-rich proteins to produce more disulfide bond cross-links might be effective in strengthening the wool fibres.

Transgenic mice have been produced with three different wool keratin fusion genes that were expressed in the hair follicles. Two of these transgenes have produced visible phenotypic changes in the hair coat (Powell and Rogers, 1990b; Powell *et al.*, 1991). Subsequently, four transgenic sheep have been produced with a wool keratin IF gene that resulted in over expression of the transgene in wool follicles (Powell *et al.*, 1994). The over expression of wool keratin IF gene in sheep resulted in substantial changes to the fibre ultrastructure with a perturbation in the normal organization of filaments and matrix. While the alterations were not positive, the structural integrity of the fibre was maintained in contrast to the deformed, brittle hair that caused premature hair loss in mice with this transgene. Additional investigations are in progress in sheep using transgenes that encode the cysteine-rich keratins and the glycine-tyrosine-rich keratins (Powell *et al.*, 1994).

IGF-I for Wool Follicle Growth

The third approach to improve wool production is to stimulate fibre growth by expression of insulin-like growth factor (IGF-I) in wool follicles. Several investigators reported that exogenous treatment of sheep with growth hormone-stimulated wool growth (Wagner and Veenhuizen, 1978; Wolfrom *et al.*, 1985; Heird *et al.*, 1988). Subsequently, Harris *et al.* (1993) reported that local infusion of sheep skin with IGF-I increased blood flow, oxygen uptake and amino acid uptake. Since IGF-I mediates many of the actions of growth hormone and has mitogenic properties, its potential as a stimulator of follicle growth in transgenic sheep was undertaken in New Zealand.

Damak *et al.* (1996) reported the production of transgenic sheep with a transgene composed of a mouse keratin promoter and ovine IGF-I cDNA. Two of five founder transgenic lambs expressed the IGF-I in their skin. The expressing transgenic ram was then bred to non-transgenic ewes and 85 lambs were born of which 43 were transgenic. When sheered at 14 months of age, the clean fleece weight of the transgenic animals was 6.2% greater ($P=0.028$) and the bulk was significantly higher ($P=0.042$) than for the non-transgenic half sibs. Other fibre characteristics were unchanged except staple strength was lower for transgenic males than transgenic and non-transgenic females. Expression of the transgene has not had any detectable negative physiological effect on these animals. If the transgenic sheep continue to have enhanced wool growth as they grow older, wool could become the first animal product resulting from improvement of a production trait by transgenesis.

IMPROVED ANIMAL HEALTH

Economic losses from diseases of farm animals have been estimated to amount to 10–20% of the total production costs (Muller and Brem, 1991). Molecular biology and genetic manipulation may be useful in augmenting conventional breeding techniques in conferring animals with improved resistance to some of these diseases and thereby reduce these costs and enhance animal welfare.

Several approaches under investigation include transfer of genes for naturally occurring disease resistance, for preformed antibodies, and for viral envelope proteins. When immunologists have a fuller understanding of the major histocompatibility complex, these genes may be extremely useful for enhancing disease resistance.

Naturally Occurring Disease Resistance

Only a few genes for disease resistance have thus far been identified (see Muller and Brem, 1994). Mice carrying the autosomal dominant Mx1 allele are resistant to influenza viruses. Transfer of the Mx1 gene into mice that lacked the Mx1 allele was successful in conferring resistance to influenza-A viruses (Arnheiter *et al.*, 1990; Kolb *et al.*, 1992). Subsequently, three Mx1 fusion genes were transferred into swine to test their effectiveness (Muller *et al.*, 1992). Two of five transgenic pigs harboring the Mx1 regulatory and structural sequences were found to respond to interferon induction of Mx1 mRNA. However, the response was insufficient to produce detectable amounts of Mx1 protein in the tissues. The other two fusion genes that were transferred into pigs were rearranged during integration, so they were not functional. In retrospect the investigators believe uncontrolled expression of Mx1 during embryogenesis was lethal, thus only animals with low levels of transgene expression of rearranged genes were produced (Muller and Brem, 1994). Once again the necessity of tight transgene regulation was crucial to the outcome, and results were not consistent for mice and pigs.

Preformed Antibodies

Genes encoding mouse α heavy and κ light chains from antibodies against phosphoryl choline (PC) were co-injected into ova to produce two transgenic pigs and three transgenic lambs (Lo *et al.*, 1991). In the transgenic pigs, the mouse immunoglobulin A (IgA) was detected in the serum despite the failure of an intact mouse κ transgene to integrate. Transgenic progeny from both founders demonstrated high levels of serum mouse IgA starting at about five weeks of age. Average levels of mouse IgA were 630 µg/ml in one line and 1293 µg/ml in the other. In both cases, IgA levels in progeny were higher than in the founders. However, mouse IgA showed little binding specificity for PC, presumably because secreted chimeric antibody included endogenous light chains with mouse heavy chains. In transgenic sheep, mouse IgA was detectable in peripheral lymphocytes but not in serum. These studies need to be expanded to obtain conclusive proof that the IgA transgene would be protective against pathogenic bacteria.

In a similar study, Weidle, Lenz and Brem (1991) produced two transgenic pigs and three transgenic rabbits that harbored mouse λ heavy and κ light chain transgenes from antibodies directed against the hapten 4-hydroxy-3-nitrophenyl-acetate. Titres of 100–300 µg IgG/ml in transgenic rabbits and up to 1000 µg IgG/ml in one transgenic pig were present in the serum of founders and transgenic progeny. Further evaluation of the antibody composition indicated xenogenic antibodies had formed by association of light chains of rabbit and pig with heavy chains of mouse.

It is clear from these recent studies that further investigations should consider using homologous regulatory sequences to inhibit formation of chimeric antibodies with low binding specificity for the target antigen.

Intracellular Immunization

A transgenic approach may be effective for producing farm animals that are genetically resistant to specific pathogenic viruses. Salter and Crittenden (1989) produced transgenic chickens that were highly resistant to infection with the subgroup A avian leukosis virus (ALV) by introducing an ALV gene that encoded a viral envelope glycoprotein. Normally, ALV enters chicken cells by attachment of the envelope glycoprotein to cell membrane receptors. However, in the transgenic chickens the subgroup A ALV virus could not enter the cells because the membrane receptors were presumably occupied with envelope protein that had been produced by the transgene. These chickens were not resistant to infection by subgroup B ALV because a different receptor is used for entry.

A similar experiment was initiated in sheep with the envelope gene from visna virus. The sheep population is widely infected with visna virus, which is an ovine lentivirus similar to equine infectious anaemia virus, caprine-arthritis encephalitis virus, and bovine, feline, simian and human immunodeficiency virus. Visna viruses are usually transmitted to lambs in colostrum or milk, where they infect the macrophages or monocytes, and establish lifelong infections. The clinical disease in sheep is ovine progressive pneumonia, arthritis, mastitis, and occasionally paralysis (Narayan and Cork, 1975). Immunizations with vaccines have not been effective in control of visna virus or other lentiviruses.

Three transgenic sheep were produced by microinjection of a visna virus fusion gene into pronuclei of sheep zygotes (Clements *et al.*, 1994). The fusion gene was composed of a visna virus LTR regulatory region fused to the coding region for visna virus envelope protein. All three lambs expressed the envelope glycoprotein in the macrophages as well as in fibroblasts isolated from the skin of the transgenic lambs. These animals have remained healthy and expression of the viral gene has had no observable detrimental effect. Two of the three sheep are producing antibodies to the envelope protein, which possibly indicates the viral gene was expressed relatively late in development and was not recognized as self-antigen. Progeny from these founders will be challenged with a virulent visna virus to test their abilities to resist infection.

Other Disease Resistance Strategies

Considerable transgenic research on modulation of immune responses with interferon and other cytokines has been conducted in mice. While some of these efforts have enhanced viral resistance (Chen *et al.*, 1988), others have resulted in deleterious side effects (Hekman *et al.*, 1988; Iwakura *et al.*, 1988). This effort has not yet been expanded into farm animals. As detailed knowledge of the various cytokines and the complexities of their interactions with various physiological states is uncovered, potential negative side effects of unwanted cytokine actions will be avoided.

Use of antisense RNA to block or inhibit RNA processing or translation in a highly specific manner has tremendous potential for use against specific pathogenic organisms. The expanding use of ribozymes in connection with antisense gene constructs should provide many new avenues for inhibiting the replication of pathogens in farm animals.

CONCLUSIONS

From the foregoing material it is clear that we are gradually making inroads toward harnessing the power of transgenic technology to improve economically important productivity traits of farm animals. In the past few years research on improved wool production and enhancement of disease resistance have brought the greatest progress. Although neither transgenic animals nor their products have reached the marketplace, it appears that wool from transgenic sheep has a good prospect to be the first (Damak *et al.*, 1996). Modification of productivity traits in dairy cattle offers considerable potential, but much of this research awaits improved efficiencies of producing transgenic cattle or development of embryonic stem cells. For many productivity traits, further progress seems highly dependent on finding more effective regulatory systems that permit precise control of transgene expression. As people search for solutions to these problems, they will make unexpected discoveries, find new approaches, and expand fundamental knowledge.

REFERENCES

Arnheiter, H., Skuntz, S., Noteborn, M., Chang, S. and Meier, E. (1990) Transgenic mice with intracellular immunity to influenza virus. *Cell*, **62**, 51–61.

Bawden, C.S., Sivaprasad, A.V., Verma, P.J., Walker, S.K. and Rogers, G.E. (1995) Expression of bacterial cysteine biosynthesis genes in transgenic mice and sheep: toard a new *in vivo* amino acid biosynthesis pathway and improved wool growth. *Transgenic Res.*, **4**, 87–104.

Bleck, G.T., White, B.R., Hunt, E.D., Rund, L.A., Barnes, J., Bidner, D. *et al.* (1996) Production of transgenic swine containing the bovine α-lactalbumin gene. *Theriogenology*, **45**, 347.

Bowen, R.A., Reed, M.L., Schnieke, A., Seidel, G.E. Jr., Stacey, A., Thomas, W.K. *et al.* (1994) Transgenic cattle resulting from biopsied embryos: Expression of c-ski in a transgenic calf. *Biol. Reprod.*, **50**, 664–668.

Brem, G., Brenig, B., Goodman, H.M., Selden, R.C., Graf, F., Kruff, B. *et al.* (1985) Production of transgenic mice, rabbits and pigs by microinjection into pronuclei. *Zuchthygiene*, **20**, 251–252.

Brem, G., Brenig, B., Muller, M., Kraublich, H. and Winnacker, E.-L. (1988) Production of transgenic pigs and possible application to pig breeding. *Occasional Publ. British Soc. Anim. Prod.*, **12**, 15–31.

Bremel, R.D. (1996) Potential role of transgenesis in dairy production and related areas. *Theriogenology*, **45**, 51–56.

Bremel, R.D., Yom, H.-C. and Bleck, G.T. (1989) Alteration of milk composition using molecular genetics. *J. Dairy Sci.*, **72**, 2826–2833.

Bounous, G., Kongshavn, P.A., Taveroff, A. and Gold, P. (1988) Evolutionary traits in human milk proteins. *Med. Hypotheses*, **27**, 133–140.

Chen, X.-Z., Yun, J.S. and Wagner, T.E. (1988) Enhanced viral resistance in transgenic mice expressing the human beta 1 interferon. *J. Virol.*, **62**, 3883–3887.

Clements, J.E., Wall, R.J., Narayan, O., Hauer, D., Schoborg, R., Sheffer, D. *et al.* (1994) Development of transgenic sheep that express the visna virus envelope gene. *Virology*, **200**, 370–380.

Coleman, M.E., DeMayo, F., Yin, K.C., Lee, H.M., Geske, R., Montgomery, C. *et al.* (1995a) Myogenic vector expression of insulin-like growth factor I stimulates muscle cell differentiation and myofiber hypertrophy in transgenic mice, *J. Biol. Chem.*, **270**, 12109–12116.

Coleman, M.E., Pursel, V.G., Wall, R.J., Haden, M., DeMayo, F. and Schwartz, R.J. (1995b) Regulatory sequences from the avian skeletal α-actin gene directs high level expression of human insulin-like growth factor-I cDNA in skeletal muscle of transgenic pigs, *J. Anim. Sci.*, **73** (Suppl. 1), 145.

Damak, S., Su, H.-Y., Jay, N.P. and Bullock, D.W. (1996) Improved wool production in transgenic sheep expressing insulin-like growth factor 1. *Bio/Technology*, **14**, 185–188.

DeBoer, A.J., Yazman, J.A. and Raun, N.S. (1994) Aminal agriculture in developing countries: technology dimensions. In *Developmental Studies Paper Series*, edited by K. Seckler, Morrilton, Arkansas: Winrock International, pp. 1–43.

Ebert, K.M., Low, M.J., Overstrom, E.W., Buonomo, F.C., Baile, C.A., Roberts, T.M. *et al.* (1988) A Moloney MLV-rat somatotropin fusion gene produces biologically active somatotropin in a transgenic pig. *Molec. Endocrinol.*, **2**, 277–283.

Ebert, K.M., Smith, T.E., Buonoma, F.C., Overstrom, E.W. and Low, M.J. (1990) Porcine growth hormone gene expression from viral promoters in transgenic swine. *Anim. Biotech.*, **1**, 145–159.

Furth, P.A., Onge, L.S., Boger, H., Gruss, P., Gossen, M., Kistner, A. *et al.* (1994) Temporal control of gene expression in transgenic mice by a tetracycline-responsive promoter. *Proc. Natl. Acad. Sci. USA*, **91**, 9302–9306.

Gerrior, S.A. and Zizza, C. (1994) Nutrient content of the U.S. Food Supply, 1909–90. *U.S. Department of Agriculture, Home Economics Research Report*, No. 52, pp. 120.

Giangiacomo, R., Nigro, F., Messina, G. and Cattaneo, T.M. (1992) Lysozyme: just an additive or a technological aid as well? *Food Additiv. and Contaminants*, **9**, 427–433.

Gossen, M., Freundlieb, S., Bender, G., Muller, G., Hillen, W. and Bujard, H. (1995) Transcriptional activation by tetracyclines in mammalian cells. *Science*, **268**, 1766–1769.

Ha, J. and Kim, K.H. (1994) Inhibtion of fatty acid synthesis by expression of an acetyl-CoA carboxylase-specific ribozyme gene. *Proc. Natl. Acad. Sci. USA*, **91**, 9951–9956.

Hammer, R.E., Pursel, V.G., Rexroad, C.E. Jr., Wall, R.J., Bolt, D.J., Ebert, K.M. *et al.* (1985) Production of transgenic rabbits, sheep and pigs by microinjection. *Nature*, **315**, 680–683.

Harris, P.M., McBride, B.W., Gurnsey, M.P., Sinclair, B.R. and Lee, J. (1993) Direct infusion of a variant of insulin-like growth factor-I into the skin of sheep and effects on local blood flow, amino acid utilization and cell replication. *J. Endocr.*, **139**, 463–472.

Heird, C.E., Hallford, F.M., Spoon, R.A., Holcombe, D.W., Pope, T.C., Olivares, V.H. *et al.* (1988) Growth and hormone profiles in fine-wool ewe lambs after long-term treatment with ovine growth hormone. *J. Anim. Sci.*, **66** (suppl. 1), 201.

Hekman, A.C., Trapman, J., Mulder, A.H., van Gaalen, J.L. and Zwarthoff, E.C. (1988) Interferon expression in the testes of transgenic mice leads to sterility. *J. Cell. Biochem.*, **49**, 325–332.

Hill, K.G., Curry, J., DeMayo, F.J., Jones-Diller, K., Slapak J.R. and Bondioli, K.R. (1992) Production of transgenic cattle by pronuclear injection. *Theriogenology*, **37**, 222.

Iwakura, Y., Asano, M., Nishimune, Y. and Kawade, Y. (1988) Male sterility in transgenic mice carrying exogenous mouse interferon-beta gene under control of the metallothionein enhancer-promoter. *EMBO J.*, **7**, 3757–3762.

Jimenez-Flores, R. and Richardson, T. (1985) Genetic engineering of the caseins to modify the behavior of molk during processing: a review. *J. Dairy Sci.*, **71**, 2640–2654.

Kolb, E., Laine, E., Strehler, D. and Staeheli, P. (1992) Resistance to influenza virus infection of Mx transgenic mice expressing Mx protein under the control of two constitutive promoters. *J. Virol.*, **66**, 1709–1716.

Krimpenfort, P., Rademakers, A., Eyestone, W., Van de Schans, A., Van den Broek, S., Kooiman, P. *et al.* (1991) Generation of transgenic dairy cattle using *in vitro* embryo production. *Bio-technology*, **9**, 844–847.

Lo, D., Pursel, V., Linton, P.J., Sandgren, E., Behringer, R., Rexroad, C. *et al.* (1991) Expression of mouse IgA by transgenic mice, pigs and sheep. *European J. Immunol.*, **21**, 1001–1006.

Maga, E.A. and Murray, J.D. (1995) Mammary gland expression of transgenes and the potential for altering the properties of milk. *Bio/Technology*, **13**, 1452–1457.

Massey, J.M. (1990) Animal production industry in the year 2000 A.D. *J. Reprod. Fertil. Suppl.*, **41**, 199–208.

McGrane, M.M., deVente, J., Yun, J., Bloom, J., Park, E., Wynshaw-Boris, A. *et al.* (1988) Tissue-specific expression and dietary regulation of a chimeric phosphoenolpyruvate carboxykinase/bovine growth hormone gene. *J. Biol. Chem.*, **263**, 11443–11451.

Mercier, J.-C. (1986) Genetic engineering: some expections. In *Exploiting New Technologies in Animal Breeding*, edited by C. Smith, J.W.B. King and J. McKay, Oxford: Oxford University Press, pp. 122–131.

Muller, M. and Brem, G. (1991) Disease resistance in farm animals. *Experientia*, **47**, 923–934.

Muller, M. and Brem, G. (1994) Transgenic strategies to increase disease resistance in livestock. *Reprod. Fertil. Dev.*, **6**, 605–613.

Muller, M., Brenig, B., Winnacker, E.-L. and Brem, G. (1992) Transgenic pigs carrying cDNA copies encoding the murine Mx1 protein which confers resistance to influenza virus infection. *Gene*, **121**, 263–270.

Murray, J.D., Nancarrow, C.D., Marshall, J.T., Hazelton I.G. and Ward, K.A. (1989) The production of transgenic Merino sheep by microinjection of ovine metallothionein-ovine growth hormone fusion genes. *Reprod. Fert. Dev.*, **1**, 147–155.

Narayan, O. and Cork, L.C. (1975) Lentiviral diseases of sheep and goats: Chronic pneumonia, leukoencephalomyelitis and arthritis. *Rev. Infect. Dis.*, **7**, 89–98.

National Research Council (1988) Current trends in consumption of animal products. In *Designing Foods: Animal Product Options in the Marketplace*, Washington D.C.: National Academy Press, pp. 18–44.

No, D., Yao, T.-P. and Evens, R.M. (1996) Ecdysome-inducible gene expression in mammalian cells and transgenic mice. *Proc. Natl. Acad. Sci. USA*, **93**, 3346–3351.

Palmiter, R.D., Brinster, R.L., Hammer, R.E., Trumbauer, M.E., Rosenfeld, M.G. and Birnberg, N.C. *et al.* (1982) Dramatic growth of mice that develop from eggs microinjected with metallothionein-growth hormone fusion genes. *Nature*, **300**, 611–615.

Polge, E.J.C., Barton, S.C., Surani, M.H.A., Miller, J.R., Wagner, T., Elsome, K. *et al.* (1989) Induced expression of a bovine growth hormone construct in transgenic pigs. In *Biotechnology of Growth Regulation*, edited by R.B. Heap, C.G. Prosser and G.E. Lamming, London: Butterworths, pp. 189–199.

Powell, B.C. and Rogers, G.E. (1990a) Hard Keratin IF and associated proteins. In *Cellular and Molecular Biology of Intermediate Filaments*. Edited by R.D. Goldman and P.M. Steinert, New York: Plenum Press, pp. 267–300.

Powell, B.C. and Rogers, G.E. (1990b) Cyclic hair-loss and regrowth in transgenic mice overexpressing an intermediate filament gene. *EMBO J.*, **9**, 1485–1493.

Powell, B.C., Nesci, A. and Rogers, G.E. (1991) Regulation of keratin gene expression in hair follicle differentiation. *Ann. N.Y. Acad. Sci.*, **642**, 1–20.

Powell, B.C., Walker, S.K., Bawden, C.S., Sivaprasad, A.V. and Roger, G.E. (1994) Transgenic sheep and wool growth: Possibilities and current status. *Reprod. Fertil. Dev.*, **6**, 615–623.

Pursel, V.G. and Solomon, M.B. (1993) Alteration of carcass composition in transgenic swine. *Food Reviews Internat.*, **9**, 423–439.

Pursel, V.G., Rexroad, C.E. Jr., Bolt, D.J., Miller, K.F., Wall, R.J., Hammer, R.E. *et al.* (1987) Progress on gene transfer in farm animals. *Vet. Immunol. Immunopathol.*, **17**, 303–312.

Pursel, V.G., Miller, K.F., Bolt, D.J., Pinkert, C.A., Hammer, R.E., Palmiter R.D. *et al.* (1989a) Insertion of growth hormone genes into pig embryos. In *Biotechnology of Growth Regulation*, edited by R.B. Heap, C.G. Prosser and G.E. Lamming, London: Butterworths, pp. 181–188.

Pursel, V.G., Pinkert, C.A., Miller, K.F., Bolt, D.J., Campbell, R.G., Palmiter, R.D. *et al.* (1989b) Genetic engineering of livestock. *Science*, **244**, 1281–1288.

Pursel, V.G., Bolt, D.J., Miller, K.F., Pinkert, C.A., Hammer, R.E., Palmiter, R.D. *et al.* (1990a) Expression and performance in transgenic swine. *J. Reprod. Fertil. Suppl.*, **40**, 235–245.

Pursel, V.G., Hammer, R.E., Bolt, D.J., Palmiter, R.D. and Brinster R.L. (1990b) Genetic engineering of swine: Integration, expression and germline transmission of growth-related genes. *J. Reprod. Fertil. Suppl.*, **41**, 77–87.

Pursel, V.G., Sutrave, P., Wall, R.J., Kelly, A.M. and Hughes, S.H. (1992) Transfer of cSKI gene into swine to enhance muscle development. *Theriogenology*, **37**, 278.

Pursel, V.G., Coleman, M.E., Wall, R.J., Elsasser, T.H., Haden, M., DeMayo, F. *et al.* (1996) Regulatory avian skeletal α-actin directs expression of insulin-Like growth factor-I to skeletal muscle of transgenic pigs. *Theriogeneology*, **35**, 348.

Pursel, V.G., Wall, R.J., Solomon, M.B., Bolt, D.J., Murray, J.D. and Ward, K.A. (1997) Transfer of an ovine metallothionein–ovine growth hormone fusion gene into swine. *J. Anim. Sci.*, **75**, 2208–2214.

Rexroad, C.E. Jr., Hammer, R.E., Bolt, D.J., Mayo, K.M., Frohman, L.A., Palmiter, R.D. *et al.* (1989) Production of transgenic sheep with growth regulating genes. *Mol. Reprod. Dev.*, **1**, 164–169.

Rexroad, C.E. Jr., Mayo, K.M., Bolt, D.J., Elsasser, T.H., Miller, K.F., Behringer, R.R. *et al.* (1991) Transferrin- and albumin-directed expression of growth-related peptides in transgenic sheep. *J. Anim. Sci.*, **69**, 2995–3004.

Rogers, G.E. (1990) Improvement of wool production through genetic engineering. *Trends Biotechnology*, **8**, 6–11.

Roshlau, K., Rommel, P., Andreewa, L., Zackel, M., Roschlau, D., Zackel, B. *et al*. (1989) Gene transfer experiments in cattle. *J. Reprod. Fertil. Suppl.*, **38**, 153–160.

Salter, D.W. and Crittenden, L.B. (1989) Transgenic chickens: insertion of retroviral vectors into the chicken germline. *Theor. Appl. Genet.*, **77**, 457–461.

Sivaprasad, A.V., Kuczek, E.S., Bawden, C.S. and Rogers, G.E. (1992) Coexpression of the *cysE* and *cysM* genes of *Salmonella Typhimurium* in mammalian cells: a step towards establishing cysteine biosynthesis in sheep by transgenesis. *Transgenic Res.*, **1**, 79–92.

Sutrave, P., Kelly, A.M. and Hughes, S.H. (1990) *ski* can cause selective growth of skeletal muscle in transgenic mice. *Genes & Develop.*, **4**, 1462–1472.

Vize, P.D., Michalska, A.E., Ashman, R., Lloyd, B., Stone, B.A., Quinn, P. *et al*. (1988) Introduction of a porcine growth hormone fusion gene into transgenic pigs promotes growth. *J. Cell Sci.*, **90**, 295–300.

Wagner, J.F. and Veenhuizen, E.L. (1978) Growth performance, carcass composition and plasma hormone levels in wether lambs when treated with growth hormone and thyrotropin. *J. Anim. Sci.*, **45** (Suppl. 1), 379.

Ward, K.A., Murray, J.D. and Nancarrow, C.D. (1989) The insertion of foreign genes into animal cells. In *Biotechnology for Livestock Production*, FAO Animal Production and Health Division, New York: Plenum Press, pp. 17–28.

Weidle, U.H., Lenz, H. and Brem, G. (1991) Genes encoding a mouse monoclonal antibody are expressed in transgenic mice, rabbits and pigs. *Gene*, **98**, 185–191.

Wieghart, M., Hoover, J.L., McCrane, M.M., Hanson, R.W., Rottman, F.M., Holtzman, S.H. *et al*. (1990) Production of transgenic swine harboring a rat phosphoenolpyruvate carboxykinasebovine growth hormone fusion gene. *J. Reprod. Fertil. Suppl.*, **41**, 89–96.

Wolfrom, G.W., Ivy, R.E. and Baldwin, C.D. (1985) Effects of growth hormone alone and in combination with Ralgro (Zeranol) in lambs. *J. Anim. Sci.*, **60** (Suppl. 1), 249.

Yom, H.-C. and Bremel, R.D. (1993) Genetic engineering of milk composition: modification of milk components in lactating transgenic animals. *Am. J. Clin. Nutr.*, **58** (Suppl), 299–306.

10. BREEDING GENETICALLY MANIPULATED TRAITS

J.P. GIBSON*

Centre for Genetic Improvement of Livestock, Department of Animal and Poultry Science, University of Guelph, Guelph, Ontario, N1G 2W1, Canada

Having created a founder transgenic animal, further development and application in commercial livestock populations follows four major components: (1) testing of transgene inheritance and effects, (2) multiplication of the number of animals carrying the transgene and creation of a nucleus or elite breeding stock, (3) dissemination of the transgene into the commercial population, (4) continued genetic improvement within the commercial population. The last only applies to those species where genetic selection usually takes place within the commercial population. The testing phase typically will include estimation of hemizygous and homozygous transgene effects on all aspects of economic merit. Difficulties at this stage can be anticipated and become a factor in determining which traits to target and in which lines or breeds to create transgenic animals. Time taken to develop a transgenic nucleus or elite breeding stock will depend on transgene effects, initial genetic lag, the risk from inbreeding depression and structure of the commercial population. Recently developed methods of statistical analysis allow accurate and unbiased estimation of transgene effects concurrent with conventional breeding values which will help in all phases of development, dissemination and utilisation. Relatively modest hemizygous transgene effects, equivalent to a 3–10% increase in performance of key traits will generally be needed to compete genetically with existing genetic improvement programs. Somewhat larger effects will be needed to cover the extra costs of transgenic programs.

KEY WORDS: transgenes; selection; breeding strategies; genetic improvement; genetic lag.

INTRODUCTION

In this chapter I consider some of the technical aspects of genetic improvement of commercial livestock when genome modification via transgenesis is utilised. Creation of transgenic animals producing very high value products such as pharmaceuticals will not involve commercial livestock production systems and is not dealt with here. The legal, social and ethical issues of producing and using transgenic livestock are only mentioned in passing where they might have direct impact on the technical requirements for a genetic improvement program. Other chapters in this book deal with creation of suitable gene constructs and achieving insertion into the germline. The introduction by Smith (*ibid.*) describes strategies of genetic improvement as currently applied in the various livestock species. I make no attempt at detailed economic assessments of transgenic programs since details are highly dependent on transgene effect, species and population structure. Hoeschele (1990) gives a useful illustrative example of economic calculations for dairy cattle. In this chapter, I start at the point where one or more transgenic animals have been born. Since every insertion event will generally be

*Tel.: (519) 824 4120 ex 3694. Fax: (519) 767 0573. E-mail: jgibson@aps.uoguelph.ca.

unique, I define as a separate transgene each insertion event irrespective of the gene construct involved.

Starting with a founder transgenic animal, there are four major components of development through to commercial application in a livestock population. The first component is the testing of transgene inheritance and effects. The second component is multiplication of the number of animals carrying the transgene and development of a transgenic nucleus or elite breeding stock. Components one and two can take place concurrently. The third component is dissemination of the transgene to the commercial population. Component four, which does not apply to all livestock species, is continued selection and genetic improvement in the commercial population in which the transgene is now segregating.

TESTING TRANSGENE TRANSMISSION AND EFFECTS

Testing Transmission

About 70% of germ-line insertion events in mice are transmitted with the expected Mendelian segregation ratios (Wall, 1996) and similar results can be expected for livestock species. Since it will be always be possible to detect genotype at the transgene locus using molecular genetic tests, departure from normal segregation ratios can be tested early among the progeny of the founder animal. Given their low reproductive capacity, it may take more than one generation to unambiguously detect aberrant segregation ratios when the founder is female. In all cases, however, it will be possible to detect marked departures from normal segregation ratios before an expensive program of testing transgene effects is entered. Where aberrant ratios are detected among the progeny of the founder, it may be preferable to delay or scale back major testing expenses until it can be determined by testing in grand-progeny whether the aberrant segregation is due to germ-line chimaerism in the founder or to other causes that will continue to cause problems in later generations.

Testing Transgene Effects

To be commercially successful, a genetic modification must have a net economic benefit for one or more segments of a livestock production industry. Since many genetically controlled traits contribute to net economic merit, each transgene will need to be tested for its effects on many traits. A given transgene will usually be targeted for a positive effect on one particular trait which prior economic assessment has indicated will have substantial economic value. Obviously, the larger the positive effects on the targeted trait the more negative effects on other traits can be tolerated. Judging the degree to which negative effects can be tolerated, however, will require a detailed bioeconomic understanding of the production system in question (see Smith, *ibid.*).

Testing Hemizygote Effects

In most cases, the effects of the transgene will need to be assessed in both the hemizygous (denoted T0) and the homozygous state (denoted TT). Given the process of multiplying the number of carriers of the gene (see below), initial testing will be of T0 versus non-transgenic 00 animals. The number of animals needed for testing in order detect transgene effects with a reasonable degree of certainty depends on the size of the effect required. This is dependant on the economic importance of the trait in question.

Table 10.1, adapted from Smith *et al.* (1987) shows the approximate number of animals to be tested for a variety of gene effects at two levels of power (probability of finding a significant effect). The gene effect (T0–00) is expressed both in phenotypic standard deviation (s.d.) units and as a percentage of the mean for three levels of coefficient of variation. The derivation assumes a random sample of T0 and 00 progeny of the founder transgenic and ignores family structure (see section on methods of estimation, below).

As an illustration of testing, imagine a transgene causing a 20% increase in growth rate and a 5% decrease in litter size inserted into a female line of pigs. Based on a recent estimate of the relative economic value of litter size versus growth rate (Gibson and VanderVoort, 1996), such a gene would have no net economic value. Growth traits typically have coefficients of variation around .10 while reproduction traits are typically around .25. Thus, only 12 animals would be required to detect the increase in growth on 80% of occasions, while 790

Table 10.1   Total number of progeny required to detect a significant ($P < 0.05$) transgene effect.[1]

Size of transgene effect [2]				Number of progeny	
In s.d. units	In percentage of mean for a coefficient of variation of			Power of test [3]	
	0.05	0.10	0.25	0.50	0.80
0.2	1	2	5	384	790
0.4	2	4	10	100	198
0.6	3	6	15	48	90
0.8	4	8	20	28	54
1.0	5	10	25	20	36
1.2	6	12	30	16	26
1.4	7	14	35	12	20
1.6	8	16	40	10	16
1.8	9	18	45	8	14
2.0	10	20	50	8	12

[1] Half progeny are carriers (T0), half not carriers (00).
[2] Effect = difference in performance between T0 and 00.
[3] Power = probability of detecting the gene effect as significant at $P \leqslant 0.05$.

animals would be required to detect the decrease in reproduction. In this situation it would be all too easy to test too few animals, fail to detect the negative effect on litter size and conclude that the gene had a large positive net economic effect. If, however, the transgene had been inserted into a sire line, this problem would not arise since litter size has almost no economic value in such lines. This argues that potential difficulties at the stage of testing transgene effects should be taken into account when deciding which traits transgenes should target, and in which lines or breeds.

A rapid assessment of transgene effects will obviously be desirable to avoid unnecessary development costs on a transgenic line that is later shown not to be commercially viable. In practice, rapid initial assessment will likely be followed by years of further testing to obtain more accurate estimates of effects. At any given time, and given a clear definition of how traits contribute to economic merit, a reasonably accurate estimate of the probability of the transgene having greater than a predefined minimum net economic effect can be estimated given the available data. Decisions on whether to increase or decrease resources to be devoted to further testing can be reviewed based on this probability in relation to the cost of further testing. The cost will vary substantially between traits. The extra information gained over time will also be useful for marketing purposes and perhaps necessary for regulatory approval.

Testing Homozygote Effects

The amount of effort required for testing homozygous transgene effects will depend on how the gene will be used in commercial production (see below). Where commercial stock are crossbred and derive entirely from breeding company stock (e.g. in poultry), the transgene might be fixed only in one parental stock such that the commercial stock is never homozygous for the transgene. In such cases the degree of dominance is irrelevant, and some deleterious homozygous effects may be tolerated in the nucleus population, provided they do not seriously interfere with nucleus breeding operations. Where homozygous animals eventually will be used in commercial production, it will be important to know in some detail how the homozygotes perform, and in particular to ensure that their net economic value is at least as high as that of non-carriers. In this latter case, the number of animals to be tested will be the same as in Table 10.1, though twice as many matings will be required since only $\frac{1}{4}$ of progeny are TT. In the former case, numbers tested can be much smaller.

One difficulty in early testing of homozygotes is the confounding effect of inbreeding depression. The earliest possible production of homozygotes is from matings between carrier (T0) progeny of the original founder. Inbreeding coefficients of the resulting homozygotes will be $F=.25$ if the parents are full-sibs, and $F=.125$ if half-sibs. Delaying production of homozygotes for a second generation of mating T0 individuals to unrelated 00, would reduce the inbreeding coefficient of TT homozygotes to $F=.06$ if first generation progeny were all full-sibs and $F=.03$ if half-sibs. Inbreeding effects are notoriously unpredictable both within and between populations, but are invariably deleterious. This suggests a two stage strategy of testing. A small number of homozygotes can be produced as early as possible, tested for consistent severe deleterious effects and the transgene eliminated if detected. Where deleterious effects appear for some animals but not others, this could be due to the effects of inbreeding rather than the transgene, particularly where $F=.25$. In such cases, a more extensive round of testing should be carried out among homozygotes produced from matings among grand-progeny of the founder, where inbreeding is small. Alternatively, the transgene might be discarded on suspicion of negative effects if other transgenes with more positive results are available.

Methods of Estimating Transgene Effects

In most cases, a reliable estimation and significance test of hemizygous effect among first generation progeny of a founder animal can be accomplished by a straight forward t test, or analysis of variance if there are full-sib families within half-sib groups. Kennedy *et al.* (1992) showed that mixed model methods accounting for genetic relationships among animals give unbiased estimates of gene effects where genotype of all animals is known. A mixed model analysis of first generation progeny, including data on all other animals in the population will give a small increase in accuracy by accounting for polygenic breeding value of mates of the founder. This will be true even if the relationship of the founder to other animals in the population is not known, which could occur if gametes or embryos used to produce transgenic founders are collected from anonymous sources, such as slaughter house oocytes. Data on the first generation of homozygotes can be included in the mixed models, but estimates of homozygote effects will in most cases remain confounded with inbreeding effects. This is because in most populations inbreeding coefficient s are relatively low so that most information on inbreeding depression will come from and be completely confounded with information on first generation homozygotes for the transgene. When data become available on second generation homozygotes, a mixed model including regression of performance on inbreeding coefficient will adequately separate homozygote effects from effects of inbreeding.

As data accumulates over generations of crossing and inter-crossing of transgenic animals, the importance of using mixed model analyses to account for genetic trend and selection (see below) will increase. Depending on the overall breeding strategy (see below) it may not be necessary or not cost effective to continue genotyping all descendants of the transgenic founder. At that point problems begin to arise with standard mixed model estimation procedures. Modifications of methods developed by Hoeschele (1988), Kinghorn *et al.* (1993) and Hofer and Kennedy (1993) proposed to deal with such situations were shown by Hofer and Kennedy (1993) to yield biased estimates. More recent methods, based on Monte Carlo Markov Chain (Gibbs sampling) methods (Pong-Wong and Woolliams, 1996) and on modified mixed model methods (Meuwissen and

Goddard, 1996) appear to give close to unbiased estimates of gene effects and polygenic breeding value in selected populations with complex pedigrees. Gibbs sampling techniques can be difficult to operate on a routine basis (e.g. Guo and Thompson, 1992) and modified mixed model methods are likely to become the method of choice if they can be shown consistently to give similar accuracy and lack of bias to Gibbs sampling procedures.

Not all animals contribute equally to estimates of gene effects. When not all animals are genotyped, Kinghorn (1996) has proposed a trigonometric method to identify which animals would contribute the most information toward estimation of gene effects were they genotyped. Combined with additional information on breeding program design, such an approach might be used to determine a cost effective strategy of genotyping in later stages of transgenic line development or commercial utilisation.

DEVELOPMENT OF TRANSGENIC STOCKS

There are many possible options for developing transgenic stocks, the choice among which will depend on the target trait, species, availability of ancillary technologies and marketing strategy of the organisation developing the transgenic stock. Smith *et al.* (1987) considered three principal options for developing transgenic stocks which cover the broad sweep of possibilities. Slightly modified, these are:

(1) to fix the transgene in a nucleus population,
(2) to develop a pool of elite breeding stock of defined transgene status,
(3) to create an interbreeding pool of transgenes and select the population for net economic merit.

Fixing Transgenes in a Nucleus

This option will be most appealing to breeding companies working with species such as chickens, turkeys and pigs, where closed nucleus breeding programs are routine. The creation of valuable transgenic animals may in itself provide the incentive to create special nucleus stocks for species such as sheep, dairy and beef cattle where nucleus breeding is traditionally less popular.

A basic scheme is outlined in Table 10.2. Founder hemizygotes are mated to non-carriers from a conventional nucleus to produce 50% T0 and 50% 00 progeny. Where natural reproductive capacity or reproductive technologies such as AI, oocyte recovery and *in-vitro* fertilisation, or embryo transfer allow, half-sib progeny would be produced in preference to full-sibs. T0 progeny would be tested for performance against 00 sibs. T0 progeny selected for economic performance would be mated to unrelated non-carriers from the conventional nucleus to produce a second generation of T0 offspring, while a few T0 progeny would be intermated to produce homozygotes for testing (see above). This cycle

Table 10.2 Breeding plan for testing and developing a purebreeding (TT) transgenic line.

Generation	Operation	Mating		Homozygote
0		Founder transgenic × Nucleus stock T0 × 00 ↙		
1	Progeny test	50% T0 half sibs ($a=1/4$) Interbreed T0 × T0 Backcross T0 × 00 from nucleus ↓	→	25% TT Test viability and economic merit ($F=12.5\%$)
2	Multiply, broaden genetic base, continue testing	50% T0 cousins ($a=1/16$) Interbreed T0 × T0 Backcross T0 × 00 from nucleus ↙	→	25% TT for further testing ($F=3\%$)
3	Continue testing, broaden base	50% T0 ($a=1/64$) Interbreed T0 × T0 ↙		
4	Develop a purebreeding TT nucleus ($F<1\%$)	25% TT Breed TT × TT individuals, selected on economic merit		

a = additive genetic relationship.
F = inbreeding coefficient.

would be repeated as required until the stock has sufficiently high genetic merit, sufficiently low potential inbreeding, and the transgene is considered sufficiently well characterised that a generation of T0∗T0 matings could be performed and the TT progeny used to found the new closed nucleus homozygous for the transgene. In Table 10.1, the T0∗T0 matings take place at generation 3, and inbreeding in the new nucleus (generation 4) attributable to the original transgenic founder is less than 1%. Carrying out the inter-se T0∗T0 matings at generation 2 would lead to an inbreeding coefficient of about 3% in the new nucleus, which would be quite acceptable in many situations.

Pigs and Poultry

Gama *et al.* (1992) examined the operation of a variety of schemes of this general type as applied to pigs. The optimum number of generations of backcrossing of the T0 stock to the conventional nucleus depended on the genetic difference in economic merit between the founder animal and the conventional nucleus, the expected severity of inbreeding depression, the rate of genetic progress in the conventional nucleus and the degree of selection for economic performance in the hemizygous stock. As a general rule, however, 3 or 4 generations of backcrossing would provide a reasonable balance between genetic lag and the desire to get a transgenic stock to market as soon as possible. Two generations of backcrossing would suffice where the transgene has a large effect on economic merit and inbreeding is not a major concern.

The new nucleus, homozygous for the transgene, is always at a lower genetic level (genetic lag) for polygenic economic merit than the conventional nucleus. Assuming that the nucleus is used to produce crossbred commercial animals, the heterozygous transgene effect would have to be equal to more than half of this polygenic lag for the transgenic nucleus to have higher overall genetic merit. For traits of low heritability, such as reproduction, the minimum transgene effect to overcome genetic lag would have to be about .15 s.d. or about 3.75% of the mean. For traits of higher heritability, such as growth traits, the minimum transgene effect was about .3–.5 s.d. or about 3.0–5.0% of the mean. Since rather modest transgene effects are required to overcome genetic lag, the primary determinant of size of transgene effect necessary for commercial success is likely to be cost of the transgenic program in relation to potential market value.

The initial genetic lag in overall merit between the founder and elite breeding stock is reduced by half each generation of backcrossing, so that it has relatively little impact on the final genetic lag if several generations of backcrossing are used. Thus, in many situations the initial source of gametes or embryos for creating founder transgenic animals need not be from animals with high genetic merit, which should substantially reduce costs of producing transgenic animals. Hospital *et al.* (1992) and Groen and Smith (1995) showed that anonymous markers could be used to speed up elimination of the genome not coming from nucleus animals, which might reduce the number of generations of backcrossing required. It would, however, be difficult to find informative marker loci if the transgene stock is closely related to the nucleus (e.g. the same breed), and gains would be very small in this situation.

Another result from the work of Gama *et al.* (1992) was that the ultimate genetic lag was not much affected by size of the transgenic population in the early generations. This suggests a strategy for simultaneously testing several transgenes in a fixed resource, sequentially and rapidly eliminating those transgenes with the least favourable effects (based on early testing results), and eventually devoting all testing and development resources to the best transgene after one or two generations of testing. Optimum strategies of resource allocation within and between different transgenes over time have not been investigated.

Similar programs have not been investigated for poultry, but poultry breeding structures are similar to those used with swine. The higher reproductive capacity of females will allow more rapid and effective testing of transgene effects. The higher rates of genetic progress in poultry (Smith, 1984) will probably cause a slight increase in genetic lag of the transgenic nucleus when compared to pigs.

Cattle

Gama and Smith (1992) presented results for introduction of a transgene into a beef cattle nucleus undergoing mass selection for growth traits. Here the principal constraint is time, given the long generation intervals for cattle. Gama and Smith found that the original nucleus could not realistically be replaced by the transgenic nucleus until about year 15 with natural mating, but as early as year 5 with use of multiple ovulation and embryo transfer (MOET). Genetic lags were substantial. Even when replacement was delayed to year 8 with MOET and year 18 with natural mating, hemizygote transgene effects of 5% and 10% respectively were required to overcome genetic lag. Time to replacement and lag could probably be reduced if techniques of oocyte recovery and *in vitro* fertilisation on prepubertal females (Duby *et al.*, 1996) can be developed to routine use.

Creation of a transgenic dairy cattle nucleus has not been investigated. In comparison to beef cattle, testing of transgene effects would take longer, due to the key dairy traits being expressed only in females after about 2 years of age. Application of female reproductive technologies would allow the same speed of backcrossing and intercrossing as for beef cattle so that the end result would probably be a minimal delay in achieving a transgenic nucleus compared to beef cattle. More detailed investigation of alternative schemes for both beef and dairy cattle would be useful. In particular, given that few cattle breeding programs are currently based on a nucleus, it would be useful to determine whether creation of transgenic cattle creates conditions that would favour development of nucleus breeding schemes.

Development of Elite Breeding Stock

This approach would apply to species where nucleus breeding schemes are not the principal means of genetic improvement, such as dairy cattle, and many populations of beef cattle and sheep. Genetic improvement in such populations typically takes place across the whole population, though in practice a portion of the population forms an elite sub-population from which much of the genetic improvement originates. Often in such populations, genetic improvement is disseminated through sale of semen and embryos from specifically identified and tested animals. I here deal exclusively with dairy cattle, though the principles would apply to other species with similar breeding structures.

A general breeding and testing scheme for dairy cattle is illustrated in Table 10.3. It is assumed that the founder is male. A founder female, having a lower reproductive rate than males would cause some delay in the multiplication and testing.

The time taken to get the transgene gene into widespread production will depend somewhat on the type of modification made, how the breeding organisation plans to capture returns, and luck. In Table 10.3 it is assumed that economic returns to the transgene program come through sale of semen and embryos. Realistically this will not commence until the organisation has produced bulls and

Table 10.3   Breeding and testing plan for transgenic dairy cattle.

Time (yrs)	Operation
0	• Founder male born
1	• Mate T0 male * 00 elite females
1.75	• Generation 1 (=G1) progeny born
2.75	• Mate T0 male progeny to 00 elite females • Mate G1 T0 * T0 (half sibs) to produce TT for testing
3.5	• G2 progeny born • First viability test for TT (F=.125)
4.00	• First reliable lactation information on T0 vs. 00 G1 animals • Progeny test EBV for founder male • Retain founder if EBV is high (enter widespread use at yr 5.75 if TT result favourable)
4.5	• Mate G2 TT × 00 elite females • Mate G2 T0 × T0 to produce TT for testing
5.25	• G3 TT and T0 progeny born
5.75	• First test of G2 TT effects on lactation available (F=.125) • Further information on T0 vs. 00 • Progeny test EBV on G1 T0 males available
7.5	• Lactation information on G3 progeny • Progeny test EBV for G2 TT available • Second test of TT performance • Best G2 TT enter widespread use
8.5	• Likely first returns from semen and embryo sales
10.5	• First large scale milk production

cows with sufficiently high total merit (EBV plus transgene effect) that dairy producers will be willing to purchase. Provided the founder bull does not have a large genetic lag behind the current elite sires, returns can reasonably be expected in year 8.5. Even if the transgenic founder bull were produced from elite parents, it would be a stroke of luck if he turned out to have an acceptable EBV. Moreover, in most countries there are likely to be extensive legislated approval processes to be met before marketing can commence, and these are unlikely to be met until G3 information becomes available at year 7.5.

Some transgenes might be aimed at substantial modifications to milk composition with the aim of developing new products, opening new markets or adding substantial value to existing markets. In such cases the organisation would likely plan to make profits through sales of the new product and create a dedicated population of cows to produce milk for them. The genetic lag for conventional economic merit between these transgene carriers and the remainder of the population is less likely to be a major concern in such situations. It would technically be feasible to use semen from either the founder bull and/or the G1 homozygotes to create a large population of commercial cows, once the performance test of G1 T0 and G2 TT was complete at year 5.75. Economic returns from sales of the new or improved dairy product would commence around year 8.75.

If the homozygote was not expected to have substantially higher economic merit than the hemizygote, the transgenic commercial population of cows could be maintained by importing hemizygote replacement progeny from the conventional commercial population. Performance of homozygotes would not be a concern, there would be no need to wait for results on testing of homozygote performance (year 5.75) and breeding to produce the transgenic commercial population could begin as early as year 4. Economic returns would commence around year 7. In practice, meeting the requirements of regulatory agencies might delay the program substantially.

Creating an Interbreeding Pool

In this situation one or more transgenes would be created, perhaps subjected to a minimal level of preliminary testing, and then put into a nucleus population subject to standard selection procedures. The segregating transgenes would increase the genetic variation in the nucleus, leading to an increased rate of response.

Saefuddin (1991) and Gibson (1994) showed by simulation that genes with moderate to large positive effects on traits under selection would rapidly increase in frequency in the nucleus. There was little extra selection response to be gained by using information on transgene genotype in such situations, and long term response actually declined slightly. With genes of smaller effect, using information on genotype was of more benefit in the short term, but caused even greater losses in response in the long term. Transgenes with negative effects on the selection criterion would rapidly be eliminated from the population.

Transgenes with favourable effects could also be lost from the nucleus through genetic drift. The probability of loss is inversely related to transgene effect and number of initial carriers introduced to the herd. Following the derivations of Robertson (1960), Smith *et al.* (1987) estimated that when introducing a transgene through use of a single breeding male, the probability of losing the gene from the nucleus was about 60% or 13% for a hemizygous transgene of effect .25 or 1.0 phenotypic s.d.. Using two males decreased probabilities of loss to 37% and 2% respectively. Most of this loss is expected to occur in the first generation (Robertson, 1960). In contrast to naturally occurring genetic polymorphisms, transgenes can be reintroduced to the nucleus if lost.

The above estimates of probability of loss assume no polygenic genetic lag between the nucleus and the carrier animals introduced to the nucleus. A substantial genetic lag could cause a dramatic increase in probability of loss. In contrast to the creation of a homozygous transgene nucleus (above), having a substantial genetic lag in the founder transgenic would be highly detrimental. When creating an interbreeding nucleus pool, therefore, founder transgenics should come directly from the nucleus to minimise genetic lag. Alternatively, a couple of cycles of backcrossing should be used to reduce any initial lag; but this would increase the time from creation of the transgenic founder to obtaining increased selection response in the nucleus.

Problems with an interbreeding nucleus pool will arise if the transgenes exhibit deleterious effects on production when homozygous. Homozygotes will begin to occur at moderate frequencies only after the transgene itself has reached a high frequency in the population. Eliminating the gene from the population would then be quite difficult, and the problem might itself take some time to be discovered if genotype information on individuals were not recorded regularly. Also, responses may be considerably less than expected if transgenes exhibit substantial dominance and negative interactions with each other. In the latter case, the population might rapidly achieve an equilibrium, exhibiting higher genetic and phenotypic variance than a conventional nucleus, but with no further selection response due to the transgenes. Moreover, there may be a need to quantify individual transgene effects and interactions for marketing and/or regulatory requirements.

The potential difficulties outlined above suggest that genotype for all transgenes should be recorded for all individuals in the interbreeding nucleus pool. The use of mixed model methods (see above) will allow estimation of direct and interaction effects among loci, with information accumulating over time, in addition to maximum accuracy of selection at any given time. As shown by Saefuddin and Gibson (1991), Gibson (1994) and Woolliams and Pong-Wong (1995), such selection leads to lower long-term responses than when not using information on genotype in the selection criterion. In practice, however, the benefits of obtaining rapid returns from the transgenic program will likely over ride any long-term considerations. Given the various uncertainties, simulation of alternative approaches to the production and use of an interbreeding nucleus pool would seem to be well worthwhile.

DISSEMINATION

Having developed a transgenic nucleus or elite breeding stock, dissemination to the commercial population can generally follow normal dissemination routes (see Smith, *ibid.*). Modifications to current marketing and distribution strategies may be necessary in some cases. Transgenes causing a new market product may be protected under patent such that the company retains sole access to the new product produced. This would lead to a separate sub-population of animals being produced and revenue generation over the long-term from product sales. Transgenes causing general enhancements of economic merit are likely to spread more widely through the whole population. It may then prove difficult or impossible for the transgenics company to maintain control over the gene once released, especially in species such as dairy cattle, where genetic improvement takes place within the commercial population rather than in nuclei. Revenue generation will then focus on sales of germplasm (animals, embryos, semen) in the short to medium term. Such transgenes also carry the greatest risk of unforeseen deleterious effects. The cost associated with such risks will need to be included in the price of the germplasm. The general risk associated with use of transgenes also argues for maintenance of existing breeding stocks as an insurance.

The optimum strategy of development and dissemination will depend on end use. Transgenes which cause impaired female reproduction when homozygous can still be used as hemizygotes in a terminal sire (TT) crossbreeding scheme. Even transgenes lethal when homozygote could be used in terminal crossbreeding, using a mixture of 00 and T0 parents in one parental line. As with conventional genetic improvement, the optimum strategy depends on the benefits expected versus the associated costs.

CONTINUED SELECTION AND GENETIC IMPROVEMENT

In species such as dairy cattle or where an interbreeding nucleus pool is created (above), genetic improvement will continue after the transgene has been released into the population. As noted above, standard mixed model methods can be used to continue to improve estimates of gene effects and to obtain maximum accuracy estimates of breeding value, provided all animals are of known genotype and the gene affects recorded traits. In large populations it is unlikely to be cost effective or even possible to genotype all animals. In such cases the Gibbs sampling approach of Pong-Wong and Woolliams (1996), or modified mixed model approaches of Meuwissen and Goddard (1996) or Kinghorn *et al.* (1993) could be used. Developments of methods proposed by Kinghorn (1996) may also become available which will help define an optimum strategy for deciding which animals it will be cost effective to genotype. Since the gains to be made by having genotype information are often fairly modest (see above), it may be that very little genotyping is warranted. Computer simulations of alternative strategies can be investigated on a case by case basis.

REFERENCES

Duby, R.T., Damiani, P., Looney, C.R., Fissore, R.A. and Rohl, J.M. (1996) Prepubertal calves as oocyte donors: promises and problems. *Theriogenology*, **45**, 121–130.
Gama, L.T., Smith, C. and Gibson, J.P. (1992) Transgene effects, introgression strategies and testing schemes in pigs. *Animal Production*, **54**, 427–440.
Gama, L.T. and Smith, C. (1992) Introgression of transgenes in cattle breeding programs. *Proceedings 43rd Annual Meeting of European Association of Animal Production*, Madrid, Spain.
Gibson, J.P. (1994) Short-term gain at the expense of long-term response with selection on identified loci. *Proceedings 5th World Congress on Genetics Applied to Livestock Production*, **21**, 201–204.
Gibson, J.P. and VanderVoort, G. (1996) Interim economic weights for swine improvement in Canada. *Report to Canadian Centre for Swine Improvement*. Mimmeo, pp. 25.
Groen, A.F. and Smith C. (1995) A stochastic simulation study of the efficiency of marker-assisted introgression in livestock. *Journal of Animal Breeding and Genetics*, **112**, 161–170.
Guo, S.W. and Thompson, E.A. (1992) A monte carlo method for combined segregation and linkage analysis. *American Journal Human Genetics*, **51**, 1111–1126.

214   J.P. GIBSON

Hoeschele, I. (1988) Genetic evaluation with data presenting evidence of mixed major gene and polymorphic inheritance. *Theoretical and Applied Genetics*, **76**, 81–92.

Hoeschele, I. (1990) Potential gain from insetion of major genes into dairy cattle. *Journal of Dairy Science*, **73**, 2601–2618.

Hoeschele, I. (1993) Elimination of quantitative trait loci equations in an animal model incorporating genetic marker data. *Journal of Dairy Science*, **76**, 1693–1713.

Hofer, A. and Kennedy, B.W. (1993) Genetic evaluation for a quantitative trait controlled by polygenes and a major locus with genotypes not or only partly known. *Genetic Selection Evolution*, **25**, 537–555.

Hospital, F., Chevalet, C. and Mulsant, P. (1992) Using markers in gene introgression breeding programs. *Genetics*, **132**, 119–1210.

Kennedy, B.W., Quinton, M. and van Arendonk, J.A.M. (1992) Estimation of effects of single genes on quantitative traits. *Journal of Animal Science*, **70**, 2000–2012.

Kinghorn, B.P., Kennedy, B.W. and Smith, C. (1993) A method of screening for genes of major effect. *Genetics*, **134**, 351–360.

Kinghorn, B.P. (1996) An index of information content for genotype probabilities derived from segregation analysis. *Genetics*, **145**, 479–483.

Meuwissen, T.H.E. and Goddard, M.E. (1996) Estimation of effects of quantitative trait loci in large complex pedigrees. *Genetics*, **146**, 409–416.

Pong-Wong, R. and Woolliams, J.A. (1996) Estimating major gene effects with partial information using Gibbs sampling. *Theoretical and Applied Genetics*, **93**, 1040–1097.

Robertson, R. (1960) A theory of limits in artificial selection. *Proceedings of the Royal Society of London B*, **153**, 234–249.

Saefuddin, A. (1990) Simulations studies of populations with transgenes under selection. *M.Sc. Thesis*. University of Guelph, Ontario, Canada.

Saefuddin, A. and Gibson, J.P. (1991) Selection response in populations with a transgene. *Journal of Animal Science*, **69** (Supplement 1), 215 (abstract).

Smith, C. (1984) Rates of genetic change in farm livestock. *Research and Development in Agriculture*, **1**, 79–85.

Smith, C., Meuwissen, T.H.E. and Gibson, J.P. (1987) On the use of transgenes in livestock improvement. *Animal Breeding Abstracts*, **55**(1), 1–10.

Wall, R.J. (1996) Transgenic livestock: Progress and prospects for the future. *Theriogenology*, **45**, 57–68.

Woolliams, J.A. and Pong-Wong, R. (1995) Short- versus long-term responses in breeding schemes. *Proceedings 46th Annual Meeting European Association of Animal Production*, Prague, p. 35 (abstract).

11. THERAPEUTIC PROTEINS FROM LIVESTOCK

IAN GARNER* and ALAN COLMAN

PPL Therapeutics, Roslin, Edinburgh, EH 25 9pp, Scotland, UK

Many therapeutic proteins are derived either from human plasma by fractionation or from recombinant systems such as large-scale cell culture. Problems exist with both approaches. Large-scale culture of bacteria, yeast and mammalian cells can produce high yields of recombinant protein. However, such processes may be hindered by cost and/or the ability of the chosen system to correctly post-translationally modify the product. Blood fractionation guarantees product quality but suffers from concerns over safety, particularly with viral contamination. In several cases, neither approach can economically meet world demand for product, particularly when this is estimated in metric tonnes. Clearly, an alternative system that could produce large quantities of usable recombinant product in a cost effective manner would be attractive. Livestock can now be genetically modified to secrete recombinant proteins in their milk. By virtue of being produced by mammalian cells *in vivo*, such products are expected to be processed in a similar manner to proteins produced in humans. The mammary gland has an impressive capacity for protein synthesis and milk can be easily harvested. This offers the possibility of producing extremely large quantities of recombinant products by simply breeding more transgenic animals. To date, high levels of expression of a number of proteins have been achieved, although none are currently in use in the clinic. The first products from this novel approach are rapidly nearing the point where companies will seek regulatory approval for their evaluation in clinical trials. Indeed, the first two products of this new technology, recombinant alpha-1-antitrypsin and anti-thrombin III are currently in clinical trials.

KEY WORDS: transgenic livestock; milk; recombinant therapeutic protein; alpha-1-antitrypsin; fibrinogen; protein C.

INTRODUCTION

Before the advent of recombinant DNA technology, therapeutic proteins had been extracted from a variety of sources over the years, including plant, animal, and human tissues or organs. Early preparations consisted of undefined elixirs containing a number of substances and were purported to be beneficial in the treatment of one or more ailments. Identification of the active ingredients in such mixtures and improvements in purity levels has increased the effectiveness of such treatments. This approach has given rise to several products such as insulin for the treatment of diabetes (Banting and Best, 1921), derived initially from dog pancreatic tissue, and more recently asparaginase for childhood leukaemia derived from the jack bean. Whilst these developments have had a major impact on patient health, the biopharmaceutical industry has continued to move ever closer to the holy grail of pure, defined products of demonstrable safety and efficacy. Advances in all areas of biology, particularly pharmacology, protein

*Corresponding author: Tel.: +44 131 440 4777. Fax: +44 131 440 4888.

chemistry and more recently molecular and cellular biology, have influenced this progression.

Current approaches to therapeutic protein production centre on the use of recombinant DNA technology to produce the desired product in a heterologous system. Large-scale culture of genetically modified bacterial or yeast cells can result in high levels of expression of a desired recombinant protein. However, inefficient or inappropriate post-translational modifications of proteins made by these systems may result in product of low biological activity and/or stability. This often limits or even precludes their clinical use. In recent years, the *in vitro* culture of mammalian cells has offered an alternative route for the production of such proteins with the promise that post-translational modifications would be performed more efficiently. Whereas it is expensive to maintain the growth requirements of such cells, these systems have proved perfectly satisfactory for some products e.g. erythropoietin which is used to treat anemia in a variety of clinical indications. In other cases, limitations in post-translational modifications, particularly at high expression levels, and low product yield result in situations where product cannot be produced in a cost effective manner in cell culture based systems e.g. protein C (Grinnell *et al.*, 1989; Yan *et al.*, 1990; Guarna *et al.*, 1995). Clearly, an alternative method of producing large quantities of complex proteins is required.

THE CASE FOR TRANSGENIC LIVESTOCK

Since the generation of the first transgenic mammal following the pronuclear injection of DNA into a single-cell mouse embryo by Gordon and colleagues (1980, 1981), the technology involved has been applied repeatedly, essentially unchanged and has been described at length (Palmiter and Brinster, 1986; Hogan *et al.*, 1994; Houdebine, 1994). Here, we will not concern ourselves with this aspect (see Chapter 8) but, rather, concentrate on the benefits it may bring and by describing the current status of therapeutic protein production in transgenic animals.

Extending the work of Gordon, the expression of recombinant proteins in the milk of transgenic livestock was pioneered by several workers, most notably by Richard Lathe, John Clark and colleagues (Lathe, 1985; Clark *et al.*, 1987). Initially, this group demonstrated that one could alter the composition of milk in a lactating animal by the introduction of a heterologous milk protein gene, the ovine β-lactoglobulin gene, into the genetic make-up of the mouse (Simons *et al.*, 1987). This demonstration of mammary gland specific expression was subsequently extended to sheep (Clark *et al.*, 1989). The resulting animals were transgenic for ovine β-lactoglobulin gene based hybrid constructs encoding either the human proteins Factor IX (FIX) or alpha-1-antitrypsin. They showed that such transgenic ewes are capable of secreting each of these recombinant human proteins into their milk upon lactation (Clark *et al.*, 1989; McClenaghar *et al.*, 1991). Although only small quantities of the recombinant proteins, were produced from these transgenic animals, the principle was established that, if higher expression levels could be attained, the use of this approach would yield a cost effective and easily expandable source of recombinant therapeutic proteins.

The same technology can be applied to other livestock species including pigs, goats and cows. Depending upon the quantities of protein required and the economic/temporal constraints of a particular potential product, one must consider the suitability of each species for the production of a given protein. Table 11.1 summarises some of the salient features of the commonly considered species.

The first of these are gestation period and time taken to attain sexual maturity. These intervals are, of course, relatively fixed and determine how long it will be before a natural lactation, and hence an appreciable amount of product, is available for analysis. The second consideration is milk volume produced per lactation. This can be supplemented by sequential lactations for species with short gestation periods. Because of its limited milk yield ($\leqslant$500 micro litre per lactation) the mouse is not considered as a producer animal. However, due to its 3 week gestation period and large litter size it provides a rapid means of evaluating the ability of a given construct to direct adequate expression of a target therapeutic protein to the milk. As such, it is used as a model system prior to large animal work to obtain information relating to expected expression level, mRNA processing and toxicity. Such experiments provide valuable information relating to the suitability of a given construct to progress to large animal work.

The rabbit can produce over a litre of milk per lactation and because of its rapid maturation and short gestation period can be bred many times in a year. With this in mind, one can harvest 8–10 litres from an individual doe during this period. The transgenic progeny produced would also be available to supplement this supply relatively quickly. The pig is capable of producing more than 100 litres of milk in a relatively short space of time but milking is labour intensive and unconventional when compared to similar sized dairy species such as the sheep and goat. These latter animals can produce very respectable milk yields in a similar time frame to the pig and are much easier to handle. Finally, thanks to years of development by the dairy industry, the ultimate milk producer is the cow

Table 11.1 Characteristics of different species.

Species	G0 birth [a]	G0 adult [a]	G1 birth [a] first natural lactation	Milk volume [b] per lactation
Cow	9 (15)[c]	23	32	>10 000
Sheep/Goat	5 (9)[c]	13	18	250–700
Pig	4	11	15	>100
Rabbit	1	6	7	~1

[a] All times are in months and relate to the starting point of microinjection.
[b] All volumes are in litres.
[c] Bracketed figures show when milk is available from induced lactation.

which is capable of producing about 10 000 litres of milk per lactation. However, this is only achieved following a nine months gestation of the original transgenic founder, a sexual maturation period of 12–15 months and then a further gestation of nine months. Where the founder animal is a bull, a second generation extends the time to milk by a further generation i.e. 21–24 months.

The ability to hormonally induce lactation in sexually immature animals allows one to obtain smaller but significant volumes of milk in a shorter time frame (Ebert et al., 1994). Although these quantities are not sufficient for production purposes they do provide enough product for early evaluation of expression levels, product characterisation and some purification process development. This early "readout" is very helpful since not all first generation transgenic animals produce high yields of the transgene product. The variability reflects the random nature of the incorporation of the transgene into the animal genome. Every founder animal has the transgene or multiples thereof integrated into a different chromosomal location.

Milk has the obvious attraction of being an easily harvestable and potentially unlimited source of recombinant proteins. For proteins needed in large amounts or whose complexity limits production to mammalian systems, this could be a considerable advantage over alternative production methods. Of particular relevance here is the fact that very often, superior expression levels to those obtained from mammalian cell culture have been achieved with complex proteins expressed in the transgenic mammary gland (see below).

THERAPEUTIC PROTEINS IN MILK

Following the work of Simons et al. (1987, 1988) and Clark et al. (1989), a flurry of activity resulted in the reporting in 1991 of three significant further developments in the transgenic livestock field. The first of these was a report from ourselves extending the work of Archibald et al. (1990). These authors described the expression of recombinant human alpha-1-antitrypsin in the milk of transgenic mice at levels of up to 7 grams per litre from a fusion of the ovine β-lactoglobulin gene promoter to genomic DNA sequence encoding human alpha-1-antitrypsin. We reported the generation of five transgenic sheep containing the same construct (Wright et al., 1991). Milk was obtained from three founder transgenic ewes and in each case shown to contain at least one gram per litre of recombinant human alpha-1-antitrypsin. One of the animals secreted milk that contained 35 grams per litre of product. This constituted 50% of the total protein content of her milk. To our knowledge, this remains to date the highest expression level achieved for a recombinant protein in this or any other system and strikingly demonstrates the power of the technology.

The second significant event was the report by Ebert and colleagues (1991) of the generation of goats transgenic for hybrid constructs consisting of either the murine Whey Acid Protein gene or the goat β-Casein gene promoters controlling the expression of a cDNA encoding a longer-acting tissue-type plasminogen activator. Milk was obtained from one founder transgenic for each construct. Expression levels were of the order of 3 milligram per litre and two to three gram per litre for these two constructs respectively.

The third significant development was the report by Krimpenfort *et al.* (1991) of the generation of cattle transgenic for a hybrid bovine αS1-Casein gene promoter and cDNA sequences encoding human lactoferrin. This work made use of embryos derived from slaughterhouse-derived oocytes, matured and fertilised *in vitro*, and demonstrated the feasibility of such an approach to generate transgenic cattle.

Since these demonstrations that one could obtain gram per litre expression levels in two dairy species and generate transgenic cattle from oocytes following IVM/IVF, many other workers have succeeded in expressing recombinant proteins, usually of human origin, via the mammary gland of transgenic livestock. Gene regulatory elements from several different milk protein genes from a number of species have been used as vectors to target expression to the mammary gland. Much of this work has been of a research and developmental nature and has made use of the mouse as producer species. To date, there have been at least twenty-six reports detailing the expression of seventeen recombinant human proteins in the milk of transgenic mice. Several other proteins have also been expressed using the transgenic murine mammary gland but these data have not been reported due to confidentiality issues. Transgenic livestock (cows, goats, sheep, pigs or rabbits) have been reported which are transgenic for one of 13 different hybrid constructs each designed to secrete one of ten recombinant therapeutic protein into their milk (Table 11.2). It is also believed that Genzyme Transgenics have generated goats transgenic for a construct designed to express a monoclonal antibody directed at colon cancer. However, at the time of writing, the details of this construct and any expression data remain confidential.

Taking the examples listed in Table 11.2, three attractive features from these reports are the range of proteins expressible, the levels attained, and the quality of the product. The examples listed include single-chain proteins [alpha-1-antitrypsin], multimeric proteins [fibrinogen] and include those requiring complex post-translational modifications such as γ-carboxylation [protein C]. In most cases, expression levels obtained in this system exceed those obtained with mammalian cell culture systems in some cases by several orders of magnitude. For example, the expression of human fibrinogen at five gram per litre is 1000-fold higher than levels obtained in *in vitro* systems (Farrell *et al.*, 1991; Hartwig and Danishefsky, 1991; Roy *et al.*, 1991; Huang *et al.*, 1993). Moreover, the transgenically derived material appears to be fully functional *in vitro* in its ability to form blood clots (Figure 11.1). Similarly, the expression of protein C at up to 1 gram per litre is significantly higher than achieved in *in vitro* systems. Product from the latter suffers from limitations to post-translational modification as expression levels increase resulting in protein with low biological activity. The transgenically derived material [at least from sheep] appears to be fully processed and is as active as plasma derived human protein C in *in vitro* anti-coagulation assays. Combined with co-ordinated breeding programmes, these high levels of expression enable the production of large quantities of a given recombinant protein.

Table 11.2   Potential therapeutic proteins in the milk of livestock.

Promoter	Protein	cg DNA	Expression level	Animal	Citation
α_{s1}-casein bovine	Lactoferrin	cDNA	Undisclosed	Cow	Krimpenfort et al. (1991)
β-casein goat	Longer acting tissue plasminogen activator	cDNA	2–3 mg ml^{-1}	Goat	Ebert et al. (1991)
β-casein goat	Antithrombin III	cDNA gDNA	6 mg ml^{-1} 10 mg ml^{-1}	Goat Goat	Genzyme Transgenics (unpublished)
WAP mouse	Longer acting tissue plasminogen activator	cDNA	3 µg ml^{-1}	Goat	Ebert et al. (1991)
WAP mouse	Protein C	cDNA	1 mg ml^{-1}	Pig	Velander et al. (1992)
α_{s1}-casein bovine	Insulin like growth factor-1	cDNA	1 mg ml^{-1}	Rabbit	Brem et al. (1994)
β-casein goat	Alpha-1-antitrypsin	gDNA gDNA	4 mg ml^{-1} 12 mg ml^{-1}	Rabbit Goat	Genzyme Transgenics (unpublished)
β-casein goat	Monoclonal antibody	cDNA	5 mg ml^{-1}	Goat	Genzyme Transgenics (unpublished)
β-casein rabbit	Interleukin-2	gDNA	$\geqslant$450 ng ml^{-1}	Rabbit	Buhler et al. (1990)
BLG sheep	Factor IX	cDNA	25 ng ml^{-1}	Sheep	Clark et al. (1989)
BLG sheep	Protein C	cDNA	300 µg ml^{-1} 750 µg ml^{-1} 750 µg ml^{-1}	Sheep (induced ewe) Rabbit Pig	PPL (unpublished)
BLG sheep	Alpha-1-antitrypsin	gDNA	35 mg ml^{-1}	Sheep	Wright et al. (1991)
BLG sheep	Fibrinogen	gDNA	5 mg ml^{-1}	Sheep	PPL (unpublished)

THE NEXT STEP

Many technical hurdles have been crossed in a relatively short space of time to develop the technology to its current status. Being able to produce large quantities of an active therapeutic protein is only half of the story. As technology progresses and expectations continue to rise, the public have come to expect that products for clinical use are guaranteed both safe and efficacious. This is an understandable state of affairs and it should not be otherwise. Over the years, procedures have been developed to ensure that such proteins progress to clinical use in a systematic manner. Before any new drug, including a therapeutic protein, is used clinically, it must, by law, satisfy the requirements of the regulatory authorities of the country/state in which it used. Procedures may vary slightly from country to country but are broadly similar. In the USA, for example, the

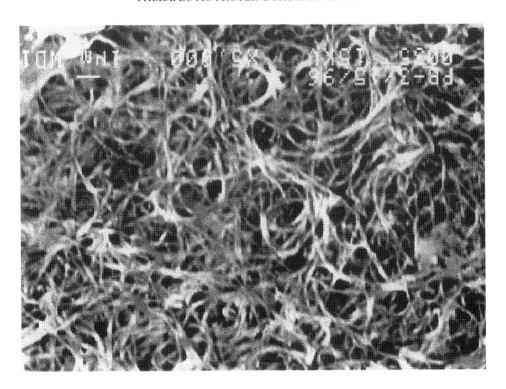

Figure 11.1   Electron Micrograph of Clot made from Transgenic Fibrinogen.

regulating authority is the "Food and Drug Administration" (FDA). Each European country has its own regulatory authority but the EU is moving towards
harmonisation with a central "Committee for Proprietary Medicinal Products"
(CPMP). This is developing a system of mutual recognition throughout the EU
similar to the system operated by the FDA. Below we will outline the procedure
required for FDA approval of a new therapy.

To gain FDA approval for a new product, one must produce the product in
compliance with satisfactory quality regulations, i.e. Good Manufacturing Practice
(GMP), and compile a profile of its properties before proceeding to tests involving human beings. Such tests are collectively called *pre-clinical trials* and they
evaluate a number of aspects of the product including toxicity, stability and
pharmacokinetic properties in animal models. These data are reviewed by the
FDA prior to them giving consent for the evaluation of the product in humans in
the form of a "Notice of Claimed Investigational Exemption for a New Drug"
(IND).

Once the IND is acquired, the properties of the product can be evaluated in
human patients in clinical trials. These take the form of a *phase I trial* on a limited
number of non-patient volunteers to determine if there are any adverse effects
such as toxicity. Initial applications of single doses are usually followed by

repeated doses in a selected number of individuals. If the product is successful at this stage it is allowed to proceed to a *phase II trial* where preliminary efficacy and safety are evaluated in a sample that usually comprises several hundred patients. Important information relating to the most appropriate dose is acquired at this stage. If successful at this point, the product is allowed to proceed to a *phase III trial* which is designed to establish if the product works for the chosen indication. Such trials may involve thousands of patients and may be conducted in general practice and/or suitable hospitals depending on the product and its proposed use or indication. Throughout this process, which may take several years, the product is compared to control groups receiving placebo or the best available current therapy treatments.

Clinical trials are legally obliged to fulfil two important criteria. Firstly, they must be approved by a relevant ethics committee as a well designed, justifiable and suitably resourced project. Secondly they can only make use of patients who have given what is referred to as "Informed Consent". Patients must be clear as to the purpose and rationale behind the trial and are free to withdraw at any time. Enrolled patients should sign a document indicating that they have given Informed Consent.

All clinical trials must be carried out to levels of competence that will satisfy the regulatory authority, referred to as Good Clinical Practice (GCP), and all information derived from them must be verifiable. This requires a high degree of monitoring and results in a mountain of paperwork. Any adverse or unexpected events must be reported immediately and it is usual to submit an annual summary of progress. Once completed, a comprehensive dossier of information is compiled containing all pertinent information. This is then submitted to the FDA as an application for a Product Licence. Only when this is obtained can a product actually begin its life as a commercial therapy. Progressing a product through such a procedure is expensive [it can cost £100 million] and is not guaranteed of success. More potential products fail this process than those that succeed. Therefore, apart from the obvious patient safety obligations we all have, it is important to adhere to the rules and regulations of this procedure so as to maximise chances of success.

Only two of the potential products listed in Table 11.2 are currently in clinical trials. Alpha-1-antitrypsin from transgenic sheep and antithrombin III from transgenic goats entered phase I clinical trials in late 1996 (see Figure 11.2). Both programmes are currently at similar stages of development. Both the FDA and CPMP have produced guideline documents covering recommendations for the use of transgenic animals in the manufacture of therapeutic products for human use. Essentially, these two documents raise the same considerations and highlight areas to which potential producers will need to pay special attention. Such topics include: a well documented history of the construct used and the generation of transgenic founders; the use of a single line of producer animals derived from a single founder animal; a well recorded genealogy of animals; excellent care and health monitoring of animals; demonstration of genetic and expression stability within a line; validation of the purification process as a means to ensure safety of

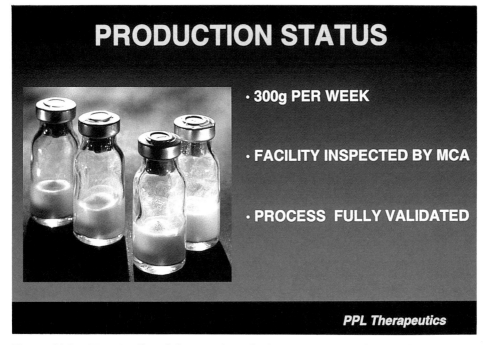

Figure 11.2 GMP Quality Alpha-1-Antitrypsin from Transgenic Sheep milk for clinical trial evaluation in human patients.

the product and extensive demonstration of the purity of the product. Below we will outline where the alpha-1-antitrypsin programme is currently in relation to the above process.

RECOMBINANT ALPHA-1-ANTITRYPSIN FROM THE MILK OF TRANSGENIC SHEEP

Following our initial demonstrations of high level expression of recombinant alpha-1-antitrypsin in the milk of transgenic sheep (Wright *et al.*, 1991) we progressed to characterising the product further. After initial purification, the transgenic protein was shown to be of a similar size and immunosensitivity (when compared with human plasma derived alpha-1-antitrypsin in a rabbit model). Bioactivity and glycosylation comparisons were also very favourable. This comparison was extended to more detailed analyses of glycosylation state, amino terminal sequencing, pI value and molecular weight determined by mass spectrometry. The transgenic protein was found to be extremely similar to human plasma derived material, except for a slight difference observed in the transgenic protein when analysed by iso-electric focussing. This is due to minor differences in terminal sialylation. The similarities between the human plasma derived and recombinant transgenic sheep milk derived alpha-1-antitrypsin prompted us to develop a production process from one of these original founder sheep. Initially we chose to target Cystic Fibrosis as the primary indication.

Before selecting the most appropriate line of animals, we investigated genetic and expression stability by breeding all founder animals and their descendants (Carver et al., 1993). This allowed us to investigate the transmission of the transgene and the expression level of the recombinant protein from generation to generation and during sequential lactations. In addition to the original five transgenic founders, we later generated another female founder animal. Of these six animals, we were unable to demonstrate transgene transmission from two females. In transgenic lineages, founder animals are referred to as G_0 (for Generation 0) and their descendants are sequentially referred to as G_1, G_2, G_3, etc. Of the others, one female produced three G_1 progeny of variable copy number. Unfortunately, she was the highest producer of recombinant alpha-1-antitrypsin of the original founder ewes. Pulse field gel electrophoresis indicated that the observed copy number differences in her progeny are the result of genetic rearrangement and not the result of segregation of two, or more, transgene integration sites. Expression levels of recombinant protein in the offspring of this founder varied with copy number. Although unsuitable as a founder animal for production of recombinant alpha-1-antitrypsin due to the observed genetic instability, this founder did demonstrate the enormous potential of the technology to produce large quantities of recombinant protein.

The three other founder animals all transmitted their transgene faithfully to their progeny demonstrating the genetic stability required for a transgenic line to be used for production purposes. One of these founder animals was a male and he enabled us to rapidly generate large numbers of direct G_1 progeny. As these had all inherited the transgene from their sire, they all contain the same integration event with the same number of transgene copies. The expression levels from this line were particularly interesting. Initially, seven transgenic G_1 ewes were generated and these all expressed human alpha-1-antitrypsin at 13–16 gram per litre in their first lactations. They subsequently expressed very similar levels during their next three lactations. Both G_2 and G_3 animals also expressed human alpha-1-antitrypsin at similar levels whilst a G_2 homozygote ewe expressed recombinant alpha-1-antitrypsin at 37.0 gram per litre in her milk. The protein produced by each animal appeared identical by a number of criteria.

These results showed for the first time that stable genetic transmission and stable expression levels could be obtained from a transgenic livestock animal. It also demonstrated that a transgenic production flock could be derived from a single founder male, or several half-brothers containing the same integrant. In the case described above, it is significant that homozygous animals are healthy. As the transgene array integrates randomly in the genome of the embryo it may disrupt a gene essential for the viability of the organism. If both genes are disrupted, the animal would not develop or may die shortly after birth. The ability to generate normal, healthy, homozygous animals confirmed that there was no insertional mutation associated with the point of transgene integration in this line. It is also noteworthy that expression levels of the recombinant protein more than doubled as the copy number increased. This would allow us to increase production by the creation of a homozygous flock. We currently have more than 600 G_2 transgenic ewes of this line. All of these animals are routinely health monitored by dedicated veterinary surgeons and a complete history of each animal is maintained.

To further satisfy the regulatory authority demands that we anticipated, we have developed a purification process and assays which allow us to produce highly pure and pathogen-free product. The process consists of a combination of skimming, filtration, viral inactivation/removal and anion/cation chromatography steps. Validation of the process allows us to conclude that the product produced benefits from up to 23 logs of clearance of viral or prion particles, should any be present. Product purity assays enable us to confirm that the product is clinical grade material suitable for clinical trials. Initially developed at a laboratory scale dealing with a maximum milk volume of hundreds of millilitres, the purification process has been scaled up to Pilot Production Plant Scale dealing with volumes of hundreds of litres. To do so, we have constructed the first facility of its type in the world in which to carry out this process and are currently producing more than 300 grams of GMP grade recombinant human alpha-1-antitrypsin each week.

THE FUTURE

Whereas the use of transgenics animals to produce recombinant proteins has progressed steadily in recent years, the future holds two major challenges. The first of these is the successful navigation of the clinical trial process and the accumulation of data that indicates that a given product is safe and efficacious in its chosen indication. The second follows on from this in that once this is achieved, one still must await marketing approval from regulatory authorities before the product can be provided to the patient population. This requires that the information accumulated earlier is reviewed favourably by the regulatory authorities concerned. We look forward to the successful conclusion of clinical trials and the subsequent use of alpha-1-antitrypsin in the clinic for the benefit of patients. Hopefully, this will soon be followed by other products produced by the transgenic mammary gland.

REFERENCES

Archibald, A.L., McClenaghan, M., Hornsey, V., Simons, J.P. and Clark. A.J. (1990) High-level expression of biologically active human α1-antitrypsin in the milk of transgenic mice. *Proc. Natl. Acad. Sci. USA*, **87**, 5178–5182.

Banting, F.G. and Best, C.H. (1921) The internal secretion of the pancreas. *The Journal of Laboratory and Clinical Medicine*, VII: **5**, 251–266.

Brem, G., Hartl, P., Besenfelder, U., Wolf, E., Zinovieva, N. and Pfaller, R. (1994) Expression of synthetic cDNA sequences encoding human insulin-like growth factor-1 (IGF-1) in the mammary gland of transgenic rabbits. *Gene*, **149**: 2, 351–355.

Buhler, T.A., Bruyere, T., Went, D.F., Stranzinger, G. and Burki, K. (1990) Rabbit β-Casein promoter directs secretion of human interleukin-2 into the milk of transgenic rabbits. Bio/Technology, 8, 140–143.

Carver, A.S., Dalrymple, M.A., Wright, G., Cottom, D.S., Reeves, D.B., Gibson, Y.H., Keenan, J.K., Barrass, D., Scott, A.R., Colman, A. and Garner, I. (1993) Transgenic livestock as bioreactors: stable expression of human alpha-1-antitrypsin by a flock of sheep. Bio/Technology, 11, 1263–1270.

Clark, A.J., Simons, P., Wilmut, I. and Lathe, R. (1987) Pharmaceuticals from transgenic livestock. Trends Biotechnol., 5, 20–24.

Clark, A.J., Bessos, H., Bishop, J.O., Brown, P., Harris, S., Lathe, R., McClenaghan, M., Prowse, C., Simons, J.P., Whitelaw, C.B.A. and Wilmut. I. (1989) Expression of human anti-hemophilic factor IX in the milk of transgenic sheep. BioTechnology, 7, 487–492.

Ebert, K.M., Selgrath, J.P., Ditullio, P., Denman, J., Smith, T.E., Memon, M.A., Schindler, J.E., Monastersky, G.M., Vitale, J.A. and Gordon, K. (1991) Transgenic production of a variant of human tissue-type plasminogen activator in goat milk: generation of transgenic goats and analysis of expression. Bio/Technology, 9, 835–838.

Ebert, K.M., Di Tullio, P., Barry, C.A., Schindelr, J.E., Ayres, S.L., Smith, T.E., Pellerin, L.J., Meade, H.M., Denman, J. and Roberts, B. (1994) Induction of human tissue plasminogen activator in the mammary gland of transgenic goats. Bio/Technology, 12, 699–702.

Farrell, D.H., Mulvihill, E.R., Huang, S., Chung, D.W. and Davie, E.W. (1991) Recombinant human fibrinogen and sulfation of the gamma' chain. Biochemistry, 30, 9414–9420.

Gordon, J.W., Scangos, G.A., Plotkin, D.J., Barbosa, J.A. and Ruddle, F.H. (1980) Genetic transformation of mouse embryos by microinjection of purified DNA. Proc. Natl. Acad. Sci. USA, 77, 7380–7384.

Gordon, J.W. and Ruddle, F.H. (1981) Integration and stable germline transmission of genes injected into mouse pronuclei. Science, 214, 1244–1246.

Grinnell, B.W., Walls, J.D., Berg, D.T., Boston, J., McClure, D.B. and Yan, S.B. (1989) Expression, characterisation and processing of recombinant human protein C from adenovirus-transformed cell lines. In: Genetics and Molecular Biology of Industrial Microorganisms. Hershberger, C.L., Queener, S.W., Hegeman, G. eds. American Society of Microbiology, Washington, DC, 226–237.

Guarna, M.M., Fann, C.H., Busby, S.J., Walker, K.M., Kilburn, D.G. and Piret, J.M. (1995) Effect of cDNA copy number on secretion rate of activated protein C. Biotechnology and Bioengineering, 46, 22–27.

Hartwig, R. and Danishefsky, K.J. (1991) Studies on the assembly and secretion of fibrinogen. J. Biol. Chem., 266, 6578–6585.

Huang, S., Mulvihill, E.R., Farrell, D.H., Chung, D.W. and Davie, E.W. (1993) Biosynthesis of human fibrinogen. Subunit interactions and potential intermediates in the assembly. J. Biol. Chem., 268, 8919–8926.

Hogan, B., Constantini, F. and Lacy, E. (1994) Manipulating the mouse embryo: a laboratory manual. Cold Spring Harbor Laboratory Press, NY.

Houdebine, L.-M. (1994) Production of pharmaceutical proteins from transgenic animals. J. of Biotechnology, 34, 269–287.

Krimpenfort, P., Rademakers, A., Eyestone, W., van der Schans, A., Van den Broek, S., Kooiman, P., Kootwijk, E., Platenburg, G., Pieper, F., Strijker, R. and de Boer, H. (1991) Generation of transgenic dairy cattle using "in vitro" embryo production. Bio/Technology, 9, 844–847.

Lathe, R. (1985) Molecular tailoring of the farm animal germline. In: ABRO Ann. Rep. HMSO. Edinburgh, 7–10.

Palmiter, R.D. and Brinster, R.L. (1986) Germ-line transformation of mice. Ann. Rev. Genet., 20, 465–499.

Roy, S.N., Procyk, R., Kudryk, B.J. and Redman, C.M. (1991) Assembly and secretion of recombinant human fibrinogen. J. Biol. Chem., 266, 4758–4763.

Simons, J.P., McClenaghan, M. and Clark, A.J. (1987) Alteration of the quality of milk by expression of sheep β-lactoglobulin in transgenic mice. Nature, 328, 530–532.

Simons, J.P., Wilmut, I., Clark, A.J., Archibald, A.L., Bishop, J.O. and Lathe, R. (1988) Gene transfer into sheep. BioTechnology, 6, 179–183.

Velander, W.H., Johnson, J.L., Page, R.L., Russell, A., Subramanian, A., Wilkins, T.D., Gwazdauskas, F.C., Pittius, C. and Drohan, W.N. (1992) High-level expression of heterologous protein in the milk of transgenic swine using the cDNA encoding human Protein C. *Proc. Natl. Acad. Sci. USA*, **89**, 12003–12007.

Wright, G., Carver, A., Cottom, D., Reeves, D., Scott, A., Simons, P., Wilmut, I., Garner, I. and Colman, A. (1991) High level expression of active human alpha-1-antitrypsin in the milk of transgenic sheep. *Bio/Technology*, **9**, 830–834.

Yan, S.B.C., Razzano, P., Chao, B., Walls, J.D., Berg, D.T., McClure, D.B. and Grinnell, B. (1990) Characterisation and novel purification of recombinant human protein C from three mammalian cell lines. *Bio/Technology*, **8**, 655–661.

12. XENOGRAFTS FROM LIVESTOCK

DAVID WHITE* and GILLIAN LANGFORD

Department of Surgery, Imutran Laboratories, 18 Trumpington Road, Cambridge CB2 2AH, UK

The world-wide shortage of organs for allotransplantation has recently led to renewed interest in the field of xenotransplantation. As the pig shares a number of anatomical and physiological similarities with man and because it can easily be bred in large numbers, it is considered as a possible source of xenografts for human transplantation. However, such discordant xenotransplantation would result in hyperacute rejection of the transplanted organ. This hyperacute rejection process is a result of the activation of the recipients complement, which leads to loss of vascular integrity, haemorrhage and thrombosis in the transplanted organ. In this chapter we describe the main strategies that are currently being employed to overcome the problem of hyperacute rejection.

One such strategy is the production of transgenic pigs expressing human regulators of complement activation such as decay accelerating factor (DAF), membrane cofactor protein (MCP) or CD59. Analysis of the different organs from pigs transgenic for human DAF showed that the transgene was expressed in all the organs analysed. Transplantation of the hearts from transgenic pigs into cynomologus monkeys resulted in a median graft survival time of 40 days. In contrast, normal pig hearts were hyperacutely rejected within 6 hours. These results demonstrate that expression of human DAF in the transgenic pigs protects them from hyperacute rejection and indicates that organs from these pigs may be suitable for clinical xenotransplantation.

An alternative strategy that is also discussed in this chapter is the modulation of the expression of the epitopes that are recognised by the xenoreactive antibodies involved in the initiation of hyperacute rejection.

KEY WORDS: xenotransplantation; hyperacure rejection; complement; transgenic; decay accelerating factor.

XENOGRAFTS FROM LIVESTOCK

As a direct result of improvements in surgical techniques and advances in immosuppressive strategies, transplantation is currently considered a viable, cost effective therapeutic solution, in many cases, to end stage organ failure. However, despite transplantation prolonging and improving the quality of patients lives, the actual number of transplant operations that can be performed is severely restricted by the limited availability of donor organs. The extent of this problem is illustrated by the fact that approximately only 10% of those patients who could benefit from a heart transplant in the United States, actually receive a heart (Evans, 1991; Evans *et al.*, 1992). Similar organ shortages occur world-wide and have led to renewed interest in the concept of transplanting organs from other species, such as non human primates or pigs, into man.

*Corresponding author: Tel.: 01223-300151. Fax: 01223-300153. E-mail: djgw@cus.cam.ac.uk.

The Choice of Donor Species for Xenotransplantation

The concept of transplanting organs between species, xenotransplantation, is not new. However, careful consideration must be given to the choice of donor species selected for xenotransplantation into man. Although non-human primates may appear·to be ideal donors because they are closely related to man, there are problems associated with such a choice. Some primates such as chimpanzees and apes are endangered species, whilst the organs from other primates such as baboons are not large enough to be transplanted into adult humans. There are also serious ethical considerations, as some cultures would regard the exploitation of animals with characteristics similar to those of man as unacceptable. Finally there are potential risks associated with the transmission of viral agents between closely related species. These factors compound to make the use of non-human primates as donors less than ideal. In contrast, the pig is currently considered to be an ideal donor species because it is easily bred, matures rapidly, and produces large numbers of offspring. In addition the organs from pigs are of a suitable size for transplanting into man and as their kidneys have a similar renal blood flow and glomerular filtration rate as man it is expected that following xenotransplantation they will be fully functional.

To date several attempts have been made to transplant organs from other species such as non-human primates or pigs into man as shown in Table 12.1. However, so far most of these operations have not met with much success. As a result of the different rates of rejection observed in these operations and in xenotransplantation experiments between different species, the different species combinations used in xenotransplantation are termed as either concordant or discordant (Calne, 1970). Transplants between concordant species, such as a chimpanzee to man, are usually rejected over a period of days, whilst grafts between discordant species, such as a pig to man, are rapidly rejected within minutes to hours.

Table 12.1 Clinical Applications of Xenotransplantation.

Year	Organ	Donor	Cases	Survival
1964	Kidney	Chimpanzee	12	<9 months
1964	Kidney	Monkey	1	10 days
1964	Kidney	Baboon	1	4.5 days
1964	Heart	Chimpanzee	1	Hours
1968	Heart	Sheep	1	Hours
1969–73	Liver	Chimpanzee	3	<14 days
1977	Heart	Baboon	1	4 weeks
1977	Heart	Chimpanzee	1	4 days
1985	Heart	Baboon	1	4 weeks
1992	Liver	Baboon	1	70 days
1992	Heart	Pig	1	24 hours
1993	Liver	Baboon	2	<71 days
1995	Bone marrow	Baboon	1	graft failed to take

Mechanisms of Discordant Xenotransplantation Rejection

The rapid rejection process seen in discordant species combinations is known as hyperacute rejection. The mechanism of this rejection process has been studied in depth and is believed to be modulated by the binding of recipient performed, naturally occurring antibodies to epitopes on the donor endothelial cells (Platt and Bach, 1991; Dalmasso et al., 1992). The major epitope recognised by the xenoreactive antibodies is a terminal galactosyl residue, Gal α1,3 Gal found on glycoproteins and glycolipids (Sandrin et al., 1994; Sandrin et al., 1995). Although this epitope is widely expressed in many animals and types of bacteria, it is not found in humans or old-world primates because they do not produce a functional form of the enzyme α1,3 galactosyl transferase, that catalyses the transfer of the terminal sugar residue to the glycoprotein or glycolipid (Galili et al., 1988). Thus, both humans and old-world primates develop antibodies to the Gal α1,3 Gal epitope which are possibly induced by gut flora.

Binding of the xenoreactive antibodies results in the activation of the complement cascade via the classical pathway (Figure 12.1) which in turn leads to the activation of endothelial cells (Platt and Bach, 1991; Dalmasso et al., 1992). This endothelial cell activation results in the cells retracting from each other and the basement membrane to which they are attached and the release of anti inflammatory enzymes and loss of coagulation inhibition. These changes result in interstitial haemorrhaging, inflammation, oedema and thrombosis (Bogman et al., 1980).

Normally, the activation of complement is modulated by a series of proteins which are either membrane bound or found in the fluid phase and are known as regulators of complement activation (Figure 12.1). The activity of these molecules is species specific, thus following discordant xenotransplantation, the donors complement regulating molecules would not be able to regulate activation of the recipients complement and thus prevent hyperacute rejection (Lachmann, 1991).

In man there are three predominant membrane bound regulators of complement activation, each of which regulates the complement cascade at a specific stage: (i) Decay accelerating factor, (DAF) which down regulates the activation of C3 by blocking the assembly of C3 convertase (Lublin and Atkinson, 1989), (ii) membrane cofactor protein (MCP) which down regulates the activation of C3 by acting as a cofactor for factor I inactivation of the convertase components (Liszewski et al., 1991) and (iii) CD59 which prevents the insertion of C9 into the lytic membrane attack complex (Rollins and Sims, 1988).

This detailed understanding of the processes involved in hyperacute rejection and the control of the complement cascade, led to the suggestion that the production of transgenic animals which express human regulators of complement activation on their cell surfaces, might result in animals whose organs are suitable for xenotransplantation into man. This hypothesis was substantiated by the observation that following transfection of human DAF or MCP cDNA into mouse fibroblasts the cells were protected from lysis by human complement (White et al., 1992).

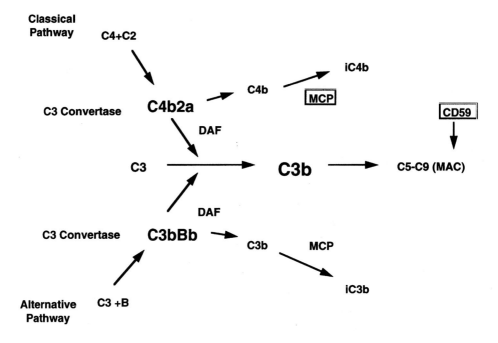

Figure 12.1   Activation and regulation of the complement cascade: Complement can be activated by either the classical or alternative pathway. Both pathways result in activation of C3 whose cleavage results in the synthesis of the membrane attack complex, which when inserted into a cell membrane leads to cell damage or lysis. The steps at which the regulators of complement activity, DAF, CD59 and MCP are activated is also indicated.

Production of Transgenic Pigs Expressing Human Decay Accelerating Factor

Several groups have reported the production of transgenic animals expressing human regulators of complement activation (Langford *et al.*, 1994; McCurry *et al.*, 1995; Fodor *et al.*, 1994). In the following section we will describe, in detail, our work involving the production and evaluation of pigs expressing the human complement regulator, DAF.

Transgenic pigs were produced by microinjection of a hDAF minigene construct (Figure 12.2) into the pronuclei of fertilised pig ova (Langford *et al.*, 1994). This procedure involved artificially inseminating mature donor gilts which had been induced to superovulate with pregnant mare's serum gonadatrophin. The pronuclear stage embryos were collected from the oviducts of the donor gilts by midventral laparotomy as described by Polge (1982). The opaque cytoplasm of pig ova, which are lipid dense, makes direct visualisation of the pronuclei, which is necessary for microinjection, impossible. However, if the ova are centrifuged the cytoplasm is stratified and it is possible to detect the pronuclei in the equatorial segment of the ova using differential interference contrast microscopy.

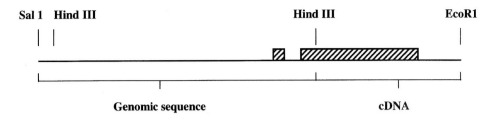

Figure 12.2 A schematic representation of the DAF minigene construct: The DAF minigene consists of approximately 4 kb of human genomic DNA between the two HindIII sites and 2 kb of cDNA between the HindIII site and the EcoR1 site. The genomic fragment includes the first exon, the 5′ untranslated region and signal peptide sequence of the DAF gene and part of the first DAF intron.

After centrifugation the visualised pronuclei were microinjected with the minigene for hDAF until their diameter increased by approximately 50% and then bilaterally transferred to the oviducts of recipient gilts.

A total of 2432 ova were microinjected and transferred to 85 recipient gilts. Forty-nine of these gilts became pregnant and produced 311 offspring. Forty-nine of the 311 offspring were identified as transgenic by slot blot analysis of DNA isolated from ear biopsy samples.

The results showed that approximately 13% of the microinjected pig ova developed into new-born pigs. This result is slightly higher than that previously reported (Pursel *et al.*, 1990) and may be attributable to several factors such as (i) differences in the developmental stage at which the ova were injected, (ii) the skill of the person microinjecting the foreign DNA, (iii) the period for which the eggs were cultured *in vitro*, (iv) the concentration of the microinjected DNA, or (v) the synchrony of the donor and recipient. If the efficiency of producing transgenic pigs is expressed as the percentage of injected ova that resulted in transgenic pigs, the efficiency of micro-injecting the hDAF minigene was 2%.

The number of copies of the hDAF minigene which incorporated into the genome of the different lines of transgenic pigs produced, ranged from 1 to 30. Similar variations in the copy number of transgenic pigs have previously been reported, for example, when the human growth hormone linked to the mouse metallothionein promoter was micro-injected into porcine ova between 1 to 490 copies of the transgene integrated into the porcine genome (Hammer *et al.*, 1985), whilst the copy number of pigs which had incorporated the porcine growth hormone linked to the mouse metallothionein promoter ranged from less than 1 to 11 (Vize *et al.*, 1988).

Expression of the Transgene

Expression of the transgene was determined at the RNA level by reverse transcriptase polymerase chain reaction (RT PCR) analysis using primers designed to span an intron/exon boundary and by Northern blot analysis. Protein expression was analysed using a double capture radio immunoassay (RIA) and by immuno-histochemistry. Northern blot analysis of ear biopsies or peripheral blood mononuclear cells showed that 67 percent of the pigs expressed the transgene in these tissues. In addition RIA showed that the transgene was expressed in each type of tissue analysed (Cozzi *et al.*, 1994). However, the level of expression was found to vary both from organ to organ within an animal and from animal to animal (Figure 12.3). Comparison of the level of hDAF protein expressed in the tissue of the different lines of transgenic pigs showed that approximately 14% of all the tissues analysed expressed hDAF at levels comparable to or greater than that seen in the equivalent human tissue.

Immunohistological analysis of the expression of hDAF showed that it was expressed in a variety of cell types, including the vascular endothelium (Rosengard *et al.*, 1995) which is the primary site of antibody and complement mediated hyperacute rejection.

Analysis of blood or ear biopsies showed that approximately 23% of the founder pigs analysed did not express the transgene. This may have been the result of integration of the transgene at an inactive chromosomal locus or changes in the sequence of the transgene that occurred during the integration process. Variations in the level of expression similar to those observed between both different lines of hDAF transgenic pigs and the organs for the same animal have previously been reported in both transgenic mice and pigs (Pursel *et al.*, 1989; Velander *et al.*, 1992; Cary *et al.*, 1993). These variations were not associated with the copy number of the animals. However, it has been suggested that expression of the transgene may be affected by the level of transcriptional activity at the site at which it integrated and the characteristics of enhancer sequences surrounding it (Pursel *et al.*, 1990).

Transmission of the Transgene

Of the 49 founder transgenic pigs produced, 36 of these pigs were bred to produce the F1 generation. Analysis of offspring produced showed that 58.5 % of the animals transmitted the transgene to approximately 50% of their offspring, indicating that they had integrated the different copies of the transgene at a single site. In contrast 19.5% of the founders transmitted the transgene to less than 10% of their offspring, suggesting that they were mosaic in their germline. The remaining 22% of the founders transmitted the transgene to more than 80% of their offspring, which along with differences in the gene copy number of the offspring suggests that these founders may have integrated the transgene on two or more different chromosomes. These results were confirmed by fluorescence *in situ* hybridisation of metaphase chromosomes which showed that those founders which transmitted the transgene to more than 50 percent of their offspring had integrated the transgene in two or more different chromosomes (Kuipers *et al.*, 1996).

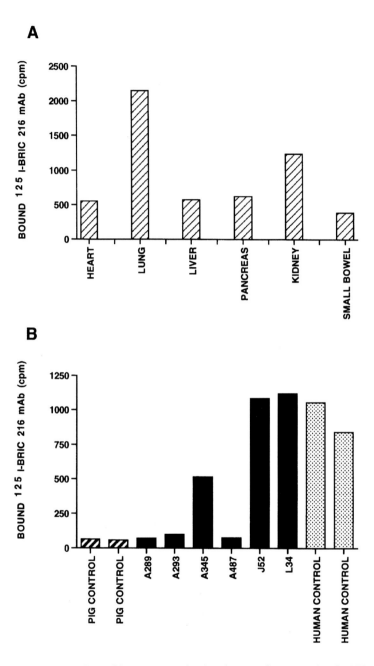

Figure 12.3 (A) Expression of human DAF in the tissues of transgenic pig J50, note the results show that the transgene is expressed at different levels in the different tissues. (B) Comparative analysis of the levels of human DAF expressed in the hearts of normal control pigs, a selection of transgenic pigs and two human controls. Note that the level of expression of human DAF in some of the transgenic pigs hearts is greater than that seen in the two human heart samples.

Protection of the Transgenic Pig Hearts from Human Complement

The efficiency of expression of the hDAF transgene in protecting porcine tissue from complement mediated damage was assessed in both *ex vivo* and *in vivo* experiments. In the *ex vivo* experiments a mock circulation was constructed in which normal and transgenic pig hearts were perfused with human blood which was then pumped around a circuit by the pig heart. Hearts were removed from 3 to 4 week old piglets via a median sternotomy and connected to the perfusion circuit. The circuit comprised of a main reservoir from which blood was pumped into the left atrium of the heart, via a paediatric oxygenator with an integrated heat exchanger. The heart then pumped the blood into an arterial reservoir which was positioned 700 mm above the heart. Overflow from this reservoir was used as a marker of cardiac output, measured as units of blood pumped per minute per gram of heart tissue against a fixed after load.

Figure 12.4 shows the cardiac output for normal pig hearts perfused with either fresh human blood or human blood which had been de-complemented using cobra venom factor. In addition, it also shows the cardiac output of transgenic pig hearts perfused with fresh blood. The results show that hearts from the transgenic pigs, which were known to express high levels of hDAF on their endothelium, performed as much work as normal pig hearts that had been perfused with decomplemented human blood, suggesting that expression of the transgene protected these hearts against complement mediated damage.

In contrast to the results obtained with transgenics hearts which expressed high levels of hDAF in their endothelium, the outputs of hearts taken from transgenic pigs which expressed little or no hDAF did not differ significantly from that of normal pigs (White *et al.*, 1995). The eventual decline in the cardiac output of either the transgenic or normal pig hearts tested is a consequence of the model used, and may result from either the build up of toxins in the circuit or the removal of essential elements.

Immunohistochemical staining for deposition of C3b in the transgenic and control pigs hearts perfused with human blood also illustrated the protective effect of the transgene (White *et al.*, 1995). If, as expected, expression of hDAF blocks the complement cascade no C3b should be formed. Histological analysis of hearts from the transgenic pigs which expressed high level of hDAF showed minimal C3b deposition, whilst high levels of C3b staining were seen in the normal pig hearts perfused with human blood.

Pig to Non-Human Primate Cardiac Xenotransplantation

In addition to the *ex vivo* model described above, the protective effect of the transgene was demonstrated by transplanting hearts from the transgenic pigs into non-human primates (White, 1996). These transplant operations were divided into two groups; one set in which the recipients of the control and transgenic hearts were immunosuppressed, and the other set in which no immunosuppression was administered. The pig hearts were implanted heterotopically into

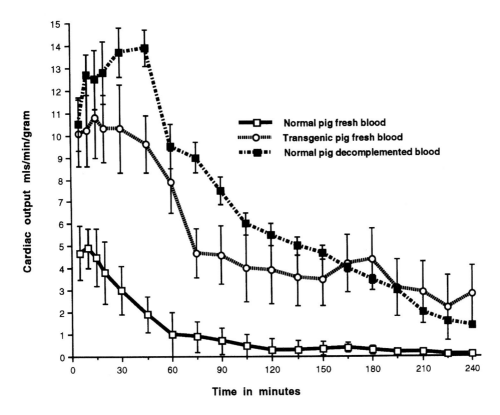

Figure 12.4 Comparison of the cardiac outputs of pig hearts perfused with human blood. Normal pig hearts were perfused with fresh human blood ($n=16$, open squares) or decomplemented human blood ($n=4$, closed squares) and transgenic pig hearts were perfused with fresh human blood ($n=5$, open circles).

the abdomen of cynomolgus monkeys. Implantation involved anastomosing the donor's aorta to the recipients aorta, and the donor's pulmonary artery to the recipients inferior vena cava. Rejection of the hearts was defined as the point at which a heart beat was not detectable by external palpitation.

Immunosuppression was based on a triple therapy of cyclosporin, cyclophosphamide and steroids. After implantation of the pig hearts, the immunosuppressive regime was based on the results obtained from monitoring clinical and immunological parameters in each animal.

The results from the group of animals which were immunosuppressed showed that the control hearts were hyperacutely rejected with a median survival of 55 minutes (range 0.1 to 6 hours). In contrast, the hearts transplanted from the 10 transgenic pigs, none of which were hyperacutely rejected, survived for a median of 40 days (range 6 to 62 days). The causes of organ failure or the reasons for terminating the experiment varied from animal to animal. However, none of the experiments were terminated because of an infection in the cynomolgus monkeys, indicating that the immunosuppressive regime used was not excessive.

In the second set of experiments, in which 8 transgenic pig hearts were transplanted heterotopically into non immunosuppressed cynomolgus monkeys, none of the transgenic hearts, which had a median survival time of 5.1 days (range 97 to 134 hours), were hyperacutely rejected. In contrast the 10 hearts from non-transgenic pigs had a median survival time of 1.6 days (range 12–104 hours). However, unlike the control animals in the immunosuppressed group, not all the control pig hearts in these experiments were hyperacutely rejected, even though histological analysis of these hearts showed that they exhibited all the characteristics lesions of hyperacute rejection. One possible explanation for this observation is that the hearts from the control animals that were not hyperacutely rejected expressed lower levels of the Gal α1,3 Gal epitope which is involved in the initiation of hyperacute rejection. Alternatively, the differences observed may be due to of differences in the expression levels of porcine proteins which could block the end stages of the human complement cascade.

The differences in the survival rates described above for transgenic or control pig hearts transplanted into non-human primates suggest that expression of hDAF by the transgenic pigs protects the organs from these animals against hyperacute rejection following xenotransplantation. Further experiments, including orthotopic xenotransplantation of transgenic pig hearts into non-human primates are necessary to further assess whether organs from these hDAF transgenic pigs could be successfully transplanted into humans. However, these preliminary experiments are seen as a positive indicator that clinical xenotransplantation using organs from these hDAF transgenic pigs may occur in the not to distant future.

The Production of Pigs Expressing Other Complement Regulating Molecules

Transgenic pigs which express human regulators of complement have also been produced by other researchers. Fodor *et al.* (1994) have described the production of transgenic pigs which express high levels of the human terminal complement inhibitor, hCD59. CD59 inhibits formation of the membrane attack complex by binding to C5b-8 and C5b-9. Production of these transgenic pigs involved microinjection of a minigene construct in which the cDNA for hCD59 was inserted into exon 1 of the murine major histocompatability complex class 1 gene H-2Kb. The design of this construct is such that the H-2Kb gene provides the necessary genomic sequences to support expression of the hCD59 cDNA. Transcription of this construct initiates at the transcriptional start site of H-2Kb and continues through the inserted CD59 cDNA and along the rest of the H-2Kb gene. Translation of the mRNA transcript starts at the ATG codon of the hCD59 gene and terminates at the stop codon of hCD59.

Analysis of tissues taken from the hCD59 transgenic pigs produced showed that the transgene was expressed in all the tissues analysed, including the vascular

endothelium. The protective effect of the transgene was demonstrated by expos-
ing transgenic or normal porcine peripheral blood mononuclear cells to human
serum containing complement and xenoreactive antibodies. The results showed
that the transgenic cells were protected from complement mediated lysis.

Transgenic pigs which express hDAF and hCD59 have also been produced
(McCurry et al., 1995). In these animals expression of the transgenic proteins is
directed by an erythroid specific promoter. The transgenic proteins expressed in
the erythrocyte cell membranes translocate to the endothelial cell membranes.
Immunofluorescence analysis of cardiac biopsies showed that both transgenic
proteins were present on the endothelium of large and small blood vessels.
Hearts from these transgenic pigs were assessed in an in vivo model in which they
were transplanted heterotopically into immunosuppressed baboons, producing a
non-working cardiac xenograft. Rejection of the transgenic pig hearts in this
model was defined as the point at which ventricular contractions ceased. The
control porcine xenografts were rejected in sixty to ninety minutes whilst the
xenografts from the transgenic pigs survived for 4, 11 and 30 hours.

It is interesting to compare the different survival times of the cardiac xenografts from the transgenic pigs which expressed hDAF and were transplanted into
immunosuppressed cynomolgus monkeys with those of the xenografts which had
hDAF and hCD59 on their vascular endothelium and were transplanted into
immunosuppressed baboons. This comparison shows that the xenogenic organs
transplanted into the baboons survived for a maximum of 30 hours whilst those
transplanted into the cynomolgus monkeys survived for a maximum of 62 days.
These differences could result from the use of different primate species or
differences in the level of expression of the transgenes.

Modulation of Epitope Expression in Transgenic Animals

In addition to the production of transgenic pigs which express human regulators
of complement activation, research has also been directed at altering the levels
of expression of the epitopes recognised by the xenoreactive antibodies in an
attempt to overcome hyperacute rejection. The major epitope recognised by the
xenoreactive antibodies has already been identified as Gal α1,3 Gal (Sandrin
et al., 1994; Sandrin et al., 1995). Two different strategies are currently being
evaluated in order to reduce expression of this epitope. The first approach
involves preventing expression of the enzyme, α1,3 galactosyl transferase, which
catalyses the transfer of the terminal galactose moiety to an N-acetyl lactosamine
acceptor substrate, and results in the formation of the terminal Gal α1,3 Gal
epitope. Expression of the galactosyl transferase could be reduced or inhibited
by the microinjection of an antisense construct against the α1,3 galactosyl
transferase. Alternatively the α1,3 galactosyl transferase enzyme could be deleted
by homologous recombination in embryonic stem cells. However, at present
deletion by homologous recombination has not yet been possible in the pig.

The second strategy to reduce expression of the Gal α1,3 Gal epitope involves
over expressing human α1,2 fucosyl transferase, an enzyme which competes for

the same substrate as the galactosyl transferase and produces a fucosylated N-acetyl lactosamine that is not antigenic in man. Transfection of the fucosyl transferase into porcine cells resulted in cells with lower levels of the Gal α1,3 Gal epitope which were more resistant to human antibody binding and human complement mediated lysis than normal pig cells (Sandrin *et al.*, 1995). Both transgenic mice and pigs which express the human fucosyl transferase gene have been produced (Sandrin *et al.*, 1995; Koike *et al.*, 1996). Analysis of tissues taken from the transgenic mice showed that they had lower levels of expression of Gal α1,3 Gal and they bound less human antibody than control mice. If similar results are seen in tissues from the transgenic pigs it is possible that organs from these animals may be resistant to hyperacute rejection and thus be suitable for xenotransplantation into man.

The results obtained from analysing transgenic animals which express either human complement regulators or reduced levels of the Gal α1,3 Gal epitope are very promising. However, it is possible that by combining both these strategies even more dramatic results may be obtained. Thus, work is currently underway to produce pigs which express both complement regulating molecules and have low levels of the Gal α1,3 Gal epitope.

The work described in this chapter in overcoming hyperacute rejection and allowing the long-term survival of pig xenografts in non-human primates suggests that clinical xenotransplantation may soon become a clinical reality. However, before any clinical xenotransplantation program can commence several important issues must be addressed. Firstly, what additional experimental data must be produced in order to justify the initiation of a clinical xenotransplantation program. It could be argued that clinical studies should not begin until all possible avenues of xenotransplantation research have been exhausted. Alternatively, it could be debated that as large numbers of patients are dying because of the limited number of organs available for allotransplantation, clinical xenotransplantation, however slim the chance of success, would be justifiable in an attempt to save lives. Obviously some kind of compromise between these two extreme viewpoints must be made. It is likely that clinical xenotransplantation may only be considered ethically acceptable when orthotopically transplanted organs from transgenic pigs have been shown to function for extended periods in non-human primates.

The second issue to address is what immunosuppressive regimes will be necessary to ensure long-term survival of patients following clinical xenotransplantation. The immunosuppressive regimes used must be designed to prevent both acute vascular rejection which occurs when the donor endothelium stimulates the production of new antibodies, and chronic rejection. However, such regimes must not result in high levels of toxicity. The third issue to address is the possible outcome of the initial clinical xenotransplantation program. It is highly probable that initiation of a clinical xenotransplantation program will result in the death of a number of the recipients. It will be essential to ensure that adverse reactions to these deaths will not impede future clinical xenotransplantation programs.

REFERENCES

Bogman, M.J.J.T., Berden, J.H.M., Hagemann, F.H.M., Maass, C.N. and Keone, R.A.P. (1980) Patterns of vascular damage in the antibody-mediated rejection of skin xenografts in the mouse. *Am. J. Path.*, **100**, 727–738.

Calne, R.Y. (1970) Organ transplantation between widely disparate species. *Trans Proc.*, **4**, 550–553.

Cary, N., Moody, J., Yannoutsos, N., Wallwork, J. and White, D. (1993) Tissue expression of human decay accelerating factor, a regulator of complement activation expressed in mice: A potential approach to inhibition of hyperacute xenograft rejection. *Transplant Proc.*, **25**, 400–401.

Cozzi, E., Langford, G.A., Richards, A., Elsome, K., Lancaster, R., Chen, P. *et al.* (1994) Expression of human decay accelerating factor in transgenic pigs. *Transplant Proc.*, **26**, 1402–1403.

Dalmasso, A.P., Vercellotti, G.M., Fischel, R.J., Bolman, R.M., Bach, F.H. and Platt, J.L. (1992) Mechanisms of complement activation in the hyperacute rejection of porcine organs transplanted into primate recipients. *Am. J. Pathol.*, **140**, 1157–1166.

Evans, R.W. (1991) Executive Summary. *The national cooperative transplantation study*. Seattle WA: *BHARC*.

Evans, R.W., Orians, C.E. and Ascher, N.L. (1992) The potential supply of donor organs: an assessment of the efficiency of organ procurement efforts in the United States. *JAMA*, **267**, 239–246.

Fodor, W.L., Williams, B.L., Matis, L.A., Madri, J.A., Rollins, S.A., Knight, J.W. *et al.* (1994) Expression of a functional human complement inhibitor in transgenic swine as an approach to prevent xenogeneic hyperacute organ rejection. *Proc. Natn. Acad. Sci. USA*, **91**, 11153–11157.

Galili, U., Shohet, S.B., Korbin, E., Stults, C.L.M. and Macher, B.A. (1988) Man, apes and Old World monkeys differ from other mammals in the expression of the α-galactosyl epitopes on nucleated cells. *J. Biol. Chem.*, **263**, 17755–17762.

Hammer, R.E., Pursel, V.G., Rexroad, C.E. Jr., Wall, R.J., Bolt, D.J., Ebert, J.M. *et al.* (1985) Production of transgenic rabbits, sheep and pigs by microinjection. *Nature, Lond.*, **315**, 680–683.

Koike, C., Kannagi, T., Muramatsu, T., Yokoyama, I. and Takagi, H. (1996) Converting (α) Gal Epitope of pig into H antigen. *Trans. Proc.*, **28**, 553.

Kuipers, H.W., Langford, G.A. and White, D.J.W. (1997) *Transgenic Research*, **6**, 253–259.

Lachmann, P.J. (1991) The control of homologous lysis. *Immun. Today*, **12**, 312–315.

Langford, G.A., Yannoutsos, N., Cozzi, E., Lancaster, R., Elsome, K., Chen, P. *et al.* (1994) Production of pigs transgenic for human decay accelerating factor. *Transplant Proc.*, **26**, 1400–1401.

Liszewski, M.K., Post, T.W. and Atkinson, J.P. (1991) Membrane cofactor protein (MCP or CD46): newest member of the regulators of complement activation gene cluster. *Annu. Rev. Immunol.*, **9**, 431–434.

Lublin, D.M. and Atkinson, J.P. (1989) Decay-accelerating factor: Biochemistry, molecular biology and function. *Annu. Rev. Immunol.*, **7**, 35–58.

McCurry, K.R., Kooyman, D.L., Alvarado, C.G., Cotterell, A.H., Martin, M.J., Logan, J.S. *et al.* (1995) Human complement regulatory proteins protect swine-to-primate cardiac xenografts from humoral injury. *Nature Medicine*, **1**, 423–427.

Platt, J.L. and Bach, F.H. (1991) Discordant xenografting: challenges and controversies. *Curr. Opin. Immun.*, **3**, 735–739.

Polge, C. (1982) Embryo transplantation and preservation. In *Control of Pig Reproduction*, edited by Cole, D.J.A. and Foxcroft, G.R. pp. 277–291. London: Butterworths.

Pursel, V.G., Pinkert, C.A., Miller, K.F., Bolt, V.G., Campbell, R.G., Palmiter, R.D. *et al.* (1989) Genetic engineering of livestock, *Science*, **244**, 1281–1285.

Pursel, V.G., Bolt, D.J., Miller, K.F., Pinkert, C.A., Hammer, R.E., Palmiter, R.D. *et al.* (1990) Expression and performance in transgenic pigs. *J. Reprod. Fert.*, **40**, 235–245.

Rollins, S.A. and Sims, P.J. (1990) The complement-inhibitory activity of CD59 resides in its capacity to block incorporation of C9 into membrane C5b-9. *J. Immunol.*, **144**, 3478–3483.

Rosengard, A.M., Cary, N.R.B., Langford, G.A., Tucker, A.W., Wallwork, J. and White, D.J.G. (1995) Tissue expression of human complement inhibitor, decay accelerating factor, in transgenic pigs — A potential approach for preventing xenograft rejection. *Transplantation*, **59**, 1325–1333.

Sandrin, M.S., Vaughan, H.A. and Mckenzie, I.F.C. (1994) Identification of Gal α1,3 Gal as the major epitote for pig to human vascularised xenografts. *Transplantn Rev.*, **8**, 134–149.

Sandrin, M.S., Fodor, W.L., Mouhtours, E., Osman, N., Cohney, S., Rollins, S.A. *et al.* (1995) Enzymatic remodelling of the carbohydrate surface of a xenogenic cell substantially reduces human antibody binding and complement-medicated cytolysis. *Nature Medicine*, **12**, 1261–1265.

Velander, W.H., Johnson, J.L., Page, R.L., Russel, C.G., Subramanian, A., Wilkins, T.D. *et al.* (1992) High-level expression of a heterologous protein in the milk of transgenic swine using cDNA encoding human protein C. *Proc. Natl. Acad. Sci. USA.*, **89**, 12003–12007.

Vize, P.D., Michalska, A.E., Ashman, R., Lloyd, B., Stone, B.A., Quinn, P. *et al.* (1988) Introduction of a porcine growth hormone fusion gene into transgenic pigs promotes growth. *J.Cell Sci.*, **90**, 295–300.

White, D.J.G., Oglesby, T., Liszewski, M.K., Tedja, I., Hourcade, D., Wang, M.W. *et al.* (1992) Expression of human decay accelerating factor or membrane cofactor protein genes on mouse cells inhibits lysis by human complement. *Transplant Proc.*, **24**, 474–476.

White, D.J.G., Langford, G.A., Cozzi, E. and Young, V.K. (1995) Production of pigs transgenic for human DAF: A strategy for xenotransplantation. *Xenotransplantation*, **2**, 213–217.

White, D.J.G. (1996) hDAF transgenic pig organs: are they concordant for human transplantation? *Xeno.*, **4**, No 3.

INDEX

Human
  alpha-lactalbumin 176
  fibrinogen 219
  genome initiative 78, 137
  lactoferrin 191, 219
  milk proteins 191
  regulators of complement
    activation 231
      plasminogen activator 218
      protein C 219
      proteins in transgenic milk 220
Hybrid vigour 5
Hyperacute rejection response 231
Hyperglycaemia 187

IGF-1
  transgenics 188
  wool follicle growth 193
Immunosensitivity of recombinant
  proteins 223
Immunosuppression 237
In vitro
  activation 25
  fertilisation 23, 174, 206
  maturation 174
Inbreeding
  coefficient 132, 203
  depression 204
  effects 205
IND 221
Inheritance
  non-additive 131
  non-Mendelian 82
  cytoplasmic 82
Insulin 215
Interbreeding pool 211
Integration locus 168
Integration frequencies 174
Introgression 124, 127
Interference 79
Iso-electric focusing 223

K88 resistance 128
Karyoplast 48
Karyotypes 150

Keratin proteins 193
kit locus 157

Lactation 172
Lactose 191
Lamins 64
Laparoscopy 32
Laparotomy 32
Linkage
  classical 92
  conservation 140
  disequilibrium 94, 109, 124
  groups 88
  human map 108
  identical by descent (IBD) 109
  likelihood ratios 79
  lodscore 79
  lodscore tables 80
  maps 121, 147
  mapping of production traits 93,
    96, 155
  multipoint 80
  multiple linked markers 93
  parametric linkage 82
  significance threshold 85
  statistical tests 79
  two point 78
Litter size 204
Locus 7
Lod score curve 81
Lysozyme 191

Malignant hyperthermia (MH) 104,
  112, 156
Mammary gland expression 216
Map(s)
  comparative maps 149
  high resolution 158
  human 145
  murine 145
  ordered gene 146
  locations 149
  position 140
  radiation hybrid 156
  reference linkage 156

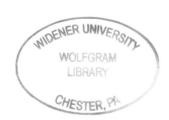